Schizophrenia: Advances and Current Management

Editor

PETER F. BUCKLEY

PSYCHIATRIC CLINICS OF NORTH AMERICA

www.psych.theclinics.com

June 2016 • Volume 39 • Number 2

ELSEVIER

1600 John F. Kennedy Boulevard • Suite 1800 • Philadelphia, Pennsylvania, 19103-2899

http://www.theclinics.com

PSYCHIATRIC CLINICS OF NORTH AMERICA Volume 39, Number 2
June 2016 ISSN 0193-953X, ISBN-13: 978-0-323-44632-7

Editor: Lauren Boyle
Developmental Editor: Kristen Helm

Psychiatric Clinics of North America (ISSN 0193-953X) is published quarterly by Elsevier Inc., 360 Park Avenue South, New York, NY 10010-1710. Months of issue are March, June, September, and December. Business and Editorial Offices: 1600 John F. Kennedy Blvd., Suite 1800, Philadelphia, PA 19103-2899. Periodicals postage paid at New York, NY and additional mailing offices. Subscription prices are $300.00 per year (US individuals), $598.00 per year (US institutions), $100.00 per year (US students/residents), $365.00 per year (Canadian individuals), $455.00 per year (international individuals), $753.00 per year (Canadian & international institutions), and $220.00 per year (Canadian & international students/residents). Foreign air speed delivery is included in all *Clinics'* subscription prices. All prices are subject to change without notice. **POSTMASTER:** Send address changes to *Psychiatric Clinics of North America*, Elsevier Health Sciences Division, Subscription Customer Service, 3251 Riverport Lane, Maryland Heights, MO 63043. **Customer Service: 1-800-654-2452 (US). From outside the United States, call 1-314-447-8871. Fax: 1-314-447-8029. E-mail: journalscustomerservice-usa@elsevier.com (for print support) and journalsonline support-usa@elsevier.com (for online support).**

Reprints. For copies of 100 or more, of articles in this publication, please contact the Commercial Reprints Department, Elsevier Inc., 360 Park Avenue South, New York, New York 10010-1710. Tel.: 212-633-3874, Fax: 212-633-3820, E-mail: reprints@elsevier.com.

Psychiatric Clinics of North America is covered in *MEDLINE/PubMed (Index Medicus)*, *Current Contents/Social and Behavioral Sciences*, *Social Science Citation Index, Embase/Excerpta Medica,* and PsycINFO.

Contributors

EDITOR

PETER F. BUCKLEY, MD
Dean, Medical College of Georgia, Augusta University, Augusta, Georgia

AUTHORS

ANTHONY O. AHMED, PhD
Assistant Professor, Department of Psychiatry, Weill Cornell Medical College, White Plains, New York

DONNA AMES, MD
Program Leader, Psychosocial Rehabilitation and Recovery Center, West Los Angeles Veterans Affairs Medical Center; Professor in Residence, David Geffen School of Medicine at University of California Los Angeles, Los Angeles, California

JOHN BARTLETT, MD, MPH
Senior Advisor, The Carter Center Mental Health Program, Atlanta, Georgia

PETER F. BUCKLEY, MD
Dean, Medical College of Georgia, Augusta University, Augusta, Georgia

ALEX BUCKNER, MS
Department of Psychiatry, Weill Cornell Medical College, White Plains, New York

SIAN M. CARR-LOPEZ, PharmD
Pharmacy Service, Veterans Affairs Northern California Health Care System, Mather, California; Clinical Professor, Department of Pharmacy Practice, University of the Pacific, Stockton, California

MARY CLARKE, MD, FRCPI, FRCPsych
Associate Clinical Professor, School of Medicine and Medical Sciences, University College Dublin; Clinical Lead, DETECT Early Intervention Services, St John of God Community Services Ltd, Dublin, Ireland

BRETT A. CLEMENTZ, PhD
Department of Psychology, University of Georgia, Athens, Georgia

ROISIN DOYLE, BA, MSc
Clinical Research Assistant, DETECT Early Intervention Services, St John of God Community Services Ltd, Dublin, Ireland

HELIO ELKIS, MD, PhD
Associate Professor, Department and Institute of Psychiatry; Director, Schizophrenia Research Program (Projesq), University of São Paulo Medical School (FMUSP), São Paulo, Brazil

GANESH GOPALAKRISHNA, MD, MHA
Assistant Professor of Clinical Psychiatry, Department of Psychiatry, University of Missouri-Columbia, Columbia, Missouri

MARY A. GUTIERREZ, PharmD, BCPP
Professor of Pharmacy Practice (Psychiatry), Chapman University School of Pharmacy, Irvine, California

KRISTIN M. HUNTER, MS
Department of Psychiatry and Health Behavior, Augusta University, Augusta, Georgia

MICHAEL Y. HWANG, MD
Adjunct Professor, Department of Psychiatry, New York Medical College, Franklin Delano Roosevelt VA Medical Center, Montrose, New York

MUAID H. ITHMAN, MD
Assistant Professor of Clinical Psychiatry, Department of Psychiatry, University of Missouri-Columbia, Columbia, Missouri

MATCHERI S. KESHAVAN, MD
Department of Psychiatry, Beth Israel Deaconess Medical Center, Harvard Medical School, Boston, Massachusetts

JOHN LAURIELLO, MD
Professor and Chairman, Department of Psychiatry, University of Missouri-Columbia, Columbia, Missouri

PAUL ALEX MABE, PhD
Professor, Department of Psychiatry and Health Behavior, Augusta University, Augusta, Georgia

RON MANDERSCHEID, PhD
Washington, DC

BRIELLE A. MARINO, MA
Department of Psychiatry, Weill Cornell Medical College, White Plains, New York

CATHERINE M. McDONOUGH, MD, MRCPsych
Consultant Psychiatrist, Cavan-Monaghan Mental Health Service, COPE Early Intervention Psychosis Service; Cavan-Monaghan Community Rehabilitation Service, St Davnet's Hospital, Monaghan, Ireland

BRIAN J. MILLER, MD, PhD, MPH
Associate Professor, Department of Psychiatry and Health Behavior, Augusta University, Augusta, Georgia

HENRY A. NASRALLAH, MD
Professor and Chairman, Department of Psychiatry, St Louis University, St Louis, Missouri

LEWIS A. OPLER, MD, PhD
Special Adjunct Research Professor, Predoctoral Program in Clinical Psychology, Long Island University, Brookville, New York

GODFREY D. PEARLSON, MD
Director, Olin Neuropsychiatry Research Center, Institute of Living, Hartford, Connecticut; Professor, Departments of Psychiatry and Neurobiology, Yale University School of Medicine, New Haven, Connecticut

JOSEPH M. PIERRE, MD
Co-Chief, Schizophrenia Treatment Unit, West Los Angeles Veterans Affairs Medical Center; Health Sciences Clinical Professor, Department of Psychiatry and Biobehavioral Sciences, David Geffen School of Medicine at University of California Los Angeles, Los Angeles, California

JENNIFER A. ROSEN, PharmD, BCPP
Pharmacy Quality Improvement Program Manager, Department of Pharmacy, Veterans Affairs Northern California Health Care System, Martinez, California; Faculty Adjunct Professor, University of the Pacific School of Pharmacy, Stockton, California; Assistant Clinical Professor, University of Southern California School of Pharmacy, Los Angeles, California

ELIZABETH ROSENTHAL, MA
Department of Psychiatry, Weill Cornell Medical College, White Plains, New York

SUSAN SHAKIB, PharmD, BCPS
Clinical Pharmacist Specialist in Mental Health, Mental Health Pharmacy Program Manager, Department of Pharmacy, Veterans Affairs Long Beach Healthcare System, Long Beach, California; Thomas J. Long School of Pharmacy and Health Sciences, University of the Pacific, Stockton, California

JOHN A. SWEENEY, PhD
Department of Psychiatry, UT Southwestern Medical School, Dallas, Texas

CAROL A. TAMMINGA, MD
Professor and Chair, Department of Psychiatry, UT Southwestern Medical School, Dallas, Texas

JOHN L. WADDINGTON, PhD, DSc
Head of Department, Molecular and Cellular Therapeutics, Royal College of Surgeons in Ireland, Dublin, Ireland; Jiangsu Key Laboratory of Translational Research and Therapy for Neuro-Psychiatric-Disorders, Department of Pharmacology, College of Pharmaceutical Sciences, Soochow University, Suzhou, China

CYNTHIA SHANNON WEICKERT, PhD
Schizophrenia Research Institute; School of Psychiatry, University of New South Wales; Neuroscience Research Australia, Randwick, New South Wales, Australia

THOMAS W. WEICKERT, PhD
Schizophrenia Research Institute; School of Psychiatry, University of New South Wales; Neuroscience Research Australia, Randwick, New South Wales, Australia

PETER J. WEIDEN, MD
Professor of Psychiatry, UIC Medical Center, Chicago, Illinois

LYNN M. YUDOFSKY, MD
Semel Institute for Neuroscience and Human Behavior, University of California Los Angeles, Los Angeles, California

SUN YOUNG YUM, MD
Department of Clinical Medical Science, Seoul National University, Seoul, South Korea

Contents

> Psychotic disorders, as defined by clinical features alone, overlap considerably in terms of symptoms, familial patterns, risk genes, outcome, and treatment response. As a result, numerous neurobiological measurements fail to distinguish patients with the most prevalent classic psychotic syndromes. Statistical methods applied to such biological measurements in large numbers of patients with psychosis yield novel categories that cut across traditional diagnostic boundaries. Such new classification approaches within psychosis hopefully represent an opportunity to transcend clinical phenomenologically defined syndromes in psychiatry with neurobiologically defined diseases that can advance drug discovery and support precision medicine approaches in psychiatry.

> Although early intervention in psychosis is clinically intuitive and theoretically feasible, the reality is that over recent decades the evidence base to support it has not advanced as much as might have been anticipated. Material benefits of early intervention in established psychosis have not been universally demonstrated and much uncertainty continues to surround the field of treatment in the prodromal phase. Undoubtedly methodological differences between studies are relevant and better understanding of different treatment models and the effectiveness of their constituent parts may yield the most benefit, particularly from a public health perspective.

> This article presents the case in favor of clinical trials of adjunctive monoclonal antibody immunotherapy in schizophrenia. Evidence for prenatal and premorbid immune risk factors for the development of schizophrenia in the offspring is highlighted. Then key evidence for immune dysfunction in patients with schizophrenia is considered. Next, previous trials of adjunctive anti-inflammatory or other immunotherapy in schizophrenia are discussed. Then evidence for psychosis as a side effect of immunotherapy for other disorders is discussed. Also presented is preliminary evidence for adjunctive monoclonal antibody immunotherapy in psychiatric

disorders. Finally, important considerations in the design and implementation of clinical trials of adjunctive monoclonal antibody immunotherapy in schizophrenia are discussed.

Medication adherence is as much of a problem today as it was 50 years ago. A major barrier to progress is that the definition emphasizes obedience to medication recommendations rather than shared outcome goals. As a result, schizophrenia patients are keenly aware of the social risks of disclosing nonadherence. Nondisclosure leads to misinformation, which in turn leads to serious errors in medication decisions. Another consequence is that adherence struggles may harm the therapeutic relationship. When nonadherence is inevitable, the strategy should shift to the use of harm reduction strategies that aim to preserve the therapeutic relationship while mitigating risks.

Although there has been more than 50 years of development, there remains a great need for better antipsychotic medications. This article looks at the recent advances in treatment of schizophrenia. New hypotheses have been suggested that may replace or complement the dopamine hypotheses. The article explores the different novel drugs that impact some of the key neurotransmitter systems currently. Phosphodiesterase 10A inhibitors and α-7 neuronal nicotinic acetylcholine receptor modulators constitute the majority. The marketing of these medications eventually may result in change about how schizophrenia is treated.

Although treatment-resistant schizophrenia (TRS) was described 50 years ago and has a gold standard treatment with clozapine based on well-defined criteria, there is still a matter of great interest and controversy. In terms of the underlying mechanisms of the development of TRS, progress has been made for the elucidation of the neurochemical mechanisms. Structural neuroimaging studies have shown that patients with TRS have significant reduction of the prefrontal cortex volume when compared with non- TRS. This article updates and enhances our previous review with new evidence mainly derived from new studies, clinical trials, systematic reviews, and meta-analyses.

Schizophrenic illness encompasses diverse clinical phenomena and consists of unclear underlying pathogeneses. For the past century, the comorbidities in schizophrenia have drawn persistent interest and debate due to its high prevalence rate and a need for better management. However, its clinical and biological diversity continue to challenge both the practicing clinicians and researchers. Emerging clinical and research evidence in the past decade suggest a distinct biopsychosocial pathogenesis and unique clinical attributes in some comorbid disorders in patients with schizophrenia. In addition, current evidence also supports improved outcomes with specific assessment and treatment of these subgroups of schizophrenia. The recent changes in DSV-5 and shift in the NIMH focus towards the *real world clinical practice and research* provide increased impetus to explore the pathogeneses and treatment of schizophrenia with comorbid disorders.

Antipsychotics are some of the most frequently prescribed medications not only for psychotic disorders and symptoms but also for a wide range of on-label and off-label indications. Because second-generation antipsychotics have largely replaced first-generation antipsychotics as first-line options due to their substantially decreased risk of extrapyramidal side effects, attention has shifted to other clinically concerning adverse events associated with antipsychotic therapy. The focus of this article is to update the nonextrapyramidal side effects associated with second-generation antipsychotics. Issues surrounding diagnosis and monitoring as well as clinical management are addressed.

The recovery model has permeated mental health systems by leading to the development of new psychiatric interventions and services and the reconfiguration of traditional ones. There is growing evidence that these interventions and services confer benefits in clinical and recovery-oriented outcomes. Despite the seeming adoption of recovery by policy makers, the transformation of mental health systems into recovery-oriented systems has been fraught with challenges.

Parity of mental health and substance abuse insurance benefits with medical care benefits, as well as parity in their management, are major ongoing concerns for adults with serious mental illness (SMI). The Mental Health Parity and Addiction Equity Act of 2008 guaranteed this parity of benefits and management in large private insurance plans and privately managed state Medicaid plans, but only if the benefits were offered at all. The Patient Protection and Affordable Care Act of 2010 extended parity to all persons receiving insurance through the state health insurance marketplaces, through the state Medicaid Expansions, and through new individual and small group plans. This article presents an analysis of how accessible parity has become for adults with SMI at both the system and personal levels several years after these legislative changes have been implemented.

Schizophrenia is a heterogeneous psychiatric illness for which the cause or causes are presently unknown. There is increasing evidence from multiple levels of research suggesting that inflammation may play an important role in the development and persistence of psychosis and cognitive impairment in a proportion of people with schizophrenia. This overview of recent literature focuses on studies of neuroinflammation that are considered to be of increasing interest in schizophrenia research and are poised to have an impact on the cause, diagnosis, and potential treatment of at least some forms or subtypes of schizophrenia.

PSYCHIATRIC CLINICS OF
NORTH AMERICA

THE CLINICS ARE AVAILABLE ONLINE!
Access your subscription at:
www.theclinics.com

Preface

Converging Perspectives on Schizophrenia

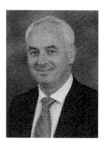

Peter F. Buckley, MD
Editor

This issue brings together an international group of stellar schizophrenia-focused clinicians and researchers to provide contemporary perspectives on the biology and treatment of schizophrenia. While the condition remains enigmatic, this issue chronicles progress in both understanding of what is, and what is not, schizophrenia and, accordingly, how best to approach care. In the opening article, Pearlson and colleagues thoroughly review and challenge symptom-based approaches to the diagnosis of schizophrenia. They describe current efforts to define neurobiological signatures between psychosis and mood disorders.

Waddington and colleagues highlight information on duration of untreated psychosis (DUP), the critical time period between the emergency of clear psychotic symptoms and the initiation of psychiatric care. They critically review extant literature, as well as highlight model programs for early intervention, on DUP from a longitudinal perspective. Turning over to biological perspectives, our colleague, Dr Miller, and I speculate on neuroinflammation and schizophrenia ... a kind of "old wine in a new bottle." There are longstanding relationships between infections, especially viruses, and schizophrenia. Recent studies now point to a more systematic pattern of immunologic disturbances in schizophrenia, thereupon, now prompting nascent attempts at novel immune-based approaches to treatment. These opportunities are highlighted in this article. While such biological theories are exciting, readers and clinicians are of course more focused on the "nuts and bolts" of clinical care and what can be done to make real improvements. To that end, medication adherence is, unquestionably, central to clinical care. Weiden reminds us just how a multifaceted and major dilemma nonadherence is in the treatment of patients with schizophrenia. This article covers recent innovations and pragmatic approaches that focus on detecting and enhancing adherence for this patient group. This article also forms the back-drop for considering innovations in clinical therapeutics. To that end, Lauriello and colleagues "take stock" of currently available antipsychotics and evaluate the potential role(s) of

Psychiatr Clin N Am 39 (2016) xiii–xiv
http://dx.doi.org/10.1016/j.psc.2016.02.001
0193-953X/16/$ – see front matter © 2016 Published by Elsevier Inc.

other putative agents that are in development. Helio Elkis and I, even in the face of the advances of psychopharmacology described by Lauriello and colleagues, also remind us that there is still a substantial minority of patients with schizophrenia who remain recalcitrant to standard treatments, up to and including clozapine. Options for clinicians are reviewed in this article as well as combinations of medications and use of old and new neuromodulatory therapies. In addition to limitations of pharmacotherapy, the extent of comorbidities and schizophrenia also complicates the care of people with schizophrenia. Comorbidities, whether they are psychiatric, physical, or a combination of both, are now more the rule than the exception among people with schizophrenia. There are many reasons that may explain this robust association, and these are detailed in the article by Hwang and colleagues.

Returning to medication nonadherence and the limitations of pharmacotherapy, we know that detecting and managing adverse effects of antipsychotic medications are key to effective care. Accordingly, Ames and colleagues describe how the complexities in adverse effects of currently available antipsychotic medications represent a substantial health care burden to the patient and a therapeutic challenge to the treating provider. Given the diverse adverse effect profiles, Ames and colleagues highlight current management strategies. Shifting gears from medications, Ahmed and colleagues focus on recovery and schizophrenia. The involvement of people in recovery from schizophrenia provides complementary and powerful synergies with "traditional" clinic-based treatment of schizophrenia. This article reviews how far we have come toward incorporating recovery principles with clinical practice. Recovery also represents a shift in health care focus, in the context of emergent health care reform. Bartlett and Manderscheid illustrate how health care reform could realize the potential of the mental health parity act that was passed several years ago. They evaluate the challenges and opportunities that could exist for the provision of services for the seriously mentally ill. Finally, our US colleagues who reside in Australia, Drs Cyndi and Tom Weickert, provide a timely and critical appraisal of the most pertinent research findings in schizophrenia. Areas that have "fallen out of favor" and/or appear to be "blind alleys" are also briefly mentioned so that the discerning reader comes away succinctly informed of "the big picture" of schizophrenia research.

Collectively, these stellar colleagues provide a cogent and comprehensive synthesis of the biology and treatment of schizophrenia. As guest editor, I express my sincerest gratitude for their efforts, which come together so nicely in this timely issue of *Psychiatric Clinics of North America*. We are also grateful to Kristen Helm, our publishing collaborator at Elsevier, for her consistency with this issue of *Psychiatric Clinics of North America*.

Peter F. Buckley, MD
Medical College of Georgia
Augusta University
1120 15th Street, AA-1002
Augusta, GA 30912, USA

E-mail address:
pbuckley@gru.edu

Does Biology Transcend the Symptom-based Boundaries of Psychosis?

Godfrey D. Pearlson, MD[a,b,c,*], Brett A. Clementz, PhD[d],
John A. Sweeney, PhD[e], Matcheri S. Keshavan, MD[f],
Carol A. Tamminga, MD[e]

KEYWORDS

- Psychosis • Biotype • Neurobiology • Reclassification • Schizophrenia
- Schizoaffective • Bipolar

KEY POINTS

- Psychotic disorders overlap considerably in terms of clinical symptoms, familial patterns, risk genes, and treatment response.
- Numerous neurobiological measurements also fail to distinguish the most prevalent classic psychotic disorders (schizophrenia, schizoaffective, and psychotic bipolar) from each other.
- Statistical methods applied to such biological measurements in large numbers of these patients result in novel classifications that cut across traditional diagnostic boundaries, to reveal "Biotypes": biologically defined entities.
- Such new types of classification approaches within psychotic illnesses hopefully represent an opportunity to move away from phenomenologically defined syndromes in psychiatry and toward neurobiologically defined diseases.

Potential Conflicts of Interest: Dr J.A. Sweeney has received support from Takeda, BMS, Lilly, Roche, and Janssen. Dr M.S. Keshavan has received support from Sunovion. Dr C.A. Tamminga has received funding from Astellas, Eli Lilly, Intracellular Therapies, Lundback, and Pure Tech Ventures. Other authors declare no financial interest in relation to the work described in this article other than National Institutes of Health grant funding.

[a] Olin Neuropsychiatry Research Center, Institute of Living, 200 Retreat Avenue, Hartford, CT 06106, USA; [b] Department of Psychiatry, Yale University School of Medicine, New Haven, CT 06520, USA; [c] Department of Neurobiology, Yale University School of Medicine, New Haven, CT 06520, USA; [d] Department of Psychology, University of Georgia, Athens, GA 30602, USA; [e] Department of Psychiatry, UT Southwestern Medical School, Dallas, TX 75390, USA; [f] Department of Psychiatry, Beth Israel Deaconess Medical Center, Harvard Medical School, Boston, MA 02215, USA
* Corresponding author. Olin Neuropsychiatry Research Center, Institute of Living, Hartford Healthcare Corporation, 200 Retreat Avenue, Hartford, CT 06106.
E-mail address: godfrey.pearlson@yale.edu

Psychiatr Clin N Am 39 (2016) 165–174
http://dx.doi.org/10.1016/j.psc.2016.01.001
0193-953X/16/$ – see front matter © 2016 Elsevier Inc. All rights reserved.

INTRODUCTION

Most clinical psychiatrists are undoubtedly confident in their ability to diagnose patients with schizophrenia correctly, and to distinguish them straightforwardly from individuals with other disorders manifesting similar symptoms. In so doing, they would likely mention *Diagnostic and Statistical Manual of Mental Disorders* (DSM) criteria, say something about a presumed unique underlying neurobiology, and invoke the name of Emil Kraepelin as having settled these distinctions more than a century ago. Because questioning our assumptions is always a useful exercise, this initial article is designed both to accomplish that aim by challenging these assumptions, as well as to provide a general conceptual lens through which some of the other articles in this issue can be viewed.

AN HISTORICAL PERSPECTIVE

Given that much of our current clinical classification within psychosis begins with Kraepelin, it is appropriate to start with a brief discussion of the great diagnostic divide that he promulgated in the late nineteenth century, a delineation that survives and is seldom challenged by clinicians today. Kraepelin made a fundamental diagnostic distinction within serious mental illnesses between those conditions that are clearly recurrent and episodic with between-episode recovery ("manic-depressive insanity") and another syndrome characterized by lack of recovery plus longitudinal deterioration of personality and intellect ("dementia precox"),[1] subsequently termed "schizophrenia" by Bleuler.[2] Most aspects of this classification are still present in our diagnostic manuals, although Kraepelin's schema has been altered in subtle ways over time.[3] For example, major depressive disorder, because it was recurrent, was certainly included within his purview of manic-depressive insanity; single episodes of mania, because they were not repeated, were not within the definition.[3] Kraepelin provided many detailed case examples of manic-depressive insanity in which patients clearly manifested psychotic symptoms, so that hallucinations, formal thought disorder, and delusions, the defining symptoms of psychosis, were certainly not limited to cases of schizophrenia; the predominant emphasis was on longitudinal course rather than cross-sectional symptoms. Although (as we will soon discuss) there are troubling problems and inconsistencies with Kraepelin's delineation, it has persisted for more than 100 years because no better diagnostic categorization system arose to replace it.

PROBLEMS WITH KRAEPELIN'S DISTINCTION

First, within much of clinical medicine there are obvious diagnostic boundaries, or "points of rarity" between distinct disorders. However, for schizophrenia and bipolar disorder, there are often areas of symptomatic overlap and substantial numbers of patients are not prototypical, with many left in a diagnostic muddle. This is due both to heterogeneity within these diagnoses and overlap between them, or as has been said, "patients don't read DSM." For example, in the realm of long-term outcome, some patients with otherwise typical bipolar disorder have clearly progressive chronic courses,[4] whereas it was recognized early that some patients with otherwise clinically typical schizophrenia show solid clinical recovery[5] and/or manifest prominent affective symptoms. These and other observations led Kasanin to propose a third diagnostic entity of "schizoaffective disorder" in 1933,[6] that many clinicians believe has served only to complicate issues, is a diagnostic evasion, and was necessitated only by a lack of clear diagnostic demarcation between many cases of schizophrenia and bipolar illness. Similar findings have been demonstrated recently.[7]

Moreover, with regard to clinical symptomatology, up to 50% of otherwise typical bipolar patients have clear-cut psychotic symptoms (hallucinations, delusions, formal thought disorder) during episodes,[8–11] as well as sharing some of the cognitive abnormalities that were thought originally only to characterize patients with schizophrenia.[12] One consequence of this is that many cases of psychosis are hard to classify, and are thereby omitted from both clinical trials and genetic analyses, inevitably skewing study outcomes. Furthermore, there is also diagnostic crossover, in that a third of patients with schizophrenia meet criteria for major depressive disorder (MDD) if the DSM exclusionary rule (a diagnosis of schizophrenia trumps one of MDD) is set aside.[13] The Kraepelinian dichotomy also has been challenged for other reasons. Ideally, as implied by early proponents of "external" validations of disease entities,[14] we would prefer distinct diseases with substantial genetic origin to "breed true" within families, to show distinct high heritability translating into the discovery of unique sets of risk genes, and, with regard to treatment, different, appropriate nonoverlapping therapies for each disorder. Last, we require diagnostic systems that differentiate patients in ways that guide illness-specific, successful, and incrementally improving treatments. However, many psychotic patients receive polypharmacy, tacitly acknowledging overlap in efficacy of "mood stabilizers" and "antipsychotics."

Unfortunately, none of these criteria hold up satisfactorily for bipolar illness and schizophrenia. Familial expression of illness crosses over diagnoses so that these illnesses fail to "breed true."[15] Although both schizophrenia and bipolar disorder are highly heritable, there is substantial overlap in the risk genes discovered to date,[16] and treatment modalities converge substantially; for example, the routine use of second-generation antipsychotics for bipolar illness, whether or not it is characterized by psychotic symptoms. These observations have led some clinicians to posit that psychosis lies on a spectrum without clear boundaries of demarcation, so that it is not possible to "carve nature at its joints."[17]

SYNDROMES VERSUS DISEASES

Kraepelin was confident that neurobiological evidence would demonstrate conclusively that the syndromes he had identified were distinct entities. He felt both that the cortical neuropathology of schizophrenia would soon be revealed, showing it to be a neurodegenerative illness and noted the strong heritability of manic-depressive illness.[18] He had cause for such confidence because his colleagues and contemporaries had recently identified microscopic brain changes associated with neurosyphilis and Alzheimer disease. Nevertheless, 100 years later we are still waiting for such conclusive neurobiological evidence to emerge; as Robins and Guze[14] stated 45 years ago, "….in the absence of laboratory tests, or a solid understanding of pathogenesis, the criteria available to psychiatry for validating those logical categories have been restricted to clinical features, outcome and family history." The consequence of this situation (as well as the lack of progress over an almost 50-year time period) cannot be too strongly emphasized. If we lack information on the basic causes and pathologic changes associated with psychosis, then we are operating in a knowledge-space defined by merely describing clinical syndromes, analogous to the fever, dropsy, seizures, or cough familiar to early medical practitioners. Stated another way, in the absence of biological tests, phenomenology as a clinical exercise describes heterogeneous syndromes in a reliable manner, but cannot identify true disease entities. Recent versions of DSM[19] represent examples of phenomenology writ large. Thus, it is no coincidence that most medications in our psychiatric armamentarium were initially identified based on chance discoveries rather than being designed as a consequence of any rational knowledge of the underlying pathology of the disorders they are intended to treat. As long as the etiology and pathogenesis of schizophrenia and other psychotic illnesses remain elusive, it is unsurprising that clinical diagnosis is not a particularly good guide to treatment response, as might be expected for heterogeneous, catchall diagnostic categories.

CAN BIOLOGICAL MEASURES HELP CLARIFY THE SITUATION?

Given this rather dismal catalog of facts, several groups have begun to explore conceptual routes to help clarify the situation by reexamining some of our conceptual assumptions, and once again turning to biological classification as a solution to our conundrum. Gathering sufficient information for the resulting data to be sufficiently powered statistically to yield meaningful and generalizable conclusions necessitates multisite efforts and research consortia. One such research group is the Bipolar-Schizophrenia Network on Intermediate Phenotypes (B-SNIP), a National Institutes of Health (NIH)-funded, multisite consortium of investigators who constructed a multimeasure approach to study stable patients with any 1 of 3 psychotic disorders (schizophrenia, schizoaffective disorder, or bipolar disorder with psychosis), plus at least 1 of their first-degree relatives and demographically matched healthy control subjects. I am familiar with this effort, as the director of 1 of the 5 currently participating sites, along with Carol Tamminga/Dallas, TX, Matcheri Keshavan/Boston, MA, Brett Clementz/Athens, GA, and Elliot Gershon/Chicago, IL, plus Gunvant Thaker and John Sweeney.

The total number of subjects assessed in the first wave of the study (B-SNIP1) is approximately 2500. Volunteers were gathered from diverse clinical settings and across multiple geographic regions to allow generalizability regarding resulting conclusions. All probands had been on stable medications for 4 or more weeks, and none was acutely ill at the time of assessment, although many were symptomatic to varying degrees. As well as carefully documenting symptoms and recording medications, basic study data consisted of standardized and reliable biological assessments conducted on the same models of equipment across the several geographically separated collection sites.

The almost 50 biological measures used were chosen based on straightforward criteria. These characteristics were that they were reliable, well-studied (defined as being found previously in multiple studies to be abnormal in association with psychotic illnesses), fully quantifiable, not strongly associated with medication status or state/stage of illness, having evidence of heritability, and having been reported to be also abnormal in unaffected close relatives of probands with the illness. This latter criterion qualified them as being *endophenotypes* (ie, markers of illness risk),[20] rather than merely *biomarkers* (indices of the presence of manifest illness). It should be emphasized that none of the measures gathered are likely specifically abnormal in patients with schizophrenia (and, by definition, their relatives); many also have been shown to be abnormal in subjects with bipolar disorder (probands and relatives), and in some cases in patients with other major mental disorders.

Examples of B-SNIP measures included those in the realms of eye movement/tracking (smooth pursuit, saccades, antisaccades), electrophysiology (resting measures and various auditory-evoked potentials), MRI (structural, diffusion-tensor imaging, and resting state functional scans), psychophysiological measures (such as pre-pulse inhibition) and assessment of multiple cognitive domains. All subjects were genotyped. A parallel study examining nonpsychotic bipolar-I volunteers is currently under way to determine whether findings from B-SNIP are specific to psychosis.

The initial questions posed by the B-SNIP1 study were straightforward: to examine these multiple biological measures across several psychotic illnesses, plus the putatively related axis II cluster-A disorders (schizotypal, schizoid, and paranoid) in nonpsychotic relatives, to determine whether these indices shared commonalities across the psychosis dimension/spectrum that might clearly separate the disorders from one another more clearly than did illness symptoms, or to discover whether or not they cross traditional diagnostic boundaries. Subsidiary questions were whether similar abnormalities to those seen in subjects with psychotic disorders occurred in their unaffected relatives across disorders (as would be expected of endophenotypes) and whether the various axis I diagnostic groups were distinguished by differences in *type* of biological abnormalities, differences in degree of *severity* of these measures, or neither of these.

MAJOR FINDINGS

Clinical symptoms evident at the time of testing did not prominently distinguish diseases based on the text revision of the fourth edition of DSM from one another, whether using the Positive and Negative Syndrome Scale for any of it subscales, the Young Mania Rating Scale, or the Montgomery-Asberg Depression Rating Scale. The Birchwood Social Functioning Scale revealed greatest impairment in subjects with schizophrenia and least in those with psychotic bipolar disorder, but again, all axis I groups appeared rather similar when compared with normalcy.[21] A novel illness rating scale (the Schizo-Bipolar Scale)[7] designed specifically to separate prototypic schizophrenia from bipolar illness along a continuum, and based on both current and historical information on typical illness symptoms, interepisode recovery, and so forth, revealed no points of separation among the 3 DSM disorders, which instead blurred into each other. Clearly then, and contrary to clinical expectation, symptom measures of various types performed very poorly in separating the DSM syndromes. Interestingly, examining proband family lineages revealed some kindreds with "pure" (ie, consistent) psychosis diagnoses, but also numerous families with mixtures of schizophrenia/bipolar diagnoses,[21] as had previously been reported by Lichtenstein and colleagues.[15]

Equally unexpectedly, all the major biological measures, while discriminating axis I subjects robustly from healthy controls, performed at best modestly for separating diagnostic groups, as summarized in Tamminga and colleagues,[22] whether the dimension chosen was cognition,[23] oculomotor,[24] structural MRI,[25] resting state functional MRI,[26] or P 300 evoked potential.[27] In many cases, abnormalities were relatively greater or lesser in one DSM-based group compared with another, but the general trend across all endophenotypes was one of only modest differences in degree of severity, marked similarity and overlap among groups, and often similar (although lesser) findings in unaffected relatives, with those meeting cluster-A criteria resembling axis I subjects more than controls. To summarize, the observed differences in biological deviation were in degree, rather than in kind (analogous to symptom distribution) and biomarkers performed modestly overall in distinguishing DSM clinical psychosis diagnoses from one another.

How are these biology-based results to be best understood? The most parsimonious explanation is that the investigators had fallen into the conceptual trap of using biology to validate existing, syndrome-based diagnostic categories, where measures show only blurred differences in degree across psychoses. Biological data, in other words, fail to validate conventional psychiatric diagnoses as a "gold standard," but instead revealed a single severity continuum, most often with schizophrenia at one end and psychotic bipolar illness at the other.

RECONCEPTUALIZATION: START WITH THE BIOLOGY

An obvious alternative strategy was for the B-SNIP investigators to start with an agnostic, bottom-up reclassification, using the same endophenotype data, but setting aside conventional, phenomenologically based, categorical diagnostic entities, to see if we could derive distinctive entities based purely on biology. This is a strategy that has been advocated for 30 or more years[28] in classifying the psychoses. An obvious recent parallel within clinical medicine is that of breast cancer, which was redefined as different disease entities with distinct treatment responses based on biological evidence.[29] Such an analysis was carried out on patients in the B-SNIP endophenotype data set[30] using multivariate taxometric analyses, and revealed 3 neurobiologically distinct biologically defined psychosis categories, termed "Biotypes," that crossed clinical diagnostic boundaries (ie, every Biotype contained subjects with all 3 conventional diagnoses). The derived Biotypes were distinctly separate from each other in a manner that was statistically vastly superior to that obtained (using the same measures) with DSM diagnoses. In addition, the Biotypes did not fit a simple severity continuum. The Biotypes appeared to be heritable, in that their unaffected first-degree relatives (who were not used in the Biotype construction) strongly resembled them on the biomarkers, and additional endophenotypes that were also not used in defining the original Biotype categories captured this statistical typology as secondary validators.[30]

Of particular interest is that some of the deviations from normal within different Biotype domains were in opposite directions; within one such domain (sensorimotor reactivity), one of the Biotype groups scored significantly less than healthy control values, whereas another scored significantly higher than these values. One can imagine that collapsing neurobiological measurements from such individuals across conventional DSM diagnoses would lead to the confusing results that have bedeviled the research field in psychosis, notably in the areas of drug and gene discovery. The obvious next step is to define the genetics and molecular biological underpinnings of each distinct Biotype, and to construct treatment trials that specifically address unique mechanisms. One of the 3 Biotypes appeared to be relatively similar to healthy controls across most neurobiological measures; patients in this category may be "phenocopies" especially sensitive to environmental psychosis risk factors.

Although these results are novel and promising, they are still preliminary, and require replication. A study funded by the National Institute of Mental Health (NIMH), B-SNIP-2, is therefore currently under way to test Biotype replicability in a new sample. Conventional schizophrenia subtypes (such as paranoid, hebephrenic) are highly unstable over time, which is one reason they were omitted from the fifth edition of DSM (DSM-5); it certainly will be necessary to demonstrate the longitudinal stability of Biotypes. Another obvious question is whether *nonpsychotic* bipolar subjects, who were not examined in B-SNIP, are biologically distinct from psychotic bipolar individuals. A separate NIMH-funded study is currently under way to address that question.

TAKE-HOME MESSAGES, AND THE FUTURE

First, there is diminishing support for the familiar, clinical phenomenology-based, classical Kraepelinian diagnostic model still used as the gold standard in DSM-5. Using multiple biological classifiers reveals an absence of true points of diagnostic rarity across the most prevalent psychotic disorders, a finding that would not be expected if these were truly distinct entities. Another problem for classic diagnostic categories, not explored in this article, is the existence of psychosis continua versus what we are accustomed to thinking of as categorical diagnoses. For example, cluster-A "personality disorders" are likely positioned on a continuum of severity with psychotic illnesses, as individuals who meet diagnostic criteria for them manifest similar if lesser biological abnormalities to patients with the disorders.[31] This is analogous perhaps to the elevated but not pathologic blood sugars found in nondiabetic relatives of patients with type 2 diabetes. There is also the phenomenon of nonpsychotic "voice-hearers," who also may belong on an extended psychosis spectrum.[32] These and allied phenomena have led some observers to argue that dimensional or spectrum concepts may describe psychotic disorders more realistically than our current categorical classifications. It also will be important to see how psychotic patients with MDD fit into any new schema (**Fig. 1**).

Available evidence shows multiple shared neurobiological signatures across the psychoses in a manner that offers very little support for conventional symptom-based diagnostic categories such as those bequeathed to us from the Kraepelinian dichotomy and instantiated today in the latest edition of the DSM. Although Kraepelin hoped that biology would ultimately validate the syndromes that he described as

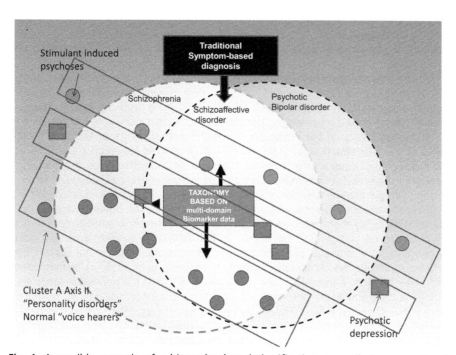

Fig. 1. A possible example of a biomarker-based classification, agnostic to conventional diagnostic categories, illustrating how dimensional or spectrum concepts might plausibly delineate psychotic disorders differently from current, symptom-based categorical classifications. Such a novel taxonomy would be based on multidomain endophenotype measures as described in the text. In addition to the 3 major diagnoses examined in B-SNIP1 (schizophrenia, schizoaffective disorder, and psychotic bipolar disorder), theoretically allied conditions are incorporated into this schema as illustrated, including psychostimulant-induced psychoses (*upper left*) and psychotic depression (*lower right*). Additional conditions portrayed include individuals who can be conceived of as existing on the mild end of a theoretic continuum with psychotic disorders, for example, persons lacking a psychiatric diagnosis but who experience phenomena allied to auditory hallucinations (so-called "voice-hearers") as well as the cluster-A "personality disorders" listed in the fourth edition of DSM (schizotypal, paranoid, and schizoid). (*Courtesy of* M. Keshavan, MD, Boston, MA.)

distinct entities, the available facts do not support his belief. An alternative means to attack the problem of classifying psychosis is an approach that uses reliable and valid neurobiological tests to derive bottom-up, statistically driven novel categories, agnostic to phenomenological symptom-based diagnostic criteria. This type of alternative taxonomic approach is necessarily based on multiple endophenotypes rather than any simple, single measure. This is not to minimize the utility of biological disease markers that are not also heritable indicators of illness predisposition. Although the latter more readily lend themselves to the discovery of disease risk genes, noninherited biomarkers may be uniquely useful for disease classifications for those illness features that lack a direct genetic antecedent.

This strategy offers promising preliminary data that suggest a means to derive a biologic redefinition of psychotic syndromes, in a manner consistent with the Research Domain Criteria[33] (RDoC), proposed by NIH.[34] This type of process is actually one that has characterized much of the history of medicine. For example, "dropsy" is now recognized not to be a distinct disease, but rather a syndrome with multiple causes, including cardiac and renal diseases and protein deficiency, each of which responds to a specific type of treatment. Perhaps a more apt example is medicine's ability to use biological tests such as chest radiographs and sputum cultures to parse a heterogeneous group of patients all presenting with the symptom of severe cough, into individuals with the diseases of viral pneumonia, pulmonary tuberculosis, and lung cancer, requiring different treatments. A salutary fact is that a substantial minority of psychotic patients are treatment-resistant, despite similar clinical presentations. Recent arguments have been made to repurpose existing drugs for the treatment of schizophrenia, based on emerging genetic and molecular biological mechanisms.[35] Logically, discovery of the molecular biological underpinnings of Biotypes would move in a similar direction, or even to novel drug designs based on a finer-grained trans-diagnostic classification scheme. The rest of medicine made the transition from syndromes to diseases many years ago, as the underlying pathology and biology of particular syndromes was discovered, but the great complexity and inaccessibility of the brain renders this enterprise a necessarily complex and daunting one for psychiatry. Previously mentioned efforts from NIMH to reclassify mental disorders as a whole based on biological observations, in their RDoC,[33] represent a parallel effort in this direction, although psychosis does not necessarily fit comfortably in this schema. Initial efforts to fit specific psychotic symptoms, such as alogia/blunted affect and hallucinations, within RDoC are being made,[36,37] and the general strategy that biological data should be gathered across current diagnostic categories is shared by both RDoC and B-SNIP.[38] The reconceptualization of psychosis categories based on biology holds the promise of new directions in disease classification and hopefully will lead to novel treatment strategies that one hopes will emerge over the next few years.

REFERENCES

1. Kraepelin E. Psychiatry: a textbook for students and physicians. 7th edition. Leipzig: Barth: McMillan; 1912.
2. Bleuler E. Dementia praecox or the group of schizophrenias. Vertex 1911;21: 394–400.
3. Pearlson GD. Etiologic, phenomenologic, and endophenotypic overlap of schizophrenia and bipolar disorder. Annu Rev Clin Psychol 2015;11:251–81.
4. Fischer BA, Carpenter WT Jr. Will the Kraepelinian dichotomy survive DSM-V? Neuropsychopharmacology 2009;34(9):2081–7.

5. Zendig E. Beitrage zur differentialdiagnose des manisch-depressiven irreseins und der dementia praecox. Allg Z Psychiatr 1909;66:932–3.
6. Kasanin J. The acute schizoaffective psychoses. 1933. Am J Psychiatry 1994; 151(Suppl 6):144–54.
7. Keshavan MS, Morris DW, Sweeney JA, et al. A dimensional approach to the psychosis spectrum between bipolar disorder and schizophrenia: the Schizo-Bipolar Scale. Schizophr Res 2011;133(1–3):250–4.
8. Coryell W, Lavori P, Endicott J, et al. Outcome in schizoaffective, psychotic, and nonpsychotic depression. Course during a six- to 24-month follow-up. Arch Gen Psychiatry 1984;41(8):787–91.
9. Keck PE Jr, McElroy SL, Havens JR, et al. Psychosis in bipolar disorder: phenomenology and impact on morbidity and course of illness. Compr Psychiatry 2003; 44(4):263–9.
10. Goodwin FK, Jamison KR. Manic-depressive illness. New York: New York: Oxford University Press; 1990.
11. Guze SB, Woodruff RA Jr, Clayton PJ. The significance of psychotic affective disorders. Arch Gen Psychiatry 1975;32(9):1147–50.
12. Glahn DC, Williams JT, McKay DR, et al. Discovering schizophrenia endophenotypes in randomly ascertained pedigrees. Biol Psychiatry 2015;77(1):75–83.
13. Majadas S, Olivares J, Galan J, et al. Prevalence of depression and its relationship with other clinical characteristics in a sample of patients with stable schizophrenia. Compr Psychiatry 2012;53(2):145–51.
14. Robins E, Guze SB. Establishment of diagnostic validity in psychiatric illness: its application to schizophrenia. Am J Psychiatry 1970;126(7):983–7.
15. Lichtenstein P, Yip BH, Bjork C, et al. Common genetic determinants of schizophrenia and bipolar disorder in Swedish families: a population-based study. Lancet 2009;373(9659):234–9.
16. Cross-Disorder Group of the Psychiatric Genomics Consortium. Identification of risk loci with shared effects on five major psychiatric disorders: a genome-wide analysis. Lancet 2013;381(9875):1371–9.
17. Crow TJ, Chance SA, Priddle TH, et al. Laterality interacts with sex across the schizophrenia/bipolarity continuum: an interpretation of meta-analyses of structural MRI. Psychiatry Res 2013;210(3):1232–44.
18. Kraepelin E. Der erschenungsformen der irreseins. [The manifestations of insanity]. Hist Psychiatry 1920;3:509–29.
19. American Psychiatric Association. Diagnostic and statistical manual of mental disorders. 5th edition. Washington, DC: American Psychiatric Association Publishing; 2013.
20. Glahn DC, Knowles EE, McKay DR, et al. Arguments for the sake of endophenotypes: examining common misconceptions about the use of endophenotypes in psychiatric genetics. Am J Med Genet B Neuropsychiatr Genet 2014;165B(2): 122–30.
21. Tamminga CA, Ivleva EI, Keshavan MS, et al. Clinical phenotypes of psychosis in the Bipolar-Schizophrenia Network on Intermediate Phenotypes (B-SNIP). Am J Psychiatry 2013;170(11):1263–74.
22. Tamminga CA, Pearlson G, Keshavan M, et al. Bipolar and schizophrenia network for intermediate phenotypes: outcomes across the psychosis continuum. Schizophr Bull 2014;40(Suppl 2):S131–7.
23. Hill SK, Reilly JL, Keefe RS, et al. Neuropsychological impairments in schizophrenia and psychotic bipolar disorder: findings from the Bipolar-Schizophrenia

Network on Intermediate Phenotypes (B-SNIP) study. Am J Psychiatry 2013; 170(11):1275–84.

24. Reilly JL, Frankovich K, Hill S, et al. Elevated antisaccade error rate as an intermediate phenotype for psychosis across diagnostic categories. Schizophr Bull 2014;40(5):1011–21.

25. Ivleva EI, Bidesi AS, Keshavan MS, et al. Gray matter volume as an intermediate phenotype for psychosis: Bipolar-Schizophrenia Network on Intermediate Phenotypes (B-SNIP). Am J Psychiatry 2013;170(11):1285–96.

26. Khadka S, Meda SA, Stevens MC, et al. Is aberrant functional connectivity a psychosis endophenotype? A resting state functional magnetic resonance imaging study. Biol Psychiatry 2013;74(6):458–66.

27. Ethridge LE, Hamm JP, Pearlson GD, et al. Event-related potential and time-frequency endophenotypes for schizophrenia and psychotic bipolar disorder. Biol Psychiatry 2014;77(2):127–36.

28. Kendell RE. Diagnosis and classification of functional psychoses. Br Med Bull 1987;43(3):499–513.

29. Curtis C, Shah SP, Chin SF, et al. The genomic and transcriptomic architecture of 2,000 breast tumours reveals novel subgroups. Nature 2012;486(7403):346–52.

30. Clementz BA, Sweeney JA, Hamm JP, et al. Identification of distinct psychosis biotypes using brain-based biomarkers. Am J Psychiatry 2015. [Epub ahead of print].

31. McCarley RW, Niznikiewicz MA, Salisbury DF, et al. Cognitive dysfunction in schizophrenia: unifying basic research and clinical aspects. Eur Arch Psychiatry Clin Neurosci 1999;249(Suppl 4):69–82.

32. Allen P, Modinos G, Hubl D, et al. Neuroimaging auditory hallucinations in schizophrenia: from neuroanatomy to neurochemistry and beyond. Schizophr Bull 2012; 38(4):695–703.

33. Insel TR, Cuthbert BN. Endophenotypes: bridging genomic complexity and disorder heterogeneity. Biol Psychiatry 2009;66(11):988–9.

34. Kapur S, Phillips AG, Insel TR. Why has it taken so long for biological psychiatry to develop clinical tests and what to do about it? Mol Psychiatry 2012;17(12): 1174–9.

35. Lencz T, Malhotra AK. Targeting the schizophrenia genome: a fast track strategy from GWAS to clinic. Mol Psychiatry 2015;20(7):820–6.

36. Ford JM, Morris SE, Hoffman RE, et al. Studying hallucinations within the NIMH RDoC framework. Schizophr Bull 2014;40(Suppl 4):S295–304.

37. Cohen AS, Najolia GM, Kim Y, et al. On the boundaries of blunt affect/alogia across severe mental illness: implications for research domain criteria. Schizophr Res 2012;140(1–3):41–5.

38. Carpenter WT. RDoC and DSM-5: what's the fuss? Schizophr Bull 2013;39(5): 945–6.

Are We Really Impacting Duration of Untreated Psychosis and Does It Matter?
Longitudinal Perspectives on Early Intervention from the Irish Public Health Services

Mary Clarke, MD, FRCPI, FRCPsych[a,b],
Catherine M. McDonough, MD, MRCPsych[c,d], Roisin Doyle, BA, MSc[b],
John L. Waddington, PhD, DSc[e,f,*]

KEYWORDS

- Duration of untreated psychosis • Outcome • Early intervention • Prodromal phase
- Public health service

KEY POINTS

- Early-intervention services are predicated on the assumption that the period of untreated psychosis can be reduced and effective interventions introduced earlier in the illness course.
- Despite nearly 3 decades in development, the evidence base supporting early intervention is not as extensive as might be expected.
- Although more is understood about the origins of prepsychotic and psychotic symptoms, the timing and constituents of optimal interventions in the prepsychotic phase is not clear.
- Methodological differences between studies hamper interpretation of the evidence and the construction of future research directions.
- These considerations may extend beyond psychotic illness to other domains of serious mental illness.

Disclosure Statement: The authors have nothing to disclose.
[a] School of Medicine and Medical Sciences, University College Dublin, Dublin 4, Ireland; [b] DETECT Early Intervention Services, St John of God Community Services Ltd, Avila House, Block 5, Blackrock Business Park, Blackrock, Co. Dublin, Ireland; [c] Cavan-Monaghan Mental Health Service, COPE Early Intervention Psychosis Service, St Davnet's Hospital, Monaghan, Co. Monaghan, Ireland; [d] Cavan-Monaghan Community Rehabilitation Service, St. Davnet's Hospital, Monaghan, Co. Monaghan, Ireland; [e] Molecular and Cellular Therapeutics, Royal College of Surgeons in Ireland, St. Stephen's Green, Dublin 2, Ireland; [f] Jiangsu Key Laboratory of Translational Research & Therapy for Neuro-Psychiatric-Disorders, Department of Pharmacology, College of Pharmaceutical Sciences, Soochow University, Suzhou, China
* Corresponding author. Molecular and Cellular Therapeutics, Royal College of Surgeons in Ireland, St. Stephen's Green, Dublin 2, Ireland.
E-mail address: jwadding@rcsi.ie

Psychiatr Clin N Am 39 (2016) 175–186
http://dx.doi.org/10.1016/j.psc.2016.01.002
0193-953X/16/$ – see front matter © 2016 Elsevier Inc. All rights reserved.

Although in many branches of medicine it is considered axiomatic that the longer an illness remains untreated the worse is long-term outcome, the concept that such a relationship might similarly apply to major mental illness has proved more challenging. The proposition that untreated psychosis has adverse consequences for brain function through some unknown pathobiological and/or psychopathological mechanism(s),[1] and the subsequent "research front" that longer duration of untreated psychosis (DUP) results in a poorer prognosis, has prompted the establishment of early-intervention (EI) services for the treatment of first-episode psychosis on a global basis, particularly in Australasia, Europe, and the United States.[2–4] It was opined that reducing DUP through early detection and the implementation of phase-specific treatments would result in improved outcomes for those traversing the emergence of psychotic illness.[5]

As clinical outcome in psychotic illness has not improved materially over recent generations, this development represented a potentially exciting step forward in the field of psychiatry. Over the past 2 decades, this proposition, that effective treatment earlier in the course of illness can improve both short-term and long-term outcome for individuals with psychosis, has been evaluated by a variety of EI services with somewhat mixed results, such that debate and indeed controversy continues as to whether these services are an effective use of resources. A key assumption underlying the implementation of EI services is that the period of untreated psychosis can be accurately identified in sufficient numbers of people so as to reduce delays to treatment, facilitate effective interventions at an earlier stage of illness, and thereby improve outcome. Although an intuitive and seemingly simple proposition, the actuality has proved more complex, with opinion ranging from doubt, through agnosticism, to proselytism.[6,7]

THE CONCEPT OF DURATION OF UNTREATED PSYCHOSIS AND ITS RELATIONSHIP TO OUTCOME
Concept of Duration of Untreated Psychosis

The concept of DUP (**Fig. 1**) refers to the period of time from the emergence of psychotic symptoms to initiation of treatment, and has been defined as the "time from manifestation of the first psychotic symptom to initiation of adequate antipsychotic treatment"[2]; thus, DUP refers to the period of active psychotic symptoms antedating initial treatment. As a concept, DUP is distinguishable from duration of untreated illness (DUI), which has the same endpoint as DUP but refers to the emergence of the first noticeable symptom.[8] The period of time between emergence of the first

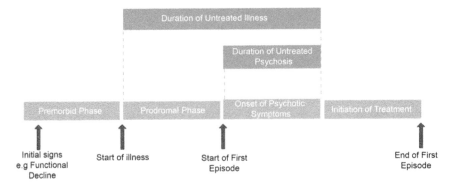

Fig. 1. Early stages of psychosis: DUI and DUP.

noticeable symptom and emergence of the first psychotic symptom is sometimes referred to as the prodrome.[9]

Measurement of Duration of Untreated Psychosis

Recent review has documented 9 instruments designed for measuring DUP. Although their interrater reliabilities were found to be adequate to excellent, with no instrument clearly outstanding relative to others, non–instrument-based, ad hoc clinical interviews remained the most common approach to measuring DUP.[10] Inevitable uncertainties as to the meaning and definition of "first noticeable symptom" and "first psychotic symptom," particularly at the interface between prodromal signs and florid, diagnostic features of psychosis, may be important contributors to differences in findings between studies.

Relationship of Duration of Untreated Psychosis to Clinical and Functional Outcome

Over the past 2 decades, the relationship between DUP and outcome has received considerable attention. Initial systematic reviews indicated shorter DUP to be associated with better outcomes in the short term across a number of domains.[2,11] Recent meta-analysis of 33 studies worldwide has reported longer DUP to be associated with poorer general symptomatic outcome, more severe positive and negative symptoms, reduced likelihood of remission, poorer social functioning and global outcomes, but not with employment, quality of life, or hospital treatment; however, those associations attaining statistical significance were modest ($r = 0.13$–0.18), indicating "a constant, subtle correlation between long DUP and poor outcome"; longer follow-up period was associated with stronger associations between DUP and negative symptoms, hospital treatment, and global outcome.[4]

A particular relationship between DUP and negative symptoms is reinforced by recent meta-analysis of 16 studies worldwide, which reported longer DUP to be associated with more severe negative symptoms at baseline and at both shorter-term (1–2 year) and longer-term (5–8 year) follow-up; however, the relationship between DUP and negative symptoms was nonlinear, with DUP longer than 9 months associated with substantially more severe negative symptoms than DUP shorter than 9 months.[12] In contrast to this relationship between DUP and negative symptoms, any relationship between DUP and cognitive dysfunction over such typical parameters of DUP and follow-up appears less clear. Although some studies have reported an association between longer DUP and poorer cognitive functioning,[13,14] reviews indicate any such relationship to be less robust than for negative symptoms.[11,15] There is evidence that some aspects of cognitive impairment predate the onset of psychotic symptoms.[15,16]

Although prospective studies and subsequent meta-analysis thereof is the "gold standard" for identifying such associations with DUP, the subtle relationships identified to date might be clearer in circumstances in which DUP is exceptionally long. Our initial studies took advantage of a naturalistic, cross-sectional experimental model that is no longer available: that of patients in whom psychosis emerged in the preneuroleptic era and who therefore experienced many years of florid psychosis before the introduction of antipsychotics. After controlling for age and for duration and continuity of subsequent antipsychotic treatment, DUP (mean 13.9 years) was a strong predictor of current negative symptoms and general cognitive impairment but not of positive symptoms or executive dysfunction, whereas duration of illness following initiation of antipsychotic treatment did not predict any measure.[17] Such extremely prolonged DUP, hopefully now encountered only rarely in the developed world, was associated specifically with severe negative symptoms and general cognitive impairment; however, executive dysfunction, although also prominent in these patients, may be "locked-in" at an earlier phase of the illness. Our subsequent study using the same naturalistic, cross-sectional experimental model (mean DUP 9.2 years) reported that as years of chronic, refractory illness accrue, psychomotor poverty, but not reality distortion or disorganization, becomes more sharply delineated and dominant within the overall structure of psychopathology and is predicted enduringly by DUP.[18]

A critical issue for contemporary prospective studies is the extent to which the initial relationships between DUP and clinical and functional indices at baseline and short-term/medium-term follow-up endure in the longer term. In our own studies, we have been able to follow an epidemiologically representative cohort of 166 persons with first-episode psychosis, with high rates of retention, from initial presentation[19] to follow-up at 4, 8, and 12 years. At 4 years, DUP (mean 17.9 months; median 5 months) predicted poorer global functioning and severity of positive and negative symptoms.[20] At 8 years, DUP predicted poorer remission status, poorer social functioning, and severity of positive symptoms; interestingly, DUI (mean 39.2 months) predicted severity of negative symptoms and poorer functional recovery between 4 and 8 years.[21] At 12 years, DUP predicted poorer remission status, poorer global functioning, poorer social functioning, severity of both positive and negative symptoms, and impaired quality of life.[22]

These sequential investigations, the longest prospective study of an epidemiologically representative inception cohort of first-episode psychosis that has examined the effect of DUP on outcome, independent of confounders, reveals the following: the relationship between DUP and poorer clinical and global functional outcome endures over at least 12 years; the relationship between DUP and negative symptoms becomes more evident with increasing duration of follow-up; path analysis indicates that the relationship between DUP and functional outcome is mediated primarily via concurrent psychopathology, particularly negative symptoms; and the lack of relationship between DUP and the real-life outcomes of independent living or gainful employment could reflect the importance of preexisting sociocultural factors, such as individual opportunity.[22]

Overall, our findings elaborate DUP as a modest but significant and potentially modifiable predictor of long-term symptomatic and general functional outcome in psychotic illness over a period that extends beyond a decade and may endure considerably thereafter. In particular, they suggest a route to reducing disability via interventions that attenuate psychopathology, particularly negative symptoms, such as EI to reduce DUP.

How Might Duration of Untreated Psychosis Influence Clinical and Functional Outcome?

The basis of these relationships involving DUP is unclear. An initial proposal[1] that untreated psychosis constitutes an active, morbid process that exerts a "biologically toxic" effect on the brain has not been substantiated on systematic review of multiple neuroimaging and neuropsychological studies; in particular, most studies that do not support the "neurotoxicity" hypothesis were larger in size and had more appropriate, longitudinal designs than the minority of studies that support this hypothesis.[23,24] Nevertheless, studies to date cannot incontrovertibly exclude some very subtle, active morbid process consequent to the underlying pathobiology of psychosis, about which we know so little,[25,26] and how this might be attenuated by early, effective intervention with antipsychotics and/or psychologically based therapies.

Alternative explanations include an effect of DUP that is mediated via one or more psychosocial process(es), such as social support,[27] or the presence of an as-yet unidentified confounding variable.[2] However, like others, we found shorter DUP also to be associated with improved overall functioning and quality of life across several standardized measures and that these associations were independent of potential confounding variables (eg, age, gender, diagnosis, premorbid adjustment, substance misuse, and years spent in education).[22] This argues against the notion that DUP may be a proxy for other factors.

FUNDAMENTAL ISSUES REGARDING EARLY INTERVENTION
Duration of Untreated Psychosis as Tractable to Early Intervention Within Public Health Services

On the basis of "a constant, subtle correlation between long DUP and poor outcome,"[4] DUP is seen as one of the few potentially modifiable determinants of outcome. EI for first-episode psychosis can be conceptualized as including one or more of an interlocking set of strategies composed of 2 main elements: (1) reducing delay to treatment, that is, reducing DUP, and the provision of more intensive intervention during the years immediately following identification of a psychotic disorder[28]; and (2) the provision of "phase-specific" interventions that are adapted specifically to patients and their families over this early course of illness.[29,30]

The focus on early identification over the past 2 decades has led to a detailed, examination of the "reverse" timeline of psychosis, beginning with the emergence of florid, diagnostic symptoms, through the prodrome, to more recent studies examining psychotic experiences in the general population, and then reconstructing prospectively the developmental timeline.[16] For many, the emergence of threshold psychotic symptoms can be identified with some clarity, but for others the situation is not as clear cut, particularly when there are comorbid conditions such as developmental disorders, Diagnostic and Statistical Manual of Mental Disorder, Fifth Edition, Axis II pathology, and/or substance misuse. Furthermore, in some but not all cases, threshold psychotic symptoms are preceded by a prodromal phase, of varying definition and duration, that appears to be associated with increased risk for threshold psychosis and can include the putative "attenuated psychosis syndrome."[31]

How Can Duration of Untreated Psychosis Be Reduced?

It has been opined that EI initiatives to shorten DUP have been expensive and have reaped relatively few substantive rewards.[6] Systematic review has identified 8 early detection initiatives: 3 variants of direct contact with general practitioners, involving various permutations of workshops, with or without information packs or follow-up/refresher sessions; service reconfiguration and establishment of an EI team with networking and community education activities; a multifocus approach, with establishment of an EI team, delivery of brochures to the general public, newspaper, radio, television and cinema advertising, and visits to schools and seminars to health professionals, including general practitioners; a multifocus approach, with the establishment of a mobile education team, educational sessions to school staff and pupils, and videos and workshops for general practitioners, school counselors, and youth workers; a multifocus approach, with public poster and leaflet campaigns, a film shown on television and university campuses, participation in school counselor meetings, and mail/telephone contacts made with general practitioners; a multifocus approach, with radio, newspaper, and poster advertising, mass postcard distribution, television docudrama and radio features, celebrity endorsement, public forums,

Web site and telephone hotline, a newsletter distributed to general practitioners and school counselors, and workshops conducted with primary health professionals.[32]

The findings suggest that broadly defined general practitioner education campaigns and dedicated EI services do not by themselves result in material reduction of DUP, whereas the evidence for multifocus initiatives is mixed. Intensive campaigns targeting the general public as well as relevant professionals may be more effective; large-scale public awareness campaigns can have a modest effect to reduce DUP, but the extent to which this exerts clinically significant impact on outcome remains inconclusive. Interestingly, at the time of the above review,[32] no published studies had systematically evaluated initiatives targeting young people or professionals from nonhealth organizations. However, a recent 1-year community awareness program providing psycho-educational workshops, EI link workers, and direct referral routes for staff in non–health service community organizations was not successful in reducing treatment delays.[33]

Our own EI services, Dublin East Treatment and Early Care Team (DETECT) and Cavan-Monaghan Overcoming Psychosis Early (COPE), involve a particular focus on engagement with primary care and indicate education campaigns to be more effective when delivered directly via continuing medical education structures than indirectly via mailed information packs.[34,35] Better links among primary care, hospital emergency departments, the criminal justice system, and psychiatric services may be important.[36] However, pathways to psychiatric care can be complex and factors such as not attributing problems to mental illness, fear of stigma, and lack of knowledge about where to access help, may compound efforts to shorten DUP.[37]

How Effective Is Reduction in Duration of Untreated Psychosis?

An initial systematic review and meta-analysis of randomized controlled trials of EI services, cognitive behavioral therapy (CBT), and family intervention for individuals with early psychosis indicated that both EI services and discrete psychological interventions improve outcome for early psychosis: EI reduced hospital admission, relapse rates, and symptom severity; used alone, family intervention reduced relapse and hospital admission rates, whereas CBT reduced symptom severity with little impact on relapse or hospital admission.[38] The investigators concluded that "on balance the evidence suggests that early intervention services are an effective way of delivering care for people with early psychosis and can reduce hospital admission, relapse rates and symptom severity while improving access to and engagement with a range of treatments."[38] A subsequent Cochrane review of EI for psychosis states that there is "some support for specialized early intervention services, but further trials are desirable, and there is a question of whether gains are maintained."[3]

How Clinically Effective Is Early Intervention?

Recent review and meta-analysis of specialized assertive EI is based primarily on one large, randomized clinical trial, the Danish OPUS study, together with 3 smaller trials, the UK Lambeth Early Onset (LEO) study, the Norwegian Optimal Treatment (OTP) study, and the UK Croyden Outreach and Assertive Support Team (COAST) study. The findings indicate positive effects on psychotic and negative symptoms, substance abuse, and user satisfaction, but the clinical effects are not sustainable when patients are transferred to standard treatment; however, the positive effects on service use and ability to live independently appear more durable. The investigators conclude, "Recommendation regarding the duration of treatment must await results of ongoing trials comparing 2 years of intervention with extended treatment periods."[39]

Interpreting the evidence is compounded by the fact that components and models of EI are complex and vary widely between different services, with many services restricted to the younger age range. Perhaps somewhat surprisingly, a detailed comparison of different service models (stand-alone/hub and spoke/integrated) has not been undertaken. Castle[6] suggests that there are material issues associated with stand-alone services, including silo effects, potential deskilling of the general mental health workforce in the area of early psychosis, and difficulty of transitions between services for patients, their families, and clinicians; he suggests that early psychosis programs have shown that "good care is good for people" but only works while it is being delivered and that gains may not be maintained in the longer term once intervention has ceased.

How Cost-Effective Is Early Intervention?

Economic evaluation of EI services has provided mixed findings, with some evidence that resources diverted into EI services are cost-effective. One review concluded that although all cost-effectiveness analyses to date suggest that it is possible to offer help early in the development of psychosis in a cost-effective manner, evaluation of the potential longer-term economic benefits of early detection and intervention is required.[40]

When "A Vision for Change," the national blueprint for mental health policy in Ireland, was published in 2007,[41] our service (DETECT) was the Irish pilot for EI in psychosis. Subsequently, we established a second EI service in Ireland (COPE). The National Clinical Mental Health Programme Plan for Ireland (2011) identified EI in psychosis as 1 of 3 initiatives for roll-out nationally,[42] and consideration is currently being given to such a national EI initiative. However, limited economic evaluation in the field of mental health in Ireland to guide service development has mirrored the previously reviewed lack of robust patient-level data. Therefore, to investigate whether the introduction of an EI service in psychosis resulted in any change to the number and duration of admissions in individuals with first-episode psychosis, we examined 2 prospective epidemiologic cohorts of individuals presenting with first-episode psychosis to an urban community mental health service (population 172,000): the historical cohort comprised individuals presenting from 1995 to 1998 and received treatment as usual (n = 132); the EI cohort presented to the same catchment area between 2008 and 2011 (n = 97) following the introduction of EI in 2005.[43]

Although we found the admission rate to decrease across these 2 time periods, reduction in rate of admission was larger in this catchment area than in the country as a whole. Introduction of the EI service was associated with reduction in DUP and the average cost of admission declined from €15,821 to €9,398 in the EI cohort. Thus, this comparison before and after EI showed cost savings consistent with some other studies internationally. Key issues are the mirror-image design of the study, focusing only on inpatient costs, and whether changes in admission pattern were due to the implementation of EI or were explained by other factors. However, examination of local and national factors indicated that the major effect was from implementation of EI. Although there are cost savings, these represent opportunity cost savings, as most costs associated with inpatient care are fixed. Studies such as this provide evidence that it is feasible to consider disinvestment strategies, such as home care, in the community.

Nevertheless, a systematic review of 11 studies concluded: "... the published literature does not support the contention that early intervention for psychosis reduces costs or achieves cost-effectiveness. Past failed attempts to reduce health costs by reducing hospitalization, and increased outpatient costs in early-intervention programmes suggest such programmes may increase costs. Future economic evaluation of early-intervention programmes would need to correctly value outpatient costs and accommodate uncertainty regarding reduced hospitalization costs, perhaps by sensitivity analysis. The current research hints that cost differences may be greater early in treatment and in patients with more severe illness."[44]

HOW "EARLY" SHOULD EARLY INTERVENTION BEGIN?
Intervention During the "High-Risk" State

Contemporary interest in EI has engendered increasing consideration of putative antecedents of florid, diagnostic symptoms, focusing initially on the prodromal period, but now extending back to psychotic experiences in the general population, including phenomena evident in childhood.[45] This then allows consideration of a developmental timeline for psychotic illness, at the levels of both psychopathology and pathobiology, that presents the challenge of how "early" EI should begin.[16]

Considerable attention has focused on the prodromal period as a window of opportunity for preventive intervention, such that identifying predictors and mechanisms of conversion to psychosis among such individuals is a critical step in the search for the "holy grail" of prevention.[46] Contemporary terminology is fluid and includes varying definitions of "clinical high risk (CHR),", "ultra-high risk (UHR)," "at-risk mental state (ARMS)," and "attenuated psychosis syndrome (APS)"; furthermore, contemporary evidence is variable as to the percentage of individuals in each category, typically 10% to 30%, who may experience subsequent conversion/transition to a psychotic episode over varying durations thereafter.[31,47]

Recent systematic reviews and meta-analyses have examined the effectiveness of a wide range of interventions during "at-risk" states, including psychological/psychosocial, pharmacologic, nutritional, and/or combinations thereof versus a variety of control procedures, to prevent or delay transition to a first-episode psychotic illness: among 11 trials, although evidence for any specific intervention was not conclusive, evidence was strongest for CBT, less so for complex psychosocial interventions, and least (but most provocative in a single, as-yet unreplicated study) for omega-3 fatty acids[48]; on meta-analysis of 10 trials of 1 year or longer, the findings were little altered, with the investigators noting with caution the paucity of evidence regarding efficacy vis-à-vis safety for antipsychotic medication, particularly in relation to metabolic adverse effects.[49]

These considerations may extend beyond psychosis to other domains of serious mental illness. Recent reviews have considered prodromal features of bipolar disorder,[50] duration of untreated mania,[51] and, more tentatively, duration of untreated depression[52] in terms of their implications for broader concepts of "at-risk" states and the effects of EI on outcome.

FUTURE DIRECTIONS: A STATE OF CLINICAL EQUIPOISE

Uncertainty in the medical community over whether an intervention will or will not be beneficial constitutes clinical equipoise, hence the evidence base for EI, whether for first-episode psychosis or, more tenuously, for "at-risk" states, would appear to typify such equipoise.[53] It has been proposed that "at-risk" states appear to predict a much broader outcome than schizophrenia or a related psychotic disorder, such that there may be broader scope in terms of prevention and heightened public health relevance for the strategy; the public health "yield" of the EI paradigm may be enhanced considerably if it is used in a more general context of mental distress predicting psychotic and/or nonpsychotic outcomes, in accordance with a broader model of staging in psychiatry that requires stage-specific treatments; these would vary from nonspecific and nonpharmacological self-management approaches through to more active psychological and/or pharmacologic treatments for more severe stages of dysfunction.[54,55]

In summary, the extent to which EI, whether for first-episode psychosis or for individuals in "at-risk" states, can be implemented on a general population basis within public health services remains challenging but not insurmountable. It is the continually evolving clinical and fiscal evidence base that will be the primary determinant of prioritization in provision of mental health care in the face of limited resources.

ACKNOWLEDGMENTS

This article is dedicated to the memory of Eadbhard O'Callaghan, who championed and pioneered the introduction of early intervention for psychosis into Irish mental health services and whose untimely death was a substantive loss to both patients and the research community. We thank Ms Angela Kearney, Librarian, St John of God Hospitaller Ministries, for her invaluable assistance.

REFERENCES

1. Wyatt RJ. Neuroleptics and the natural course of schizophrenia. Schizophr Bull 1991;17(2):325–51.
2. Marshall M, Lewis S, Lockwood A, et al. Association between duration of untreated psychosis and outcome in cohorts of first-episode patients: a systematic review. Arch Gen Psychiatry 2005;62(9):975–83 [Systematic Review/Meta-analyses].
3. Marshall M, Rathbone J. Early intervention for psychosis. Cochrane Database Syst Rev 2011;(6):CD004718. [Systematic Review/Meta-analyses].
4. Penttila M, Jaaskelainen E, Hirvonen N, et al. Duration of untreated psychosis as predictor of long-term outcome in schizophrenia: systematic review and meta-analysis. Br J Psychiatry 2014;205(2):88–94 [Systematic Review/Meta-analyses].
5. Wyatt RJ, Henter I. Rationale for the study of early intervention. Schizophr Res 2001;51(1):69–76.
6. Castle DJ. The truth, and nothing but the truth, about early intervention in psychosis. Aust N Z J Psychiatry 2012;46(1):10–3.
7. McGorry PD. Early intervention in psychosis: obvious, effective, overdue. J Nerv Ment Dis 2015;203(5):310.
8. Norman RM, Townsend L, Malla AK. Duration of untreated psychosis and cognitive functioning in first-episode patients. Br J Psychiatry 2001;179:340–5.
9. Miller TJ, McGlashan TH, Rosen JL, et al. Prodromal assessment with the structured interview for prodromal syndromes and the scale of prodromal symptoms: predictive validity, interrater reliability, and training to reliability. Schizophr Bull 2003;29(4):703.
10. Register-Brown K, Hong LE. Reliability and validity of methods for measuring the duration of untreated psychosis: a quantitative review and meta-analysis. Schizophr Res 2014;160(1–3):20–6 [Systematic Review/Meta-analyses].
11. Perkins DO, Gu H, Boteva K, et al. Relationship between duration of untreated psychosis and outcome in first-episode schizophrenia: a critical review and meta-analysis. Am J Psychiatry 2005;162(10):1785–804 [Systematic Review/Meta-analyses].
12. Boonstra N, Klaassen R, Sytema S, et al. Duration of untreated psychosis and negative symptoms-a systematic review and meta-analysis of individual patient data. Schizophr Res 2012;142(1–3):12–9 [Systematic Review/Meta-analyses].

13. Amminger GP, Edwards J, Brewer WJ, et al. Duration of untreated psychosis and cognitive deterioration in first-episode schizophrenia. Schizophr Res 2002;54(3): 223–30.

14. Lappin JM, Morgan KD, Morgan C, et al. Duration of untreated psychosis and neuropsychological function in first episode psychosis. Schizophr Res 2007; 95(1–3):103–10.

15. Rapp C, Studerus E, Bugra H, et al. Duration of untreated psychosis and cognitive functioning. Schizophr Res 2013;145(1–3):43–9.

16. Waddington J, Hennessy R, O'Tuathaigh C, et al. Schizophrenia and the lifetime trajectory of psychotic illness: developmental neuroscience and pathobiology, redux. The origins of schizophrenia. New York: Columbia University Press; 2012.

17. Scully PJ, Coakley G, Kinsella A, et al. Psychopathology, executive (frontal) and general cognitive impairment in relation to duration of initially untreated versus subsequently treated psychosis in chronic schizophrenia. Psychol Med 1997; 27(6):1303–10.

18. Meagher DJ, Quinn JF, Bourke S, et al. Longitudinal assessment of psychopathological domains over late-stage schizophrenia in relation to duration of initially untreated psychosis: 3-year prospective study in a long-term inpatient population. Psychiatry Res 2004;126(3):217–27.

19. Browne S, Clarke M, Gervin M, et al. Determinants of quality of life at first presentation with schizophrenia. Br J Psychiatry 2000;176:173–6.

20. Clarke M, Whitty P, Browne S, et al. Untreated illness and outcome of psychosis. Br J Psychiatry 2006;189(3):235–40.

21. Crumlish N, Whitty P, Clarke M, et al. Beyond the critical period: longitudinal study of 8-year outcome in first-episode non-affective psychosis. Br J Psychiatry 2009; 194(1):18–24.

22. Hill M, Crumlish N, Clarke M, et al. Prospective relationship of duration of untreated psychosis to psychopathology and functional outcome over 12 years. Schizophr Res 2012;141(2–3):215–21.

23. Rund BR. Does active psychosis cause neurobiological pathology? A critical review of the neurotoxicity hypothesis. Psychol Med 2014;44(8):1577–90.

24. Anderson KK, Rodrigues M, Mann K, et al. Minimal evidence that untreated psychosis damages brain structures: a systematic review. Schizophr Res 2015; 162(1–3):222–33 [Systematic Review/Meta-analyses].

25. Howes OD, Kambeitz J, Kim E, et al. The nature of dopamine dysfunction in schizophrenia and what this means for treatment. Arch Gen Psychiatry 2012; 69(8):776–86.

26. Slifstein M, van de Giessen E, Van Snellenberg J, et al. Deficits in prefrontal cortical and extrastriatal dopamine release in schizophrenia: a positron emission tomographic functional magnetic resonance imaging study. JAMA Psychiatry 2015;72(4):316–24.

27. Norman RM. Are the effects of duration of untreated psychosis socially mediated? Can J Psychiatry 2014;59(10):518–22.

28. Joseph R, Birchwood M. The national policy reforms for mental health services and the story of early intervention services in the United Kingdom. J Psychiatry Neurosci 2005;30(5):362–5.

29. McGorry PD, Edwards J, Mihalopoulos C, et al. EPPIC: an evolving system of early detection and optimal management. Schizophr Bull 1996;22(2):305–26.

30. Srihari VH, Shah J, Keshavan MS. Is early intervention for psychosis feasible and effective? Psychiatr Clin North Am 2012;35(3):613–31.

31. Carpenter WT, Schiffman J. Diagnostic concepts in the context of clinical high risk/attenuated psychosis syndrome. Schizophr Bull 2015;41(5):1001–2.

32. Lloyd-Evans B, Crosby M, Stockton S, et al. Initiatives to shorten duration of untreated psychosis: systematic review. Br J Psychiatry 2011;198(4):256–63 [Systematic Review/Meta-analyses].

33. Lloyd-Evans B, Sweeney A, Hinton M, et al. Evaluation of a community awareness programme to reduce delays in referrals to early intervention services and enhance early detection of psychosis. BMC Psychiatry 2015;15:98.

34. Renwick L, Gavin B, McGlade N, et al. Early intervention service for psychosis: views from primary care. Early Interv Psychiatry 2008;2(4):285–90.

35. Nkire N, Sardinha S, Nwosu B, et al. Evaluation of knowledge and attitudes among primary care physicians in Cavan-Monaghan as 'gatekeepers-in-waiting' for the introduction of Carepath for Overcoming Psychosis Early (COPE). Early Interv Psychiatry 2015;9(2):141–50.

36. Bhui K, Ullrich S, Coid JW. Which pathways to psychiatric care lead to earlier treatment and a shorter duration of first-episode psychosis? BMC Psychiatry 2014;14:72.

37. Tanskanen S, Morant N, Hinton M, et al. Service user and carer experiences of seeking help for a first episode of psychosis: a UK qualitative study. BMC Psychiatry 2011;11:157.

38. Bird V, Premkumar P, Kendall T, et al. Early intervention services, cognitive-behavioural therapy and family intervention in early psychosis: systematic review. Br J Psychiatry 2010;197(5):350–6 [Systematic Review/Meta-analyses].

39. Nordentoft M, Ramussen JO, Melau M, et al. How successful are first episode programs? A review of the evidence for specialized assertive early intervention. Curr Opin Psychiatry 2014;27(3):167–72.

40. Valmaggia LR, McGuire PK, Fusar-Poli P, et al. Economic impact of early detection and early intervention of psychosis. Curr Pharm Des 2012;18(4):592–5.

41. Department of Health. A vision for change: report of the expert group on mental health policy. Dublin (Ireland): Stationery Office; 2006. Available at: http://health.gov.ie/wpcontent/uploads/2014/03/vision_for_change.pdf.

42. Health Service Executive. National mental health programme plan consultation document. 2011. Available at: http://health.gov.ie/wp-content/uploads/2014/04/National_Mental_Health_Programme_Plan_Nov2011_draft.pdf. Accessed October 9, 2015.

43. Behan C, Cullinan J, Kennelly B, et al. Estimating the cost and effect of early intervention on in-patient admission in first episode psychosis. J Ment Health Policy Econ 2015;18(2):57–62.

44. Amos A. Assessing the cost of early intervention in psychosis: a systematic review. Aust N Z J Psychiatry 2012;46(8):719 [Systematic Review/Meta-analyses].

45. Linscott RJ, van Os J. An updated and conservative systematic review and meta-analysis of epidemiological evidence on psychotic experiences in children and adults: on the pathway from proneness to persistence to dimensional expression across mental disorders. Psychol Med 2013;43(6):1133–49 [Systematic Review/Meta-analyses].

46. Addington J, Heinssen R. Prediction and prevention of psychosis in youth at clinical high risk. Annu Rev Clin Psychol 2012;8:269–89.

47. Nieman DH, McGorry PD. Detection and treatment of at-risk mental state for developing a first psychosis: making up the balance. Lancet 2015;2(9):825–34.

48. Stafford MR, Jackson H, Mayo-Wilson E, et al. Early interventions to prevent psychosis: systematic review and meta-analysis. BMJ 2013;346:f185 [Systematic Review/Meta-analyses].

49. van der Gaag M, Smit F, Bechdolf A, et al. Preventing a first episode of psychosis: meta-analysis of randomized controlled prevention trials of 12 month and longer-term follow-ups. Schizophr Res 2013;149(1–3):56–62 [Systematic Review/Meta-analyses].

50. Howes OD, Falkenberg I. Early detection and intervention in bipolar affective disorder: targeting the development of the disorder. Curr Psychiatry Rep 2011; 13(6):493–9.

51. Malhi GS, Bargh DM, Coulston CM, et al. Predicting bipolar disorder on the basis of phenomenology: implications for prevention and early intervention. Bipolar Disord 2014;16(5):455–70.

52. Bukh JD, Bock C, Vinberg M, et al. The effect of prolonged duration of untreated depression on antidepressant treatment outcome. J Affect Disord 2013;145(1):42–8.

53. Clarke M, O'Callaghan E. Is earlier better? At the beginning of schizophrenia: timing and opportunities for early intervention. Psychiatr Clin North Am 2003; 26(1):65–83.

54. McGorry P, van Os J. Redeeming diagnosis in psychiatry: timing versus specificity. Lancet 2013;381(9863):343–5.

55. Fusar-Poli P, Yung AR, McGorry P, et al. Lessons learned from the psychosis high-risk state: towards a general staging model of prodromal intervention. Psychol Med 2014;44(1):17–24.

The Case for Adjunctive Monoclonal Antibody Immunotherapy in Schizophrenia

CrossMark

Brian J. Miller, MD, PhD, MPH[a],*, Peter F. Buckley, MD[b]

KEYWORDS

- Schizophrenia • Psychosis • Immune • Inflammation • Cytokine
- Monoclonal antibody • Treatment • Adjunct

KEY POINTS

- There is robust evidence that schizophrenia is associated with immune system dysfunction throughout the lifespan.
- There is need to more extensively evaluate the hypothesis that immune dysfunction may be involved in the pathophysiology of schizophrenia.
- Monoclonal antibodies act by directly neutralizing cytokines or by binding cytokine receptors.
- Monoclonal antibodies do not have any off-target effects; therefore, improvements in psychopathology in response to these agents would further directly implicate inflammatory pathways in the pathophysiology of schizophrenia.
- Overall, there is a compelling rationale for well-designed, carefully conducted trials of monoclonal antibody immunotherapy in schizophrenia.

INTRODUCTION

In a recent seminal finding in neuroscience, two independent studies found functional lymphatic vessels lining the dural sinuses of dissected mouse brain meninges—that is, a "direct connection" between the brain and immune system.[1,2] The presence of a functional and classical lymphatic system in the central nervous system (CNS) is a paradigm-shifting finding that challenges basic assumptions in neuroimmunology and how clinicians perceive brain-immune interactions. If confirmed in humans, it may follow that dysfunction of meningeal lymphatic vessels contributes to the pathophysiology of a variety of CNS disorders associated with immune system involvement,

Disclosure Statement: The authors have nothing to disclose.
[a] Department of Psychiatry and Health Behavior, Augusta University, 997 Saint Sebastian Way, Augusta, GA 30912, USA; [b] Medical College of Georgia, Augusta University, 1120 15th Street, AA-1006, Augusta, GA 30912, USA
* Corresponding author.
E-mail address: brmiller@gru.edu

including schizophrenia, and would enable a more mechanistic approach to the study of the neuroimmunology of these disorders.

The investigation of immune system abnormalities in schizophrenia, although ongoing for decades, has more recently become a popular area of research. This interest has been at least partially stimulated by increased understanding of the interactions that occur between the immune system and the brain in other chronic medical disorders, and furthered by the recent discovery of meningeal lymphatic vessels. Schizophrenia is associated with immune system dysfunction throughout the lifespan. Advances in genetics have led to the identification of associations between genes involved in the regulation of the immune system and increased risk of schizophrenia.[3] Prenatal maternal infection with a variety of different infectious agents is a replicated risk factor for the development of schizophrenia in the offspring,[4] and may act synergistically with family history of psychosis on schizophrenia risk.[5] An association between schizophrenia and infections seems to be bidirectional: hospital contact for infection during childhood or adolescence is associated with an increased risk of schizophrenia in adulthood,[6] and schizophrenia is also a risk factor for infections.[7] Patients with schizophrenia have immune abnormalities in the blood, cerebrospinal fluid, and CNS, including immune cell numbers, inflammatory markers, and antibody titers.[8] Acutely ill patients with schizophrenia seem to have an increased prevalence of certain comorbid infections (eg, lower urinary tract infections).[9,10] Schizophrenia is also associated with increased mortality from infectious diseases, including pneumonia and influenza.[11,12]

Presently, all approved antipsychotics for the treatment of schizophrenia are antidopaminergic agents. Although these medications are effective for many patients, particularly positive symptoms, many other patients have some degree of treatment resistance. Thus, there is a great impetus to identify other effective pharmacologic treatments for schizophrenia, especially for negative symptoms and cognitive dysfunction. Several trials have also found that treatment with nonsteroidal anti-inflammatory drugs (NSAIDs) or agents with anti-inflammatory properties, including aspirin, celecoxib, estrogen, and N-acetylcysteine, in adjunct with antipsychotics, may be associated with significant improvement in psychopathology in schizophrenia.[13,14] Importantly, in two studies, baseline blood levels of cytokines, key signaling molecules of the immune system that regulate inflammation, predicted response to adjunctive NSAID treatment.[15,16] Essentially, patients who had evidence in the blood of increased inflammation baseline were more likely to improve with NSAIDs. Taken together, these findings suggest a need for more extensively evaluation of the hypothesis that immune dysfunction may be involved in the pathophysiology of schizophrenia.

This evidence, energy, and enthusiasm, coupled with advances in molecular biology, has afforded the field an unparalleled opportunity to investigate this immune hypothesis, toward identifying new potential treatments to alleviate symptoms and improve quality of life in patients with schizophrenia. Currently, several humanized monoclonal antibodies are approved for the treatment of autoimmune disorders and cancers. These antibodies act by directly neutralizing cytokines or by binding cytokine receptors. Cytokines are key signaling molecules of the immune system that exert effects in the periphery and brain. They are produced by immune and nonimmune cells, and exert their effects by binding specific receptors on a variety of target cells. Cytokine receptors also exist in soluble forms, which can inhibit (eg, soluble interleukin-2 receptor [sIL-2R]) or enhance (eg, sIL-6R) the biologic activity of cytokines. There are endogenous cytokine receptor antagonists (eg, IL-1 receptor antagonist [IL-1RA]) that compete with cytokines for membrane receptors. Cytokines are key regulators of acute and chronic inflammation, a complex but vital biologic response that impacts all organ systems. Cytokines help coordinate the function of the innate immune system and components of the immune system and a host of other physiologic processes throughout the body.[17,18]

This article presents the case in favor of clinical trials of adjunctive monoclonal antibody immunotherapy in schizophrenia. First, we highlight evidence for prenatal and premorbid immune risk factors for the development of schizophrenia in the offspring. We then consider key evidence for immune dysfunction in patients with schizophrenia. Next, we discuss previous trials of adjunctive anti-inflammatory or other immunotherapy in schizophrenia. We then discuss evidence for psychosis as a side effect of immunotherapy for other disorders. We also present preliminary evidence for adjunctive monoclonal antibody immunotherapy in psychiatric disorders. Finally, we discuss important considerations in the design and implementation of clinical trials of adjunctive monoclonal antibody immunotherapy in schizophrenia.

PRENATAL AND PREMORBID IMMUNE RISK FACTORS FOR SCHIZOPHRENIA

A comprehensive review of prenatal and premorbid immune risk factors for the development of schizophrenia in the offspring is beyond the scope of this article, and the reader is referred to several previous reviews on the topic.[4,19,20] Prenatal maternal infections with a variety of viral and bacterial agents are a replicated risk factor for schizophrenia.[4] Given the myriad of different infectious agents associated with schizophrenia, the inflammatory response to infection has been posited as a potential common mediator of these associations. Animal models of maternal immune activation with adjuvants in the absence of a specific pathogen (including synthetic double-stranded ribonucleic acid; poly [I:C], which induces an antiviral inflammatory response; lipopolysaccharide, which mimics bacterial infection; and cytokines [eg, IL-6]) have been investigated. In these animal models, changes in behavior, neurocognition, brain morphology, blood cytokine levels, and neurotransmitter function with homology to schizophrenia have been observed in adult offspring. There is some parallel evidence in humans that alterations in maternal cytokines during pregnancy are associated with increased risk of schizophrenia in the offspring; that inflammation is a potential common mediator of known risk factors for schizophrenia; and that prenatal exposure to inflammation is associated with abnormalities in immune function, neurocognition, brain morphology, and gene expression in adult patients with schizophrenia.[19] These findings support the hypothesis that prenatal inflammation may alter fetal brain development, thereby increasing vulnerability to schizophrenia.

However, although prenatal maternal infections are a robust risk factor for schizophrenia in the offspring, most exposed persons do not subsequently develop schizophrenia. This observation suggests that interactions with genetic, epigenetic, or other environmental risk factors may interact and may mitigate schizophrenia. Indeed, recent large, genome-wide association studies have found that genes involved in the development and regulation of the immune system, including the major histocompatibility complex, are associated with increased risk of schizophrenia.[3] Furthermore, there is evidence that maternal infection during pregnancy may act synergistically with family history of psychosis on schizophrenia risk.[5]

Immune-based premorbid risk factors for schizophrenia also seem to extend beyond the prenatal period to include childhood and adolescence. This association seems to be bidirectional: hospital contact for autoimmune disorders and/or infections during childhood or adolescence is associated with an increased risk of schizophrenia in adulthood,[6] and schizophrenia is also a risk factor for autoimmune disorders and infections.[7] Furthermore, the presence of an autoimmune disorder and hospital contact for infections may act synergistically on subsequent risk of schizophrenia.[21] As posited for prenatal maternal infections, inflammation may be a common mediator of these associations. In a cohort study of about 4500 individuals, blood IL-6 levels at age 9 were associated with risk of psychotic experiences and fulminant psychotic disorder at age 18.[22] Furthermore, higher IL-6 levels in childhood were associated with risk of psychotic experiences in a dose-dependent fashion. Taken together, these findings implicate the immune system as a risk factor for schizophrenia with effects that may persist into adulthood.

IMMUNE DYSFUNCTION IN SCHIZOPHRENIA

A comprehensive review of immune dysfunction in schizophrenia (**Box 1**) is beyond the scope of this article, and the reader is referred to several previous reviews on the topic.[23–26]

There is evidence that patients with schizophrenia have immune abnormalities in the blood, cerebrospinal fluid, and CNS, including immune cell numbers, inflammatory markers, and antibody titers.[8] Two important themes emerge from these studies. First, inflammatory abnormalities are present in subjects with first-episode psychosis (FEP) compared with control subjects, suggesting an association that may be independent of the effects of antipsychotic medications. Second, the concentrations of some immune markers may vary with the clinical status of patients: there seems to be separate groups of state and trait markers. The state-related cytokines include IL-1β, IL-6, and transforming growth factor-β. Patients with schizophrenia have higher blood levels of these cytokines than control subjects during an exacerbation of symptoms, but levels significantly decrease with antipsychotic treatment of acute illness.[23] By contrast, the cytokines IL-12, interferon (IFN)-γ, and tumor necrosis factor (TNF)-α seem to be trait markers. Blood levels of these cytokines are higher in patients with FEP and in patients with chronic illness, during both periods of symptomatic worsening and during periods of clinical stability, than in control subjects.[23] There is also evidence that specific blood

---

Box 1
Summary of evidence for immune system dysfunction in schizophrenia

- Genes involved in the regulation of the immune system are associated with an increased risk of schizophrenia.

- Prenatal maternal infection, with a variety of different infectious agents, is a replicated risk factor for the development of schizophrenia in the offspring.

- The association between schizophrenia and infections seems to be bidirectional: hospital contact for infection is associated with an increased risk of schizophrenia, and schizophrenia is also a risk factor for infections.

- Some patients with schizophrenia have evidence of immune abnormalities in the blood, cerebrospinal fluid, and central nervous system, including immune cell numbers, inflammatory markers, and antibody titers.

- Acutely ill patients with schizophrenia seem to have an increased prevalence of certain comorbid infections.

- Schizophrenia is also associated with increased mortality from infectious diseases, including pneumonia and influenza.

- Several trials have found that anti-inflammatory agents, given in adjunct to antipsychotics, are associated with significant improvement in psychopathology in schizophrenia.

lymphocyte populations may also segregate into state and trait markers.[25] Patients with schizophrenia also have significant elevations in the acute-phase reactant C-reactive protein (CRP), which is synthesized by the liver in response to inflammation.[24] Patients with FEP also have an increased prevalence of positive anticardiolipin IgG and N-methyl-D-aspartate receptor autoantibody titers, and patients with chronic schizophrenia have an increased prevalence of a myriad of autoantibodies, although their relevance to the pathophysiology of schizophrenia remains unclear.[26] Additional evidence for potential state-related markers in schizophrenia has been reviewed elsewhere.[27] Important limitations of this literature include inadequate consideration of potential confounding factors (eg, body mass index and smoking), and that only a subset of studies explored relationships between immune markers and psychopathology. It should also be emphasized that there is significant heterogeneity in the literature regarding findings for markers of immune dysfunction in schizophrenia, including negative studies, although alterations in some markers (eg, IL-6) have been frequently replicated. An important potential explanation for these heterogeneous findings is that immune system dysfunction occurs in only a subset of patients with schizophrenia.

PREVIOUS TRIALS OF ADJUNCTIVE ANTI-INFLAMMATORY OR IMMUNOMODULATORY AGENTS IN SCHIZOPHRENIA

Two recent meta-analyses have explored the efficacy of adjunctive anti-inflammatory agents in schizophrenia. Nitta and colleagues[13] performed a meta-analysis of eight studies (N = 774 patients with schizophrenia) of adjunctive NSAIDs (six trials of celecoxib and two trials of aspirin), including three unpublished reports. They found that NSAIDs were associated with a small effect size (ES) reduction in Positive and Negative Syndrome Scale (PANSS) total score at the trend level (ES = -0.24; $P = .06$), and a small, significant ES reduction in PANSS positive subscale score (ES = -0.19; $P = .04$). Importantly, they also found that significant superiority of NSAIDs over placebo for PANSS total scores was moderated by treatment with aspirin, inpatient and first-episode status, and lower baseline PANSS negative subscale scores. That inpatient and first-episode status moderated the efficacy of adjunctive NSAIDs in this meta-analysis is broadly consistent with our findings of associations between abnormal immune markers and clinical status (ie, state vs trait markers in patients with acute-psychosis or FEP).

In another meta-analysis of 26 double-blind trials of various anti-inflammatory agents, including aspirin, celecoxib, davunetide, fatty acids, estrogens, minocycline, and N-acetylcysteine, Sommer and colleagues[14] found significant effects for aspirin (N = 270; ES = 0.30), estrogens (N = 262; ES = 0.51), and N-acetylcysteine (N = 140; ES = 0.45), but not celecoxib, davunetide, fatty acids, or minocycline. An important potential explanation for these heterogeneous findings is that immune system dysfunction occurs in only a subset of patients with schizophrenia, which influences the likelihood of response to this treatment approach. This is supported by the two previous studies, which found that baseline blood levels of cytokines predicted response to adjunctive NSAID treatment.[15,16]

Studies of other immunomodulatory treatments in schizophrenia have been limited. Levine and colleagues[28] reported a trial of adjunctive treatment with the immunosuppressant azathioprine in two parallel groups (totaling 11 patients) with treatment-resistant schizophrenia and high titers of antiplatelet autoantibodies. The first group received a 7-week course of oral azathioprine, 150 mg daily; the second group received two 7-week courses, separated by 6 weeks. Two of the eleven patients had significant improvements in symptoms: a 51-year-old man with a 27-year history of schizophrenia whose PANSS total score reduced from 101 to 44 over 7 weeks, and a 41-year-old man with a 23-year history of schizophrenia whose PANSS total score reduced from 132 to 114 over the second 7-week course of treatment. Seven of the eleven patients had significant reductions in the level of antiplatelet autoantibodies. Despite the small size and open-label nature of the trial, findings suggest that immune-based treatment may be helpful in a subset of patients with schizophrenia. A recent protocol for a 12-week trial of adjunctive methotrexate in schizophrenia has also been described.[29] That treatment with anti-inflammatory agents is associated with improvements in psychopathology and provides important empirical support for a pathophysiologic role for inflammation in some patients with schizophrenia.

PSYCHOSIS AS A SIDE EFFECT OF IMMUNOTHERAPY

Cytokine-based immunotherapy is often used in the treatment of certain cancers and chronic diseases, including hepatitis C, malignant melanoma, and multiple sclerosis. This has included treatment with IFN-α and IFN-β, and IL-2, either as monotherapy or in combination with IFN-α. These treatments have been associated with a broad range of neuropsychiatric adverse effects, most commonly depression, but also psychosis. In a retrospective study of 943 patients in Japan treated with IFN for hepatitis C, Hosoda and colleagues[30] reported four patients (0.4%) developed psychosis (auditory hallucinations and persecutory delusions, primarily in the context of mood symptoms). Psychotic symptoms resolved within 3 months of discontinuation of IFN and treatment with antipsychotic medication. In another study of 11,241 patients in Italy also treated with IFN for hepatitis C, Fattovich and colleagues[31] reported 10 patients (0.1%) developed psychosis that resolved following discontinuation of IFN and treatment with psychotropic medication. To our knowledge, all other reports of psychosis as an adverse effect of treatment with IFN-α (with or without IL-2) have been case reports or case series (reviewed elsewhere[32,33]). Outside of IFN-α-induced psychosis, one study of 10 patients with advanced cancers found that after 3 months of chronic treatment with recombinant IL-2, six (60%) had significant increase in the schizophrenia scale of the Minnesota Multiphasic Personality Inventory.[34] There are also several case reports of IFN-β-induced psychosis in patients with multiple sclerosis.[35,36] Of course, it is challenging to establish a causal link between emergent psychosis and cytokine-based treatment, versus another cause (eg, new-onset psychiatric disorder, illicit drug use, or a brain lesion attributable to multiple sclerosis). However, that immunotherapy with certain cytokines may be associated with psychosis (albeit rarely) indirectly supports the plausibility that immunotherapy with other different cytokines may be a potential treatment of psychosis.

EVIDENCE FOR ADJUNCTIVE MONOCLONAL ANTIBODY IMMUNOTHERAPY IN PSYCHIATRIC DISORDERS

In a seminal study, Raison and colleagues[37] performed a trial of adjunctive infliximab, a monoclonal antibody against the inflammatory cytokine TNF-α, versus placebo in 60 patients with treatment-resistant depression. Although they did not find an overall difference in the change in Hamilton Scale for Depression scores between treatment groups, there was a significant time by group interaction favoring infliximab-treated patients with elevated baseline levels of the inflammatory marker CRP greater than 5 mg/L. Furthermore, infliximab-treated patients with elevated CRP also had improved sleep continuity compared with infliximab-treated patients with low inflammation.[38] In an analysis of peripheral blood mononuclear cells from patients in this trial, infliximab responders (defined as 50% reduction in depressive symptoms at any point during the

12-week trial) demonstrated inhibition of genes related to apoptosis through TNF signaling at 6 and 24 hours after the first infusion.[39] This study found evidence for a pathophysiologic role for inflammation in some patients with depression, and that TNF-α antagonism may improve treatment-resistant depressive symptoms in patients with high baseline inflammatory biomarkers. These findings highlight another important limitation of previous trials of adjunctive anti-inflammatory agents in schizophrenia. Namely, evidence of inflammation in the peripheral blood was not an inclusion criterion, which may have decreased the signal-to-noise ratio for this study.

To date, two small studies of cytokine-based immunotherapy in schizophrenia have been published, although several other larger trials are ongoing. The first is a case series of two patients with treatment-resistant paranoid schizophrenia who had significant improvement in total psychopathology during open-label adjunctive treatment with recombinant human IFN-γ1b, 0.5 mL subcutaneously weekly for 4 weeks, and then tapered down over 2 to 3 weeks.[40] One patient, a 47-year-old man with a 26-year history of psychosis, had a 22% decrease in PANSS total score (from 119 to 93) after 7 weeks. The other patient, a 36-year-old man with a 13-year history of psychosis, had a 27% decrease in PANSS total score (from 132 to 96) after 6 weeks. One patient had a transient doubling of liver enzymes after 2 weeks, which normalized by week 4. Otherwise IFN-γ1b treatment was well tolerated by both patients.

Our research group recently published an 8-week open-label trial of adjunctive tocilizumab (an anti-IL-6 receptor monoclonal antibody) in six patients with Diagnostic and Statistical Manual of Mental Disorder-IV schizophrenia or schizoaffective disorder.[41] Subjects were age 18 to 55, taking a nonclozapine antipsychotic, and had no psychiatric hospitalizations in the past 3 months and stable psychotropic medications for greater than or equal to 1 month. We excluded subjects with scheduled immunomodulatory agents, immune disorder history, illicit drug use in the past month, unstable medical conditions, active or chronic infections, pregnancy, breastfeeding, or reproductive-age women not using contraception. Subjects received 4 mg/kg tocilizumab intravenously at baseline and again at 4 weeks. Five subjects completed the trial; one was removed (psychiatric hospitalization caused by psychosocial stressors). Infusions were well tolerated without clinically significant adverse effects. Compared with baseline, there was significant improvement in Brief Assessment of Cognition in Schizophrenia verbal fluency at 4 weeks (0.6 standard deviation [SD] improvement); digit symbol coding at 2, 4, and 8 weeks (1.0-SD improvement); and composite score at 4 and 8 weeks (0.7-SD improvement). There were no significant changes in psychopathology, although subjects were clinically stable at study entry. Taken together, these three trials support the feasibility and potential efficacy of adjunctive monoclonal antibody immunotherapy in improving psychopathology.

CONSIDERATIONS IN CLINICAL TRIALS OF ADJUNCTIVE MONOCLONAL ANTIBODY IMMUNOTHERAPY IN SCHIZOPHRENIA

There are several potential advantages of monoclonal antibody immunotherapy (**Box 2**) over NSAIDs or other anti-inflammatory agents. Perhaps most importantly, NSAIDs have relevant off-target (ie, nonimmune) effects. For example, aspirin may modulate N-methyl-D-aspartate receptors[42] and celecoxib may impact glucocorticoid receptors.[43] By contrast, monoclonal antibodies do not have any off-target effects, only acting on specific inflammatory cytokines. Therefore, improvements in psychopathology in response to monoclonal antibody immunotherapy would further (and directly) implicate inflammatory pathways in the pathophysiology of schizophrenia.

Box 2
Considerations for adjunctive monoclonal antibody immunotherapy in schizophrenia

Advantages

No relevant off-target (ie, nonimmune) effects.

More potent anti-inflammatory properties than other agents.

Intravenous route of administration obviates issues of medication adherence that may confound findings in research clinical trials.

Disadvantages

Serious potential adverse effects because of profound immunosuppression, including life-threatening infections, demyelinating disorders, ulcers, and malignancy.

High cost (potentially >$1000 per dose) may limit more widespread use.

Intravenous route of administration poses a myriad of logistical issues for patients and clinicians.

Monoclonal antibodies permit direct testing of the hypothesis that inflammation plays a causal role in schizophrenia symptomatology.

Compared with other anti-inflammatory agents, monoclonal antibodies also have more potent anti-inflammatory properties. Indeed, NSAIDs have minimal efficacy in conditions with significant inflammation (eg, autoimmune disorders). In schizophrenia, adjunctive anti-inflammatory agents have been associated with small-to-moderate ESs for improvements in psychopathology. Although this most likely reflects that fact that immune system dysfunction occurs in only a subset of patients with schizophrenia, another possibility is that more potent anti-inflammatory agents are needed for more robust effects. This may also help explain why treatment studies that have targeted inflammation in schizophrenia have yielded mixed results.

Another important issue regarding monoclonal antibody immunotherapy is route of administration. Presently, most of these agents are administered by intravenous infusion (although some agents can be given subcutaneously or orally), typically once monthly. From a purely research perspective, this is advantageous in terms of obviating issues of medication adherence that may confound findings.

Despite these potential advantages, there are other important considerations regarding the clinical use of adjunctive monoclonal antibody immunotherapy. There are several serious potential adverse effects (see **Box 2**) caused by profound immunosuppression, which include life-threatening infections, demyelinating disorders, ulcers, and malignancy. Although side effects of NSAIDs are generally more benign, there is increased risk of gastrointestinal bleeding and cardiovascular mortality with prolonged use of these agents. The high cost of adjunctive monoclonal antibody immunotherapy (potentially >$1000 per dose) is another important factor that may limit use. Furthermore, the route of administration of many monoclonals poses a myriad of logistical issues for patients and clinicians in terms of the necessary time, facilities, and equipment to perform intravenous infusions, and monitoring for patient safety (eg, risk of anaphylaxis during and after the infusion).

Several other important considerations in the design and implementation of clinical trials of adjunctive monoclonal antibody immunotherapy include selection of the therapeutic target, patient selection, timing of therapy during the course of the disorder, and the duration of treatment. Unfortunately, many previous studies did not explore associations between cytokine levels and psychopathology or cognition in schizophrenia, which limits the available data on which to make decisions regarding the most promising therapeutic targets. Overall, previous studies suggest that immune dysfunction in schizophrenia is manifested by a decrease in anti-inflammatory cytokines and an increase in proinflammatory cytokines, including IL-1β, IL-6, and TNF-α. There is some evidence for correlations between levels of these proinflammatory cytokines and psychopathology, most notably for IL-6, and monoclonal antibodies that antagonize these cytokines are available and approved by the Food and Drug Administration for other disorders. There is also evidence from the previous case series that targeting IFN-γ may also be a viable therapeutic strategy.[40] Thus, at this time IL-1β, IL-6, TNF-α, and IFN-γ represent the most promising initial therapeutic targets. Regarding patient selection, the study of infliximab by Raison and colleagues[37] suggest that it would behoove the field to conduct trials of adjunctive monoclonal antibody immunotherapy exclusively in patients with evidence of inflammation in the peripheral blood. This treatment approach will increase the likelihood of response and the signal-to-noise ratio in such a trial.

Another important consideration is the timing of adjunctive anti-inflammatory therapy during the course of the disorder. In several meta-analyses, we found that some inflammatory and immune parameters may be abnormal (vs controls) during periods of acute psychosis (including the first-episode), but not clinical stability.[23,25] By contrast, other immune and inflammatory parameters may be abnormal regardless of clinical status. That inpatient and first-episode status moderated the efficacy of adjunctive NSAIDs in the meta-analysis by Nitta and colleagues[13] is broadly consistent with these observations. Thus, studies of adjunctive monoclonal antibody immunotherapy should consider acutely ill (eg, hospitalized) and clinically stable patients separately. There is strong evidence for cognitive impairment in prodromal psychosis[44] and FEP,[45] and gray matter loss before the onset of psychosis.[46] Given this premorbid decline in cognition, illness phase is an important consideration. Is it pragmatic to expect improved cognition in patients with chronic illness? Our preliminary study of tocilizumab was associated with significant improvements in cognitive function in patients with chronic schizophrenia (mean illness duration, >10 years).[41] However, future studies could consider immunotherapy in earlier phases of illness.

Duration of treatment is also an important consideration. Most of the previous trials of adjunctive NSAIDs were of shorter duration (<12 weeks) and in acutely ill patients. Thus, it is not clear whether adjunctive anti-inflammatory treatments help patients reach a new, lower baseline level of symptomatology, or rather if they accelerate the speed of response to antipsychotic medications during periods of acute psychosis. The risk of long-term treatment, including increased gastrointestinal bleeding and cardiovascular mortality associated with anti-inflammatory therapy, and demyelinating disorders, ulcers, and malignancy with monoclonal antibody immunotherapy, must also be considered.

SUMMARY

Overall, there is a compelling rationale for well-designed, carefully conducted trials of monoclonal antibody immunotherapy in schizophrenia. A confluence of evidence supports an association between prenatal inflammation and risk of schizophrenia. Some patients with schizophrenia have immune abnormalities in the blood, cerebrospinal fluid, and CNS, including immune cell numbers, inflammatory markers, and antibody titers. The efficacy of previous trials of adjunctive NSAIDs provides important empirical support for a pathophysiologic role for inflammation in some patients with schizophrenia. Certain immune-based therapies may cause psychosis as an adverse effect. Preliminary trials support the feasibility of trials of adjunctive monoclonal antibody immunotherapy for psychiatric symptoms. Despite potential limitations and important trial design considerations, monoclonal antibody immunotherapy does not have nonimmune effects, thereby permitting direct testing of the hypothesis that inflammation plays a causal role in schizophrenia symptomatology.

For many chronic diseases, polypharmacy is the rule rather than the exception. But a common feature of this polypharmacy is the use of medications with different mechanisms of action. Furthermore, the medication "cocktail" is often rationally tailored to the individual patient based on comorbidities. So, for example, a patient with essential hypertension plus comorbid congestive heart failure might be treated with an antihypertensive regimen consisting of a β-blocker. All approved antipsychotics for the treatment of schizophrenia are antidopaminergic agents. Thus, the study of adjunctive monoclonal antibody immunotherapy represents a step toward "rational polypharmacy" for patients with schizophrenia. Monoclonal antibody immunotherapy is likely best suited for a subgroup of patients with schizophrenia and evidence of immune dysfunction. Thus far, although there is evidence in general terms of immune dysfunction among patients with schizophrenia, research to date has not clearly identified features of a distinct subgroup, and the causes of immune dysfunction are likely multifactorial. Furthermore, although there are considerable ongoing efforts, there is not yet a single biomarker (or group of biomarkers) to distinguish patients with schizophrenia from healthy control subjects, or patients with schizophrenia with or without comorbid immune dysfunction. Such studies, regardless of outcome, will provide valuable insights into the role of the immune system in schizophrenia, and represent an important potential step toward more personalized medicine for patients with schizophrenia.

REFERENCES

1. Louveau A, Smirnov I, Keyes TJ, et al. Structural and functional features of central nervous system lymphatic vessels. Nature 2015;523:337–41.
2. Aspelund A, Antila S, Proulx ST, et al. A dural lymphatic vascular system that drains brain interstitial fluid and macromolecules. J Exp Med 2015;212:991–9.
3. Schizophrenia Working Group of the Psychiatric Genomics Consortium. Biological insights from 108 schizophrenia-associated genetic loci. Nature 2014;511: 421–7.
4. Brown AS, Derkits EJ. Prenatal infection and schizophrenia: a review of epidemiologic and translational studies. Am J Psychiatry 2010;167:261–80.
5. Clarke MC, Tanskanen A, Huttunen M, et al. Evidence for an interaction between familial liability and prenatal exposure to infection in the causation of schizophrenia. Am J Psychiatry 2009;166:1025–30.
6. Nielsen PR, Benros ME, Mortensen PB. Hospital contacts with infection and risk of schizophrenia: a population-based cohort study with linkage of Danish national registers. Schizophr Bull 2014;40(6):1526–32.
7. Benros ME, Pedersen MG, Rasmussen H, et al. A nationwide study on the risk of autoimmune diseases in individuals with a personal or a family history of schizophrenia and related psychosis. Am J Psychiatry 2014;171:218–26.
8. Kirkpatrick B, Miller BJ. Inflammation and schizophrenia. Schizophr Bull 2013;39: 1174–9.
9. Miller BJ, Graham KL, Bodenheimer CM, et al. A prevalence study of urinary tract infections in acute relapse of schizophrenia. J Clin Psychiatry 2013;73:271–7.
10. Laney D, Philip N, Miller BJ. Recurrent urinary tract infections in acute psychosis. Schizophr Res 2015;164:275–6.

11. Saha S, Chant D, McGrath J. A systematic review of mortality in schizophrenia: is the differential mortality gap worsening over time? Arch Gen Psychiatry 2007;64: 1123–31.

12. Brown S, Kim M, Mitchell C, et al. Twenty-five year mortality of a community cohort with schizophrenia. Br J Psychiatry 2010;196:116–21.

13. Nitta M, Kishimoto T, Müller N, et al. Adjunctive use of nonsteroidal anti-inflammatory drugs for schizophrenia: a meta-analytic investigation of randomized controlled trials. Schizophr Bull 2013;39:1230–41.

14. Sommer IE, van Westrhenen R, Begemann MJ, et al. Efficacy of anti-inflammatory agents to improve symptoms in patients with schizophrenia: an update. Schizophr Bull 2014;40:181–91.

15. Laan W, Grobbee DE, Selten JP, et al. Adjuvant aspirin therapy reduces symptoms of schizophrenia spectrum disorders: results from a randomized, double-blind, placebo-controlled trial. J Clin Psychiatry 2010;71:520–7.

16. Muller N, Ulmschneider M, Scheppach C, et al. COX-2 inhibition as a treatment approach in schizophrenia: immunological considerations and clinical effects of celecoxib add-on therapy. Eur Arch Psychiatry Clin Neurosci 2004;254:14–22.

17. Florencio-Silva R, Sasso GR, Sasso-Cerri E, et al. Biology of bone tissue: structure, function, and factors that influence bone cells. Biomed Res Int 2015;2015: 421746.

18. Ingman WV, Robertson SA. The essential roles of TGFB1 in reproduction. Cytokine Growth Factor Rev 2009;20:233–9.

19. Miller B, Culpepper N, Rapaport M, et al. Prenatal inflammation and neurodevelopment in schizophrenia: a review of human studies. Prog Neuropsychopharmacol Biol Psychiatry 2013;42:92–100.

20. Meyer U. Prenatal poly(i:C) exposure and other developmental immune activation models in rodent systems. Biol Psychiatry 2014;75:307–15.

21. Benros ME, Waltoft BL, Nordentoft M, et al. Autoimmune diseases and severe infections as risk factors for mood disorders: a nationwide study. JAMA Psychiatry 2013;70:812–20.

22. Khandaker GM, Pearson RM, Zammit S, et al. Association of serum interleukin 6 and C-reactive protein in childhood with depression and psychosis in young adult life: a population-based longitudinal study. JAMA Psychiatry 2014;71:1121–8.

23. Miller B, Buckley P, Seabolt W, et al. Meta-analysis of cytokine alterations in schizophrenia: clinical status and antipsychotic effects. Biol Psychiatry 2011; 70:663–71.

24. Miller BJ, Culpepper N, Rapaport MH. C-reactive protein levels in schizophrenia: a review and meta-analysis. Clin Schizophr Relat Psychoses 2014;7:223–30.

25. Miller B, Gassama B, Sebastian D, et al. Meta-analysis of lymphocytes in schizophrenia: clinical status and antipsychotic effects. Biol Psychiatry 2013;73:993–9.

26. Ezeoke A, Mellor A, Buckley P, et al. A systematic quantitative review of blood autoantibody elevations in schizophrenia. Schizophr Res 2013;150:245–51.

27. Miller BJ, Buckley P. Is relapse in schizophrenia an immune-mediated effect? Focus 2012;10:115–23.

28. Levine J, Gutman J, Feraro R, et al. Side effect profile of azathioprine in the treatment of chronic schizophrenic patients. Neuropsychobiology 1997;36:172–6.

29. Chaudhry IB, Husain N, ur Rahman R, et al. A randomised double-blind placebo-controlled 12- week feasibility trial of methotrexate added to treatment as usual in early schizophrenia: study protocol for a randomised controlled trial. Trials 2015; 16:9.

30. Hosoda S, Takimura H, Shibayama M, et al. Psychiatric symptoms related to interferon therapy for chronic hepatitis C: clinical features and prognosis. Psychiatry Clin Neurosci 2000;54:565–72.
31. Fattovich G, Giustina G, Favarato S, et al. A survey of adverse events in 11,241 patients with chronic viral hepatitis treated with alfa interferon. J Hepatol 1996;24:38–47.
32. Myint AM, Schwarz MJ, Steinbusch HW, et al. Neuropsychiatric disorders related to interferon and interleukins treatment. Metab Brain Dis 2009;24:55–68.
33. Silverman BC, Kim AY, Freudenreich O. Interferon-induced psychosis as a "psychiatric contraindication" to hepatitis C treatment: a review and case-based discussion. Psychosomatics 2010;51:1–7.
34. Pizzi C, Caraglia M, Cianciulli M, et al. Low-dose recombinant IL-2 induces psychological changes: monitoring by Minnesota Multiphasic Personality Inventory (MMPI). Anticancer Res 2002;22:727–32.
35. Lamotte G, Cogez J, Viader F. Interferon-β-1a-induced psychosis in a patient with multiple sclerosis. Psychiatry Clin Neurosci 2012;66:462.
36. Manfredi G, Kotzalidis GD, Sani G, et al. Persistent interferon-β-1b-induced psychosis in a patient with multiple sclerosis. Psychiatry Clin Neurosci 2010;64:584–6.
37. Raison CL, Rutherford RE, Woolwine BJ, et al. A randomized controlled trial of the tumor necrosis factor antagonist infliximab for treatment-resistant depression: the role of baseline inflammatory biomarkers. JAMA Psychiatry 2013;70:31–41.
38. Weinberger JF, Raison CL, Rye DB, et al. Inhibition of tumor necrosis factor improves sleep continuity in patients with treatment resistant depression and high inflammation. Brain Behav Immun 2015;47:193–200.
39. Mehta D, Raison CL, Woolwine BJ, et al. Transcriptional signatures related to glucose and lipid metabolism predict treatment response to the tumor necrosis factor antagonist infliximab in patients with treatment-resistant depression. Brain Behav Immun 2013;31:205–15.
40. Grüber L, Bunse T, Weidinger E, et al. Adjunctive recombinant human interferon gamma-1b for treatment-resistant schizophrenia in 2 patients. J Clin Psychiatry 2014;75:266–1267.
41. Miller BJ, Dias JK, Lemos HP, et al. An open-label, pilot trial of adjunctive tocilizumab in schizophrenia. J Clin Psychiatry, in press.
42. Senol N, Ceyhan BM, Ersoy IH, et al. Aspirin increases NMDA receptor subunit 2A concentrations in rat hippocampus. J Recept Signal Transduct Res 2012;32:17–21.
43. Hu F, Wang X, Pace TW, et al. Inhibition of COX-2 by celecoxib enhances glucocorticoid receptor function. Mol Psychiatry 2005;10:426–8.
44. Fusar-Poli P, Deste G, Smieskova R, et al. Cognitive functioning in prodromal psychosis: a meta-analysis. Arch Gen Psychiatry 2012;69:562–71.
45. Mesholam-Gately RI, Giuliano AJ, Goff KP, et al. Neurocognition in first-episode schizophrenia: a meta-analytic review. Neuropsychology 2009;23:315–36.
46. Bhojraj TS, Sweeney JA, Prasad KM, et al. Gray matter loss in young relatives at risk for schizophrenia: relation with prodromal psychopathology. Neuroimage 2011;54:S272–9.

Redefining Medication Adherence in the Treatment of Schizophrenia

How Current Approaches to Adherence Lead to Misinformation and Threaten Therapeutic Relationships

 CrossMark

Peter J. Weiden, MD*

KEYWORDS

- Schizophrenia • Outcome • Patient acceptance of health care • Relapse
- Physician-patient relations • Harm reduction • Communication

KEY POINTS

- If there were an easy answer to improving adherence to antipsychotic medication, we would have found it. New approaches are needed that reevaluate the current concept of adherence.
- The current focus on following a clinician's recommendation should be changed toward identification or preventing of disruptions in continuity of antipsychotic treatment for any reason.
- The indirect consequences of adherence problems may be just as severe as direct consequences, and includes misinformation about the medication regimen and that the way adherence problems are handled is a threat to the therapeutic relationship.
- Changing the way adherence challenges are addressed can reduce errors from misinformation, and also can be adapted to strengthen rather than harm the therapeutic relationship.

Disclosure Statement: The author has at present and/or has had within the past 12 months, the following affiliation with one or more. Consultant: Alkermes, Delpor, Forum, Johnson & Johnson (Janssen Pharmaceuticals), Lundbeck, Otsuka, Neurocrine, Sunovion, Teva, Vanda; Research Support: AbbVie, Alkermes, Forum, Forest Laboratories, Genentech, Johnson & Johnson (Janssen Pharmaceuticals), Otsuka, Neurocrine, Novartis, Reckitt Benckiser Pharmaceuticals, Takeda; Speaker's Bureau: Alkermes, Forum, Johnson & Johnson (Janssen Pharmaceuticals), Lundbeck, Otsuka, Novartis, Sunovion; Stockholder: Delpor.
This article was supported by NIMH Medication Adherence in Schizophrenia: Development of a CBT-based Intervention (R34 MH080978) and the Katie Ganaway foundation.
Department of Psychiatry, UIC Medical Center, Chicago, IL 60611, USA
* Uptown Research, 2012 West Lawrence Avenue, Chicago, IL 60640.
E-mail address: pweiden@uptownresearch.com

Psychiatr Clin N Am 39 (2016) 199–216
http://dx.doi.org/10.1016/j.psc.2016.01.004
0193-953X/16/$ – see front matter © 2016 Elsevier Inc. All rights reserved.

psych.theclinics.com

INTRODUCTION

Insanity: doing the same thing over and over again and expecting different results.
—Albert Einstein

If there were an easy answer that would solve the problem of nonadherence to antipsychotic medication, we would have found it by now.[1] There have been many advances in the treatment of schizophrenia over the past few decades, but improved adherence is not one of them. This is not to say that our understanding of issues has stood still; we better understand the forces at play that comprise many of the determinants of adherence challenges for patients with schizophrenia.[2–4] Nonetheless, disruptions in antipsychotic treatment continue to be an enormous challenge, and remain a major obstacle to achieving better outcomes from currently available treatments.

There are many excellent general reviews available for readers who are interested in a more traditional risk factor and intervention approach to this topic.[5–8] It is the goal of this review to move beyond some of the traditional approaches to adherence problems and offer another perspective on how to better address this vexing problem.

The central hypothesis of this review is that the current definition of adherence is fundamentally flawed, and these flaws then create insolvable problems that limit the effectiveness of adherence management in current practice. If this hypothesis is true, then the solution will go beyond "improving adherence." There are many other ways in which outcome can improve from different approaches, even for patients who remain nonadherent. Even then, clinicians can target indirect complications of nonadherence that also harm outcome. Examples include reducing the degree to which misinformation about the medication regimen leads to downstream complications, and focusing on strengthening the therapeutic alliance even when there is a disagreement about the role of medication, and, finally reducing the harmful consequences when medication discontinuation has occurred or seems inevitable. Notice that all of these are important therapeutic goals in their own right over and above any adherence improvements. Only then, with a broader, holistic perspective, can we recalibrate the goals of any adherence intervention.

The starting point is to carefully review the standard definition of adherence, and review how this definition actually leads to more assessment failures, complicates the therapeutic relationship, and ironically limits the potential benefits of interventions hoping to improve adherence.

DEFINITION OF ADHERENCE

According to the World Health Organization (WHO), adherence is defined as

The extent to which a person's behavior—taking medication, following a diet, and/ or executing lifestyle changes, corresponds with agreed recommendations from a health care provider[9]

Maybe you are asking yourself, "So, what's wrong with that?" or, "What's the clinical relevance of how adherence is defined?" The language of adherence and nonadherence is such a familiar part of medical training and day-to-day practice that it is easy to forget the tacit and unspoken meaning of the term. The following 2 case vignettes illustrate the problems in the way adherence is defined when it comes to working with patients with schizophrenia.

Adherence Definition Does Not Include Medication Attitude or Intent

---

Case 1: Mary and the hurricane blowing away adherence

Mary has schizophrenia and generally goes to the clinic and picks up her medication prescriptions at her appointment, and gets the medications filled at a local pharmacy on her way back home. However, a hurricane caused flooding, and the clinic was closed on the day of her appointment. Over the next weeks, although public transportation services were disrupted, phone lines were working. Mary confirms her next appointment. Mary did not contact the pharmacy to see how she could get her medications, and her medications ran out for a month between appointments.

Using the WHO definition, Mary was not adherent to her medication for a month after the hurricane struck. She could have been adherent. All she had to do was call her clinic or her pharmacy for refills. However, most of us would feel uneasy about calling Mary a "nonadherent patient"; her history is one of a patient who is generally adherent and cooperative with treatment recommendations. We would think of Mary's nonadherence in the larger context of its occurrence, in the aftermath of a natural disaster that disrupted her routine. And, examined more closely, there probably was an interaction between the disruption caused by a hurricane and her persistent symptoms of schizophrenia. It is likely that cognitive or negative symptoms of schizophrenia were obstacles that prevented her from coming up with an adaptive solution to her medications running out. The answer is to broaden the adherence definition into distinguishing between adherence behavior (were medications taken/not taken?) and adherence attitude (does the person want to take/not take medication?). This is very relevant to an illness such as schizophrenia, an illness that often affects the ability and the willingness to take medication.

The Definition of Adherence Is Silent About Efficacy of the Intervention

---

Case 2: John and seeking treatment for attention-deficit/hyperactivity disorder (ADHD)

John has had 2 psychotic episodes while at college and has met diagnostic criteria for schizophrenia. John does not agree and believes that the psychotic episodes were caused by academic stress. He responds very well to antipsychotic medication, but he told his outpatient psychiatrist he will stop his medication, especially because he is now frustrated by cognitive difficulties making it much harder to study than before he got ill. He was surprised that his cognition did not get better after he stopped his antipsychotic, so he went online and now believes his problems are better explained by a diagnosis of ADHD, not schizophrenia. He seeks out several second opinions, and one of the consultants agrees that ADHD is the primary problem. John changes psychiatrists, starts on a stimulant for ADHD. He is very diligent about his appointments and is taking ADHD medication exactly as prescribed.

Using the WHO definition, John was adherent, but the adherence was to ADHD treatment, not his schizophrenia treatment. Of course, John found a clinician who agreed with his own beliefs, so his previous nonadherence to antipsychotic medication is not relevant. However, this does not feel right because stimulants without antipsychotic medication are likely to cause an exacerbation of schizophrenia. The root cause of the problem is that adherence is defined *only* as an agreement between the patient and the clinician. The definition is silent about being effective. By omitting efficacy, the focus of the term is on whether the patient's behavior deviated from an agreement with the doctor. This omission has had unfortunate consequences in that it emphasizes on agreement at the expense of emphasizing efficacy. The definition places too much focus on obedience (does the patient follow the recommendation?) and too little on outcome (does the difference between recommended and taken matter?). The adverse consequences of this omission are particularly problematic in schizophrenia in light of some of the public debates about effectiveness of antipsychotic medication, as well as the current emphasis focused on shared decision making in serious mental illness.

The rest of the review discusses some of the consequences of the current adherence approach and how redefining adherence can offer new ways to mitigate the detrimental effects of adherence challenge on outcome.

DIRECT AND INDIRECT CONSEQUENCES OF NONADHERENCE

There are a multitude of long-term studies comparing stabilized patients with schizophrenia who remain on antipsychotic medications with those who discontinue antipsychotics that show that medication discontinuation is associated with worse outcome.[10-14] Rather than dwell on what is already known, this review focuses on other aspects of the adherence problem that are less understood.

These include the following:

1. Better understanding of dose-response aspects of nonadherence[13]
2. Impact of poor quality of information on outcome
3. How adherence issues can harm the therapeutic relationship

Regardless of whether medication cessation was part of a research study or whether it was based on a patient decision against clinical advice, the consequences have been that those discontinuing antipsychotics, when compared with those who remain on antipsychotics, will be on the whole more symptomatic and will have a greatly increased chance of relapse (see summary in **Box 1**).

ESTABLISHING EFFICACY: WHAT IS THE "DOSE-RESPONSE" CURVE OF MEDICATION GAPS?

The problem with "nonadherence" is that it covers a broad swath of medication behaviors, ranging from complete cessation to transient medication gaps to taking a lower dose than prescribed.[22,23] A closer look shows that some kinds of nonadherence are more problematic than others. Patients who consistently take less antipsychotic

---

Box 1
Summary of role of long-term antipsychotic medication

- Once a diagnosis of schizophrenia is established, all treatment guidelines strongly endorse continuous antipsychotic therapy[15]

- The recommendation for continuous antipsychotic is not changed by duration of illness, time on antipsychotic, or relative response[16,17]

- Dose-reduction approaches have been successful; therefore, using an efficacy approach to defining nonadherence, it is very difficult to evaluate whether patient decision to take less than prescribed represents "nonadherence"[18,19]

- Strategies that have tried to discontinue antipsychotics under careful medical supervision have found the following:
  - Episodic, targeted medication discontinuation ("drug holidays") should not be recommended even when carefully monitored
  - Patients should be advised of the risks of even relatively brief medication gaps[15]

- Despite recommendations otherwise, medication gaps are very common and frequently unreported and unrecognized in clinical practice[20-22]

- The adverse impact of medication gaps on symptoms and relapse risk are not affected by the cause of the medication gap; therefore, the basic problem is not as much "nonadherence" as it is "disruption of continuous medication therapy"

Data from Refs.[15-22]

medication than prescribed are also "nonadherent" despite the possibility that there is not any worse outcome associated with dose reduction. Complete medication cessation is associated with serious consequences in terms of relapse risk. Temporary medication discontinuation ("medication gaps") have an intermediate effect, but are clearly associated with greater level of symptoms and relapse risk.

Some authors have criticized the universality of the recommendations of maintenance antipsychotic treatment by invoking research that a small minority of patients with a diagnosis of schizophrenia seem to be able to exit the mental health system, and go on and live their lives without taking medication. However, is not possible to prospectively identify those individual patients in advance, and the overwhelming majority of patients with schizophrenia in the clinical practice setting benefit from staying on long-term antipsychotic medication.

MISINFORMATION AS AN INDIRECT COMPLICATION OF RELUCTANCE TO DISCLOSE NONADHERENCE

Moving on from the *direct* consequences of disruptions of continuity of antipsychotic medication, there are serious *indirect* consequences that are complications of the overall adherence problem. One of these is the frequency with which clinicians are misinformed because of lack of accurate information about the degree to which their patients have not followed their recommendations.[4] There often is a wide discrepancy between what the clinician has *prescribed* and what was actually *taken*, but then the clinician bases follow-up recommendations based on the belief that what was actually *taken* is the same as what was *prescribed*.[24] **Tables 1** and **2** show the way in which misinformation adds to safety risks and also causes errors in subsequent medication recommendations.[5] Therefore, better recognition of medication gaps is an important goal in its own right regardless of whether or not anything can be done to reduce those gaps.

ADHERENCE AS A THREAT TO THE THERAPEUTIC RELATIONSHIP

Perhaps the most pernicious indirect consequence of the current approach to adherence is that it is likely that the way it is currently handled in clinical practice is harmful to the therapeutic relationship. Recall that adherence is defined as not following a treatment recommendation. As such, the "outcome" from an adherence perspective is based on whether or not the patient did what was recommended within a context of a treatment relationship. Within the social ecology of psychiatric treatment, failure to

Table 1	
Potential safety risks due to misinformation	
Increased risk of medication toxicities	When a medication regimen is continued after hospital admission and causes toxicity due to excessively rapid reexposure of medication(s) that had been prescribed but not taken
Increased risk of tardive dyskinesia	Intermittent treatment from medication gaps is a risk factor for withdrawal and tardive dyskinesia
Increased risk of antipsychotic withdrawal problems	Patients who go on and off prescribed medications are at risk (depending on specific medication) of withdrawal dyskinesia, rebound extrapyramidal symptoms or akathisia, antihistamine withdrawal, or anticholinergic withdrawal

Table 2	
Errors in treatment decisions due to misinformation	
Misclassification of adherence problems as treatment resistance	Unrecognized medication gaps causing persistent symptoms lead to multiple changes in antipsychotic medication
Misclassification of treatment resistance as an adherence problem	Patients attributed to adherence problems, but the adherence problems arise from persistent symptoms caused by insufficient efficacy
Erroneous information about prior medication history	Unrecognized medication gaps may affect decisions based on history of relative response to medication

follow the recommendation is socially undesirable. Although social desirability of adherence is hardly unique to mental health services, the schizophrenia population is relatively disenfranchised or socially isolated, thereby elevating the relative importance of the therapeutic relationship with his or her clinicians. Also, it is well established that patients with schizophrenia are particularly sensitive to hostile and critical comments. Assuming that disclosure of intentional nonadherence is likely to elicit, at best, negative feedback from many clinicians, it follows that patients may find these responses stressful and difficult.[25] Even if well intended, the way clinicians react to information of recent or intended medication discontinuation may be perceived as patronizing, insensitive, or as being a personal criticism (see **Box 2** for summary).

The Adherence Interview: Better Information, Better Alliance

If patients' concerns and complaints about problems with medication are dismissed or trivialized, then the patients will be frustrated and feel that their opinions do not matter. Clinicians may also react with frustration because the patient seems to be ignoring recommendations and will likely suffer serious consequences as a result. However, it will not help the therapeutic relationship if the clinician's frustration appears to be based on annoyance that the patient is not obeying the medication recommendation rather than true concern for the patient's well-being. Once the patient has experienced these kinds of interactions, the patient will be more likely to take adherence matters into his or her own hands, and decide it is not in the patient's best interests to disclose

Box 2
Ways in which adherence is a threat to the therapeutic relationship
• The "obedience" aspect of how adherence is defined can hurt the therapeutic relationship
• The patient may not feel that it is emotionally safe to disclose not taking medications as prescribed
• Either party may believe that not following a recommendation signifies being a "bad" patient
• The clinician may view adherence as a matter of "trust," so nonadherence is perceived as a betrayal of trust
• Or, there may be avoidance of the topic, "don't ask, don't tell" because of negative experiences from disagreeing or disclosing nonadherence

his or her true beliefs and decisions about the recommended medication regimen. Another aspect of any therapeutic relationship is trust.[26] Trust arises over time, and is based on expectations of honesty, integrity, and predictability.[27] Trust as it pertains to adherence issues is that the treatment recommendation will be congruent with expected outcomes.[28] Although it is essential for the clinician to clearly articulate the benefits of antipsychotic medication for successful treatment, and the importance of staying on continuous antipsychotic therapy for long-term treatment, it is also important to be honest about limitations of current therapies.

Glass Half Full or Empty? The Dangers in "Overselling" Medication Benefits

Because the focus is on benefits, it is easy to minimize limitations. Clinicians use as a frame of reference the relative benefits of antipsychotic medication. The basis of comparison will be the differences between the patient's clinical state before receiving antipsychotics and the degree to which those symptoms are reduced or eliminated by medication. Then, the clinician will do his or her best to educate the patient that the improvements are attributed to medication, and that stopping medication will cause relapse and return of symptoms. The natural tendency is to emphasize the positive aspects of medication, but in doing so, there is the risk of going overboard and imply that the medications are fully effective and restorative. The patient's frame of reference is quite different. Their basis of comparison is the difference between their current condition and the way they were (and felt) before the onset of their mental illness. In other words, patients want to be "normal" and will have a natural expectation that when told, "Medications are effective!" or "You will get better by taking medication," that medications will return them to a premorbid, "normal" condition. When antipsychotic medications are "oversold," it may be make it harder for patients to trust future medication recommendations (**Fig. 1**).

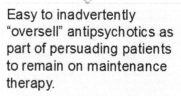

Clinicians and Patients Differ in Expectations of Response
Potential Impact on Trust and Credibility

Clinician Calibration	Patient Calibration
Antipsychotics can be very effective relative to being off medication	Antipsychotics are not effective because medications do not restore the person to premorbid state; "I am still not normal!"
Easy to inadvertently "oversell" antipsychotics as part of persuading patients to remain on maintenance therapy. "This will make you better!"	Patients become skeptical of being told that medications are helpful and then are disappointed. "I've heard that before!"

Fig. 1. Calibration of response: it depends who you ask!

ADHERENCE INTERVENTIONS

There are a range of specific interventions and approaches for adherence problems. Some of the common elements of interventions include identifying the specific risk factors on an individual patient basis, and then matching the type of intervention with the specific risk factor. One example is that using cell phones as conduits for medication reminders is effective only for patients with cell phones, is unlikely to be helpful for patients who decide to stop medication, but might be very helpful for patients who have trouble with following a medication routine. Some other basic aspects that are well described in the literature on adherence in schizophrenia are summarized in **Table 3**.

The rest of this article continues to focus on the conceptual concerns alluded to earlier in this article. These include the following:

- Adapting the understanding of the consequences of medication gaps to inform which adherence problems are most clinically relevant
- Reducing the likelihood of lack of information and misinformation
- Addressing adherence challenges in ways that strengthen the therapeutic relationship

Table 3
Some universal recommendations for addressing adherence challenges

After a diagnosis of schizophrenia[29,30]	• Educate patient and family about need for ongoing antipsychotic medication • Anticipate nonadherence is likely to occur
Assessing adherence status[31,32]	• Routine screen for adherence problems • Assessment should include adherence attitudes as well as behaviors • Clinicians need to be aware that they will not detect most adherence problems • Ancillary sources include family members, case managers, and pharmacy refill records, as indicated
Therapeutic relationships	• Maintain therapeutic alliance • Continuity of care whenever possible
Use of long-acting formulations[33–36]	• Probably underused • May improve adherence and outcome for some patients • Better for monitoring adherence
Management of side effects[2]	• Individualize antipsychotic choice • Use lowest effective dose • Proactively address distress from side effects
Adherence problems arising from cognitive or negative symptoms[2]	• Simplify medication regimen • Medication supervision, if available • Use behavioral cues and reminders • Use a long-acting antipsychotic formulation
Lowering barriers to medication access	• Ensuring medication access • Reducing cost barriers • Facilitating transportation and other concrete services
Dealing with stigma	• Use Cognitive-Behavioral Therapy (CBT)-oriented approaches that can address problems without relying on a diagnostic model

Data from Refs.[2,29–36]

REDUCING FREQUENCY OF MEDICATION GAPS

The importance of carefully assessing and trying to uncover medication gaps cannot be overemphasized. Many of these gaps occur in patients who are not fundamentally opposed to antipsychotic medication. Therefore, if discovered, they often lend themselves to relatively straightforward solutions once they are recognized. The recommendations follow the evidence. In particular, clinicians need to be more concerned about the potential risks of medication gaps than the risks of lowing the dose, as long as the dose lowering is gradual and does not include episodes of complete discontinuation. The risks of dose lowering and dose discontinuation do not seem to depend on the reason behind the change (eg, whether it was the result of an intentional decision or was due to a disruption in routine). This can be incorporated into discussions about safety and efficacy of antipsychotic medication. Invoking medication safety is useful in that safety messages are more likely to be accepted, even for patients who intentionally stop their medication.

Work on Establishing Medication Routines

Having schizophrenia greatly increases the likelihood of "accidental" or "unintentional" medication gaps. Introducing and monitoring medication routine can reduce the likelihood of medication gaps and also improve the chances of discovering them when things go awry. One way to reduce the likelihood of an inadvertent medication gap while improving the chances of detection when they occur is to carefully review and establish medication routines. For example, Velligan and colleagues[37,38] have shown in a series of studies that behavioral approaches are effective, but the intervention needs to be focused on details of the medication routine. An example is the use of home visits to help patients organize where medications are stored and to link their medication routine with other automatic habits such as brushing teeth. (If a case manager is not available for home visits, it may be helpful for a friend or family member to do a home review.) Other methods include working with a pharmacy that will communicate any delays in picking up medications as well as reduce any other obstacles that get in the way of access.[39]

SHIFT THE EMPHASIS TO THE IMPORTANCE OF ACCURATE INFORMATION

When clinicians are not aware of medication gaps, they may conclude that the medication regimen is less effective than it could be if taken continuously. The misinformation has consequences. Without knowing full information, the clinician will make medication decisions that are at best futile and may even be harmful. The intervention goal here is to find ways to improve the accuracy of treatment information. Because the consequences of misinformation go beyond the consequences of nonadherence, it should be managed as a separate problem.

Making It Safe to Disclose Adherence Challenges

Clinicians know what medications they have prescribed, but they frequently do not know which medications were taken. The literature is very clear that clinicians frequently underestimate the frequency and magnitude of nonadherence occurring in their own practice. One of the causes of this detection gap arises from patients withholding (or not volunteering) nonadherence between visits. It is important to make it easier and safer for patients to disclose adherence issues between visits.

There are many reasons why a patient with schizophrenia would want the clinical team to believe that medications are taken as prescribed. Patients with schizophrenia may be relatively susceptible to social desirability factors ranging from passive acquiescence to fear (real or imagined) of disappointing their treatment team (eg, being thought of as a "bad" patient). Also, patients with schizophrenia may reasonably fear real-life consequences of disclosing nonadherence, such as hospitalization or losing housing benefits.

The goal is to help the patient understand that accurate reporting of medication status is a safe harbor and hopefully dispel anxiety or wariness. Given that medication discontinuation is so common to be almost universal, the patient might find it reassuring to hear that medication discontinuation is a common part of day-to-day practice and is not taken personally. Of course, these statements can be adapted or modified to correspond to your clinical style and philosophy. Unless done ahead of time, patients will not know how you might react to hearing about their adherence challenges (or their use of substances!). Asking for honest disclosure also means discussing and alleviating any concerns. Patients may be worried about whether disclosing nonadherence will have treatment repercussions (eg, "Will you hospitalize me?") or other life consequences ("Will you tell my parents?" "Will you tell my school?"). It is only fair that you disclose how you would handle these concerns. Assuming that the priority is accuracy of treatment information, it is sensible to protect privacy of disclosure concerns as much as possible. (It may not always be possible to guarantee complete confidentiality after disclosing nonadherence, but then the patient is more apt to withhold the adherence information. Is that better?).

The rationale of how the team will respond to disclosing medication deviations and discontinuations is shown in **Table 4**.

Follow-up visits should include a brief review of what happened with the medication since the last visit. Clinicians who wait for their patients to take the initiative to disclose nonadherence often have to wait for a long time. Disclosing nonadherence can be stressful, and may be easier to respond to a gentle question than bringing it up without prompting. The discussion can be prefaced by reminding the patient about the importance of having accurate information about the medication regimen as taken; for example, "You know, I know what I have prescribed but I don't know what you've

Table 4
Creating a "Safe Harbor" atmosphere to facilitate disclosure

Action	Rationale	Example Statement
Orient new patients about the importance of disclosing medication deviations or discontinuations	Anticipating that many patients withhold critical adherence information	"It is really common for patients to stop medications...but I tell all my patients ahead of time that it is really important to let me know."
Explain that prompt disclosure is important for safety reasons	Patients might be reluctant disclose without having an important and understandable reason	"It is safer for you if I know what you are actually taking, not what I think you are taking."
Advanced reassurance that honest disclosure is safe and will be treated respectfully	Commons reason for withholding information is fear of being thought of as a "bad" patient	"Sometimes patients worry about what will happen after telling me they have stopped their medication. Well, I want you to know ahead of time that it happens all the time and I don't take it personally."

actually taken. It is really important for your care that I really know what's been taken, which makes it safer for you and more likely that I will 'get it right' for medication adjustments later on." Afterward, the most important point for follow-up questions is that it is emotionally safe, with gentle questions and reassuring tone, for the patient to respond honestly.

The other aspect to this assessment is to ask about any potential disruptions in routine that may have resulted in disruption of medication continuity. The patient may not think of these kinds of medication gaps as being problems, or it may be that some jogging of memory is needed. Instances of disruption of medication routine may include going on trips, comings and goings of family (eg, parents leaving on a vacation may result in missed doses), or whether there were any problems with medications running out and not getting filled. Another common situation is when a medication routine is disrupted because of intermittent substance use "My friends were in town and we went out partying and I did not take my medications with me."

Greater Use of Long-acting Antipsychotics as a Better Information Platform

Long-acting formulations are often recommended for "nonadherence." However, long-acting formulations do not always guarantee adherence because once on a long-acting medication, patients can (and do) stop their long-acting antipsychotics just as they stop their oral medication. The most reliable way in which long-acting formulations are better than their oral counterparts is the enormous improvement in the quality of information available. One example of the difference in information for monitoring comes from a multicenter randomized controlled trial (RCT) comparing motivational interviewing (MI) with health education in 114 patients with schizophrenia selected based on history of nonadherence,[40] with 75% of the sample on oral and 25% on a long-acting formulation. Despite the smaller number of subjects on long-acting medication, an unexpected finding was that significant benefits of MI were observed only in the long-acting subgroup. Another RCT on paying patients to accept medication was restricted to individuals who were not consistent with their long-acting regimen.[41] This study would not have been feasible (either for patient selection or for outcome assessment) with oral formulations. One way of understanding the findings is that long-acting status makes adherence assessments accurate.

In clinical practice, once the patient has been stabilized on the long-acting antipsychotic, it is usually very easy to know whether the patient has received antipsychotic medication without any interruption. Likewise, any delays or interruptions are known right away, and allow for prompt response to resume a regular schedule. Should the patient decide to stop taking antipsychotic medication, the clinicians will be informed right away. The advantages of reliable information are always there, even when there are shortcomings in efficacy or adherence. For example, when patients continue to experience significant symptoms despite therapeutic doses of a long-acting formulation, covert nonadherence is eliminated as a potential nonpharmacologic reason for poor response (although substance abuse or medical comorbidities still need to be evaluated). Should the patient decide to stop taking antipsychotic medication, that person's decision will be apparent in "real time," allowing for a review and discussion of the pertinent issues right away.

ADDRESSING ADHERENCE TO STRENGTHEN THE THERAPEUTIC RELATIONSHIP

There is no reason why adherence challenges have to threaten a therapeutic relationship. Most of the time patients want to feel better and do better, and most clinicians want their patients to achieve the best outcomes possible.[42–44] If there are differences in how to achieve those goals, it does not automatically follow that it has to be a source of acrimony, alienation, or mistrust. Most patients, if given the chance, feel better when they feel safe to disclose their true feelings about the difficulties posed by their condition. They would feel a sense of relief if their clinician could really understand how disappointing and frustrating it is to have to take medications that do not fully restore the individual back to his or her premorbid condition. Most patients would find it liberating to feel like they are allowed to openly discuss ambivalence to medication without getting cutoff midsentence to be told to stay on medication. Active listening without interruption will make it easier for patients to articulate concerns that are counterintuitive but important. Examples include reports of nonadherence because of rapid *improvement*,[45] or concern that psychotic symptoms represent *side effects* rather than benefits of antipsychotics.[44] Most patients would like to be honest with their clinicians and feel safe that they will not be thought of as a "bad patient" if they admit to stopping medication. Most patients will find it reassuring when their clinicians provide guidance as to how they can feel better, even if that guidance is not immediately accepted.[46]

Differences of opinion that are respected are easier to accept than when verbalizing those differences leaves someone feeling chastised. Clinicians can learn that listening and acknowledging feelings does not represent colluding or abandoning the process of making strong recommendations with conviction. Acknowledging the obvious, that treatment recommendations are often not followed, does not mean resignation or willingness to accept suboptimal outcomes. The central thesis is that clinicians are better off realizing that the road to improving adherence is often through the therapeutic relationship.[47] McCabe and colleagues[48] have shown how conversations can be repaired toward common goals, and that this is associated with better adherence. If well-meaning, but futile, attempts to "stop" nonadherence results in damaging the therapeutic relationship, then it has defeated its purpose.

Assessing Patient Experience with Adherence Issues with Other Clinicians

We often work with individuals who have already had years of interactions with other clinicians. When meeting a patient for the first time, it is naïve to believe that the initial interactions will be a "blank slate." A more realistic assumption is that the patient's initial relationship with any new clinician will be, for better or worse, largely shaped by the cumulative experiences from his or her past treatment encounters. It is also reasonable to assume a large part of those encounters will have medication-focused interactions. The patient will likely have formed opinions on the truthfulness and trustworthiness of prescribing clinicians when it comes to medication recommendations. Likewise, patients will have expectations, good, bad, or ugly, about the kinds of responses if and when they inform clinicians about concerns about medication. It is also likely that the patient has formed his or her own beliefs about the underlying motivations of clinicians for their emphasis on pharmacologic treatments.

Therefore, the initial assessment is an excellent time to do a detailed assessment of the interactions concerning therapeutic relationships and prescribed medications. The information provided in **Box 3** is used as a guide as to how to manage medication issues, including adherence, in ways that might improve rather than threaten the therapeutic relationship. In the likely event that the patient reports disappointment, frustration, or anger at previous clinicians, it is helpful to withhold judgment or blame. It is better to discuss how negative experiences can be avoided, especially when there are differences of opinion regarding medication

---

Box 3
Initial assessment: prior experience with adherence discussions

Impact of medication management on prior relationships with clinicians

- Why did your clinician(s) recommend medication?

- Did you worry whether there were any hidden reasons for recommending medication that are not explained to you?

- Did you tell your prescribing clinician(s) about any side effects? How do they handle your concerns? Have some clinicians been more worried about your side effects than others?

- In the past, was there anything your clinician did that made it easier for you to stay with medication?

- How about anything that "turned you off" to the idea of taking medication?

Differences of opinion between you and your clinicians about medication

- Do you feel like you can be honest about reporting any medication problems?

- Did you ever stop your medication on your own?

- If so, did you tell your clinician? How was the reaction? Were you treated any differently? Did you get into trouble? Or, was their response helpful?

- Did you ever keep it [stopping medication] to yourself? If so, were you worried about what would happen if they knew you stopped?

---

recommendations, and also use reports of positive experiences as a guide for future interactions.

Harm Reduction Approaches When Intentional Nonadherence Is Likely

Up until now, much effort has been placed in developing therapeutic approaches that try to "stop" nonadherence. These have included patient-based psychoeducation (this refers to patient-based psychoeducation only; please note that psychoeducation including families has been shown to be effective for improving adherence and outcome[49–51]),[52,53] "compliance therapy,"[54–56] and MI.[40,57] None of these strategies have been effective. It is time to shift to other therapeutic approaches that accept the reality that sometimes patients will stop no matter what. This section covers how to introduce harm-reduction strategies once it is apparent that further discussion is futile.

Responding When Nonadherence Is Being Considered

The clinician or treatment team needs to clearly articulate that medication cessation is not recommended due to relapse risk, and review the evidence for this. It is helpful to review the patient's life goals and to ask about whether a symptom exacerbation would be disruptive, and whether it is worth the risk. It is also helpful to ask permission to speak with family members and others involved in the patient's care. If the patient seems to reject going back to the full therapeutic regimen, it may be helpful to discuss a "compromise" between patient and clinician (eg, postponing the decision, or agreeing on a dose reduction rather than discontinuation).

Responding When Recent Nonadherence has Happened and Now Is Disclosed

When the patient discloses medication deviations, discontinuations, or differences, the clinician needs to uphold his or her part of the agreement and make sure that the response makes good on the earlier promise of emotional safety. It may be

Table 5
Harm reduction after disclosure of intent to stop medication

Advantages of Harm-Reduction Approach	Potential Concerns or Limitations When Considering Harm Reduction
May facilitate honest reporting of intent to stop medication	There may be concern that pre-disclosure of harm-reduction strategy might encourage nonadherence
Makes it easier for patient to be honest about intent to stop medication	Some clinicians may not feel comfortable with using a harm-reduction approach regardless of its potential merits
Makes it possible to have collaborative treatment plan despite clinician opposition to discontinuation	Harm-reduction approach not possible if the patient has already stopped medication or disengaged with treatment
A slow down-titration schedule that is acknowledged and monitored is less risky than abrupt medication discontinuation without guidance	Not feasible to set up a collaborative discontinuation plan when medication is given under coercion
May allow for earlier identification of symptom exacerbation before full discontinuation	Misunderstanding of clinician's disagreement with patient decision
After a relapse and resuming medication, it may be easier to review "lessons learned" to facilitate the learning process	Patient may tell others that the clinician recommended discontinuation, omitting that this was not initiated by clinician

See text for details of the clinical circumstances for considering this approach.

appropriate to thank the patient for having the courage to disclose nonadherence, especially if the patient struggled with the decision, and that even if the clinician does not agree with the patient 's decision, the clinician can voice appreciation of prompt disclosure. If the patient does not feel safe for having disclosed, it is unlikely that there will be any more voluntary disclosure later on.

Responding When the Patient Intends to Stop Medication No Matter What

This section covers the situation of when the patient has made a decision to stop antipsychotic medication sometime *in the near future*, and that nothing is going to change his or her mind. The only question is how to respond to the decision. The harm-reduction approach uses principles based on similar models of substance abuse interventions, to focus on reducing the future risks and also facilitating honest reporting of adherence behavior.[58,59] It is the author's belief that the standard approach to always try to "stop" nonadherence has created strong resistance to using harm reduction in clinical practice as well as lost research opportunities to evaluate the potential for this approach to improve long-term outcomes (**Table 5**).

SUMMARY

Adherence challenges remain a basic and crucial aspect of treatment of schizophrenia. Although adherence is a challenge across all disease areas, there are reasons why nonadherence is an even bigger problem in this condition. The illness starts in young adulthood, a developmental period that always brings challenging problems with acceptance of any disease. Medications are only partly effective, leaving the patient and clinicians with vastly different impressions of whether medications "work." The relative loss of autonomy and independence that is associated with this illness means that for most patients the therapeutic relationship takes on primary importance, yet often relationships are transient within many of our treatment services. The illness creates psychological reasons to stop medication, and also manifests symptoms that often lead to inadvertent or accidental medication gaps. Because the definition of adherence does not allow for full understanding of these challenges, the field has been at an impasse for some time. Focusing on obedience rather than disruptions in outcome does not work. Trying to "stop" nonadherence when it is going to happen no matter what is a bad idea. It does not work and there is no reason to believe it will ever work. It is time to redefine our goals and objectives. This review suggests that the primary goal is to reduce medication gaps and discontinuities as much as possible regardless of cause. Also, even when these gaps happen, it is possible to minimize collateral damage from misinformation by focusing on better detection and disclosure. For patients who are ambivalent or opposed to antipsychotic medication, our belief is that it is best to take a longer term, developmental perspective. The road to better adherence may take a while, and in the long-run it is more effective to focus on the therapeutic relationship. This can be accomplished through dropping adversarial or imperious responses to patients' concerns, and focus on understanding those concerns before responding. Finally, when nonadherence is a choice and seems inevitable, then it is best to stop trying to "stop" nonadherence, and rather to focus on coming up with a collaborative harm-reduction strategy to try to mitigate the risks and consequences of medication discontinuation.

ACKNOWLEDGMENTS

The author would like to acknowledge Vasiliki Weiden for her comments and review of the article.

REFERENCES

1. Weiden P. Understanding and addressing adherence issues in schizophrenia: from theory to practice. J Clin Psychiatry 2007;68(Suppl 14):14–9.
2. Velligan DI, Weiden PJ, Sajatovic M, et al. Strategies for addressing adherence problems in patients with serious and persistent mental illness: recommendations from the expert consensus guidelines. J Psychiatr Pract 2010;16:306–24.
3. Sajatovic M, Velligan DI, Weiden PJ, et al. Measurement of psychiatric treatment adherence. J Psychosom Res 2010;69:591–9.
4. Velligan D, Sajatovic M, Valenstein M, et al. Methodological challenges in psychiatric treatment adherence research. Clin Schizophr Relat Psychoses 2010;4: 74–91.
5. Turkington D: Assessment and management of medication nonadherence in schizophrenia P, Weiden. In: Lieberman JA, Murray RM, editors. Comprehensive care of schizophrenia: a textbook of clinical management. 2nd edition. Oxford: Oxford University Press; 2013. p. 219–43.
6. Byerly MJ, Nakonezny PA, Lescouflair E. Antipsychotic medication adherence in schizophrenia. Psychiatr Clin North Am 2007;30:437–52.
7. Velligan DI, Weiden PJ, Sajatovic M, et al. Assessment of adherence problems in patients with serious and persistent mental illness: recommendations from the expert consensus guidelines. J Psychiatr Pract 2010;16:34–45.
8. Fenton WS, Blyler CR, Heinssen RK. Determinants of medication compliance in schizophrenia: empirical and clinical findings. Schizophr Bull 1997;23:637–51.
9. World Health Organization. Available at: www.who.int/chp/knowledge/publications/adherence_Section1.pdf. Accessed June 10, 2015.

10. Leucht S, Heres S, Kissling W, et al. Evidence-based pharmacotherapy of schizo-phrenia. Int J Neuropsychopharmacol 2011;14:269–84.
11. Ascher-Svanum H, Faries DE, Zhu B, et al. Medication adherence and long-term functional outcomes in the treatment of schizophrenia in usual care. J Clin Psychiatry 2006;67:453–60.
12. Perkins DO. Predictors of noncompliance in patients with schizophrenia. J Clin Psychiatry 2002;63:1121–8.
13. Cramer JA, Roy A, Burrell A, et al. Medication compliance and persistence: terminology and definitions. Value Health 2008;11:44–7.
14. Claxton AJ, Cramer J, Pierce C. A systematic review of the associations between dose regimens and medication compliance. Clin Ther 2001;23:1296–310.
15. Buchanan RW, Kreyenbuhl J, Kelly DL, et al, Schizophrenia Patient Outcomes Research Team (PORT). The 2009 schizophrenia PORT psychopharmacological treatment recommendations and summary statements. Schizophr Bull 2010;36:71–93.
16. Kane JM, Leucht S, Carpenter D, et al. The expert consensus guideline series: optimizing pharmacologic treatment of psychotic disorders. J Clin Psychiatry 2003;64:1–100.
17. Weiden PJ, Preskorn SH, Fahnestock PA, et al. Translating the psychopharmacology of antipsychotics to individualized treatment for severe mental illness: a roadmap. J Clin Psychiatry 2007;68(Suppl 7):1–48.
18. Schooler NR, Keith S, Severe J, et al. Relapse and rehospitalization during maintenance treatment of schizophrenia: the effects of dose reduction and family treatment. Arch Gen Psychiatry 1997;54:453–63.
19. Schooler NR. Maintenance medication for schizophrenia. Strategies for dose reduction. Schizophr Bull 1991;17:311–24.
20. Mojtabai R, Lavelle J, Gibson PJ, et al. Gaps in use of antipsychotics after discharge by first-admission patients with schizophrenia, 1989-1996. Psychiatr Serv 2002;53:337–9.
21. Weiden PJ, Kozma C, Grogg A, et al. Partial compliance and risk of rehospitalization among California Medicaid patients with schizophrenia. Psychiatr Serv 2004;55:886–91.
22. Valenstein M, Blow FC, Copeland LA, et al. Poor antipsychotic adherence among patients with schizophrenia: medication and patient factors. Schizophr Bull 2004;30:255–64.
23. Valenstein M, Ganoczy D, McCarthy JF, et al. Antipsychotic adherence over time among patients receiving treatment for schizophrenia: a retrospective review. J Clin Psychiatry 2006;67:1542–50.
24. Velligan DI, Lam YW, Glahn DC, et al. Defining and assessing adherence to oral antipsychotics: a review of the literature. Schizophr Bull 2006;32:724–42.
25. Sellwood W, Tarrier N, Quinn J, et al. The family and compliance in schizophrenia: the influence of clinical variables, relatives' knowledge and expressed emotion. Psychol Med 2003;33:91–6.
26. Jaeger S, Weisshaupt S, Flammer E, et al. Control beliefs, therapeutic relationship, and adherence in schizophrenia outpatients: a cross-sectional study. Am J Health Behav 2014;38:914–23.
27. Weiden P, Havens L. Psychotherapeutic management techniques in the treatment of outpatients with schizophrenia. Hosp Community Psychiatry 1994;45:549–55.

28. Misdrahi D, Petit M, Blanc O, et al. The influence of therapeutic alliance and insight on medication adherence in schizophrenia. Nord J Psychiatry 2012;66: 49–54.

29. Perkins DO, Gu H, McEvoy JP, et al. Predictors of treatment discontinuation and medication nonadherence in patients recovering from a first episode of schizophrenia, schizophreniform disorder, or schizoaffective disorder: a randomized, double-blind, flexible-dose, multicenter study. J Clin Psychiatry 2008;69(1): 106–13.

30. Weiden PJ, Buckley PF, Grody M. Understanding and treating "first-episode" schizophrenia. Psychiatr Clin North Am 2007;30:481–510.

31. Riley W, Velligan D, Sajatovic M, et al. Adherence to psychiatric treatments. CML - Psychiatry 2009;20(4):89–96.

32. Velligan DI, Wang M, Diamond P, et al. Relationships among subjective and objective measures of adherence to oral antipsychotic medications. Psychiatr Serv 2007;58:1187–92.

33. Alphs L, Benson C, Cheshire-Kinney K, et al. Real-world outcomes of paliperidone palmitate compared to daily oral antipsychotic therapy in schizophrenia: a randomized, open-label, review board-blinded 15-month study. J Clin Psychiatry 2015;76:554–61.

34. Subotnik KL, Casaus LR, Ventura J, et al. Long-acting injectable risperidone for relapse prevention and control of breakthrough symptoms after a recent first episode of schizophrenia: a randomized clinical trial. JAMA Psychiatry 2015; 72(8):822–9.

35. Weiden PJ, Roma RS, Velligan DI, et al. The challenge of offering long-acting antipsychotic therapies: a preliminary discourse analysis of psychiatrist recommendations for injectable therapy to patients with schizophrenia. J Clin Psychiatry 2015;76:684–90.

36. Weiden P, Solari H, Kim S, et al. Long-acting injectable antipsychotics and the management of nonadherence. Psychiatr Ann 2011;41:271–8.

37. Velligan D, Mintz J, Maples N, et al. A randomized trial comparing in person and electronic interventions for improving adherence to oral medications in schizophrenia. Schizophr Bull 2013;39:999–1007.

38. Velligan DI, Mueller J, Wang M, et al. Use of environmental supports among patients with schizophrenia. Psychiatr Serv 2006;57:219–24.

39. Valenstein M, Kavanagh J, Lee T, et al. Using a pharmacy-based intervention to improve antipsychotic adherence among patients with serious mental illness. Schizophr Bull 2011;37:727–36.

40. Barkhof E, Meijer CJ, de Sonneville LM, et al. The effect of motivational interviewing on medication adherence and hospitalization rates in nonadherent patients with multi-episode schizophrenia. Schizophr Bull 2013;39:1242–51.

41. Priebe S, Yeeles K, Bremner S, et al. Effectiveness of financial incentives to improve adherence to maintenance treatment with antipsychotics: cluster randomised controlled trial. BMJ 2013;347:f5847.

42. Shea SC. The "medication interest model": an integrative clinical interviewing approach for improving medication adherence-part 2: implications for teaching and research. Prof Case Manag 2009;14:6–15 [quiz: 16–7].

43. Shea SC, Barney C. Teaching clinical interviewing skills using role-playing: conveying empathy to performing a suicide assessment: a primer for individual role-playing and scripted group role-playing. Psychiatr Clin North Am 2015;38: 147–83.

44. Weiden PJ. The adherence interview: better information, better alliance. Psychiatr Ann 2011;41:279–85.

45. Moritz S, Hunsche A, Lincoln TM. Nonadherence to antipsychotics: the role of positive attitudes towards positive symptoms. Eur Neuropsychopharmacol 2014;24:1745–52.

46. Tranulis C, Goff D, Henderson DC, et al. Becoming adherent to antipsychotics: a qualitative study of treatment-experienced schizophrenia patients. Psychiatr Serv 2011;62:888–92.

47. Lencer R, Harris MSH, Weiden PJ, et al. When psychopharmacology is not enough: using cognitive behavioral therapy techniques for persons with persistent psychosis. Boston: Hogrefe Publishing; 2011.

48. McCabe R, Healey PG, Priebe S, et al. Shared understanding in psychiatrist-patient communication: association with treatment adherence in schizophrenia. Patient Educ Couns 2013;93:73–9.

49. Kopelowicz A, Zarate R, Wallace CJ, et al. The ability of multifamily groups to improve treatment adherence in Mexican Americans with schizophrenia. Arch Gen Psychiatry 2012;69:265–73.

50. Dixon L, Adams C, Lucksted A. Update on family psychoeducation for schizophrenia. Schizophr Bull 2000;26:5–20.

51. Pitschel-Walz G, Bauml J, Bender W, et al. Psychoeducation and compliance in the treatment of schizophrenia: results of the Munich Psychosis Information Project Study. J Clin Psychiatry 2006;67:443–52.

52. Zygmunt A, Olfson M, Boyer CA, et al. Interventions to improve medication adherence in schizophrenia. Am J Psychiatry 2002;159:1653–64.

53. Vreeland B, Minsky S, Yanos PT, et al. Efficacy of the Team Solutions Program for educating patients about illness management and treatment. Psychiatr Serv 2006;57:822–8.

54. Gray R, Wykes T, Gournay K. From compliance to concordance: a review of the literature on interventions to enhance compliance with antipsychotic medication. J Psychiatr Ment Health Nurs 2002;9:277–84.

55. Byerly MJ, Fisher R, Carmody T, et al. A trial of compliance therapy in outpatients with schizophrenia or schizoaffective disorder. J Clin Psychiatry 2005;66:997–1001.

56. Schulz M, Gray R, Spiekermann A, et al. Adherence therapy following an acute episode of schizophrenia: a multi-centre randomised controlled trial. Schizophr Res 2013;146:59–63.

57. Nieuwlaat R, Wilczynski N, Navarro T, et al. Interventions for enhancing medication adherence. Cochrane Database Syst Rev 2014;(11):CD000011.

58. Staring AB, Van der Gaag M, Koopmans GT, et al. Treatment adherence therapy in people with psychotic disorders: randomised controlled trial. Br J Psychiatry 2010;197:448–55.

59. Staring AB, van der Gaag M, Koopmans GT, et al. Individually-tailored intervention promotes treatment adherence in psychotic patients: an RCT. Ned Tijdschr Geneeskd 2011;155:A3135 [in Dutch].

Update on New and Emerging Treatments for Schizophrenia

Ganesh Gopalakrishna, MD, MHA*, Muaid H. Ithman, MD,
John Lauriello, MD

KEYWORDS

- Schizophrenia • Advances • Antipsychotics • Cognition • Negative symptoms

KEY POINTS

- Review of recent advances in treatment of schizophrenia including discussion of various neurotransmitter systems.
- Review newly Food and Drug Administration–approved medications and formulations in the treatment of schizophrenia.
- Examine the evidence for of novel drugs tested in schizophrenia.

INTRODUCTION

The serendipitous discovery in the 1950s that the phenothiazine, chlorpromazine (Thorazine) was an effective antipsychotic is often touted as one of the greatest advances of 20th-century medicine and dramatically changed the treatment and outcome of schizophrenia.[1] It set in motion a wave of drug discovery over the following 2 decades resulting in 15 approved antipsychotics in United States and 40 worldwide. Despite a concern over agranulocytosis, clozapine was reintroduced in the United States as the first second-generation antipsychotic (SGA) in the 1990s and is still the only antipsychotic shown to be effective in treatment-resistant patients. Its mechanism, which deemphasizes monodopamine blockage spurred the introduction of

Disclosure Statement: Equity ownership, profit-sharing agreements, royalties, patents: None; Research or other grants from private industry or closely affiliated nonprofit funds: Alkermes Event Monitoring Event Board—Contract paid to the University of Missouri; Advisory Panel: None; Speakers Bureau: None; Pharmaceutical CME Activity honoraria or other CME activity: RMEI LLC CME program funded through unrestricted educational grant from Janssen Scientific Affairs, LLC and Alkermes; Travel funds: None. (J. Lauriello). There is no conflict of interest to report for (G. Gopalakrishna, M.H. Ithman).
Department of Psychiatry, University of Missouri-Columbia, One Hospital Drive, Columbia, MO 65212, USA
* Corresponding author.
E-mail address: gopalakrishnag@health.missouri.edu

Abbreviations and Acronyms	
AMPA	Alpha-amino-3-hydroxy-5-methyl-4- isoxazolepropionic acid
cAMP	Cyclic adenosine monophosphate
FDA	Food and Drug Administration
mGluR	Metabotropic glutamate receptor
nAChR	Nicotinic acetylcholinergic receptor
NMDA	N-methyl-d-aspartate
PAM	Positive allosteric modulator
PANSS	Positive and Negative Syndrome Scale
PDE	Phosphodiesterase
SGA	Second-generation antipsychotic

other SGAs, which have much lower hematologic risk, but lack the exceptional efficacy.[2] Comparison studies of the first-generation antipsychotics and SGAs have demonstrated similar efficacy with the SGAs, as a group, tending to be better tolerated (especially in neurologic effects) and thus considered first-line treatment for schizophrenia.[3] Another recent advancement in treatment of schizophrenia has been the introduction of long-acting injectable (LAI) antipsychotics of some of the SGAs. Although LAIs have been available since the 1980s, the accessibility of SGA as LAIs, with fewer extrapyramidal side effects, has resulted in a renewed interest in their use. Despite the prodigious number of new antipsychotics in the previous century, only about 36% of the patients with schizophrenia reach remission.[4] About one-third of patients diagnosed with schizophrenia are considered to be treatment resistant after 2 or more adequate trials with antipsychotics.[5] So, although there has been more than 50 years of development, there remains a great need for more efficacious and better tolerated antipsychotic medications, as well as compounds that improve other impacted areas in schizophrenia (ie, cognition). This article looks at the recent advances in treatment of schizophrenia. We review newly Food and Drug Administration (FDA)–approved medications and formulations, examine the evidence for a number of novel drugs being tested in schizophrenia and describe promising compounds in the pharmaceutical pipeline.

Recently Approved Medications for Schizophrenia

In 2015, 2 newly approved antipsychotics came to market, the first with a potentially breakthrough delivery method, the other a long-awaited second in class option. We review both of these drugs with the understanding that at the time of writing this article, there is limited postmarketing evidence available about their efficacy, safety, and tolerability (**Table 1**).

Three-month paliperidone palmitate (Invega Trinza)

Paliperidone is the 9-OH metabolite of risperidone, first made available as LAI paliperidone palmitate in the United states for acute and maintenance treatment of schizophrenia in adults in 2009 under the trade name Invega Sustenna.[6] Paliperidone palmitate is the palmitate ester of paliperidone, in an aqueous-based nanosuspension with very low water solubility, facilitating slow dissolution after intramuscular injection.[7] In November 2014, paliperidone palmitate was approved by the FDA in the United States to treat schizoaffective disorder as monotherapy or adjunctive therapy.[8] Pivotal trial studies and subsequent postmarketing studies have shown that paliperidone palmitate to be an efficacious, safe, and well-tolerated SGA LAI that could significantly improve adherence, reduce relapse rates, enhance the rate of remission, and ultimately improve clinical outcomes in schizophrenia.[9,10]

Table 1
Newly approved medications for schizophrenia

Agent	Mechanism of Action	Significant Results from Research	Phase of Development
Three-month paliperidone palmitate (Invega Trinza)	Blockade of both 5-HT2A and dopamine 2 receptors	Double-blind multicenter randomized trial showed reductions in relapse and safety compared with placebo	Available in the market as of May 2015
Brexpiprazole (Rexulti)	Partial agonist at 5-HT1A and D2 receptors and strong antagonist at 5-HT2A	Double-blind multicenter randomized phase III trial improved PANSS scores compared with placebo	Available in the market as of May 2015
Cariprazine (Vrylar)	D2 and D3 receptors antagonist-partial agonist properties, with greater affinity to D3 and 5-HT1B receptor antagonism	Three 6-week double blind multinational, multicenter phase III trials demonstrating efficacy and safety	Available in the market as of September 2015
LAI of aripiprazole lauroxil (Aristada)	Prodrug of aripiprazole; D2 and 5-HT(2A) receptor antagonism, partial D2 agonist and significant 5-HT(1A) agonist actions	A 12-week multicenter, randomized, double-blind, placebo-controlled trial demonstrating evaluated the efficacy, safety and tolerability	Available in the market as of October 2015

Abbreviations: 5-HT1A, 5-hydroxytryptamine 1A; 5-HT2A, 5-hydroxytryptamine 2A; LAI, long-acting injection; PANSS, Positive and Negative Syndrome Scale.

In May 2015, the US FDA approved the 3-month paliperidone palmitate injection (Invega Trinza) to treat schizophrenia.[11] Approval was based on the results of a long-term maintenance trial designed to evaluate the efficacy and safety of the 3-month formulation of paliperidone palmitate versus placebo in delaying the time to relapse in schizophrenia symptoms in patient previously treated with once monthly paliperidone palmitate for at least 4 months.[12] The multicenter trial was conducted in 8 countries between April 2012 and April 2014. The study consisted of 4 phases: a screening phase for 3 weeks, a flexible dose open-label transition phase for 17 weeks, an open-label maintenance phase for 12 weeks, and an open-ended double-blind phase. There were 506 patients between the ages of 18 and 70 years old with the diagnosis of schizophrenia enrolled in this study; 305 patients were randomized either to 3-month paliperidone palmitate (n = 160) or placebo (n = 145). The study results showed significant difference in relapse rate in favor of the paliperidone palmitate group over the placebo group (*P*<.001). The study concluded that 3-month paliperidone palmitate significantly delayed first time relapse for at least 4 months in schizophrenic patients initially treated with once monthly paliperidone palmitate.[12] The

3-month formulation was well-tolerated compared with placebo. Of 305 patients, 183 experienced side effects (62% in the paliperidone group vs 58% in the placebo group), which included headaches (9% vs 4%), (weight gain 9% vs 3%), nasopharyngitis (6% vs 1%), and akathisia (4.5% vs 1%). Also, overall the side effect profile of the 3-month paliperidone palmitate was not much different than other marketed paliperidone formulations.

Brexpiprazole (Rexulti)

Brexpiprazole (Rexulti) developed by Otsuka and Lundbeck was recently approved by the US FDA as a monotherapy for the treatment of adults diagnosed with schizophrenia, in addition for use as an adjunctive to an antidepressant medication to treat adults with major depressive disorder.[13] Brexpiprazole exhibits a high affinity for serotonin, dopamine, and noradrenalin receptors, acting as a partial agonist at serotonin 5-HT1A and dopamine D2 receptors, and is a strong antagonist at serotonin 5-HT2A and noradrenalin α1B and α2C receptors.[14] It is the second in the class of partial agonist antipsychotics the first being aripiprazole (Abilify) also developed by Otsuka. The efficacy of brexpiprazole as a monotherapy in treatment of adults with schizophrenia was studied in a pivotal multicenter, randomized, double-blind, controlled phase III trial of fixed dose of brexpiprazole over 6 months. The study consisted of a pretreatment screening phase, a 6-week double-blind treatment period and a 30-day follow-up phase. Patients were randomized (2:3:3:3) into 1 of 4 treatment groups (1, 2, or 4 mg brexpiprazole, or placebo). The primary endpoint for this study was change from baseline to week 6 in the Positive and Negative Syndrome Scale (PANSS) Total Score with secondary outcomes of changes in Clinical Global Impressions—Severity, Personal and Social Performance scale; PANSS positive and negative subscales; PANSS excited component and Marder Factor cores, Clinical Global Impressions—Improvement score at week 6, response rate, and discontinuation rate for lack of efficacy.[15]

There were 1005 patients aged 18 to 70 years who were screened at 64 centers in different countries, and 674 patients were randomized to double-blind treatment. In the brexpiprazole groups, 68% (n = 458) completed the study, compared with 64.1% (n = 118) in the placebo group. The most common reasons for dropping out of the treatment across all the treatment groups were withdrawal of consent to participate (12.5%), lack of efficacy (9.8%), and emergence of adverse effects (8.5%).

The study result showed that 4 mg brexpiprazole significantly improved the primary endpoint of the study compared with placebo (treatment difference, −6.47; $P = .0022$), and had similar impact to the key secondary endpoint, namely, Clinical Global Impressions—Severity versus placebo (treatment difference, −0.38; $P = .0015$). Brexpiprazole 1 and 2 mg also showed numerical improvement versus placebo, although the result was not statistically significant ($P>.05$).

The most common side effects included headache, insomnia, and agitation; the brexpiprazole groups showed lower incidence of akathisia compared with placebo (4.2%–6.5% vs 7.1%). Moderate weight gain was observed at week 6 of treatment (1.23–1.89 kg) for brexpiprazole group compared with 0.35 kg for the placebo group.

This study established the efficacy and tolerability of brexpiprazole 4 mg for the treatment of acute schizophrenia in adults, and confirmed the result of another multicenter randomized, double-blind, placebo-controlled trial. The study from Correll and colleagues[16] included patients with acute exacerbation of schizophrenia, who were randomly assigned to daily brexpiprazole at 0.25 mg, 2 mg, or 4 mg, or placebo for period of 6 weeks. The completion rate for 0.25 mg, 2 mg, and 4 mg brexpiprazole were 62%, 68%, and 67%, respectively compared with 59% for placebo group. At week 6, patients treated with 2 mg and 4 mg of brexpiprazole showed statistically significant decrease in PANSS total score (treatment difference of -8.72 and -7.64, respectively) and CGI severity score (treatment difference of -0.33 and -0.38) compared with the placebo group. The most common side effects for brexpiprazole group was akathisia (2 mg, 4.4%; 4 mg, 7.2%; placebo, 2.2%), moderate weight gain (1.45 kg for the 2 mg group and 1.28 kg for the 4 mg group compared with 0.42 kg for the placebo group at week 6). Lipids, glucose level, and extrapyramidal symptoms rating did not show any clinical or statistically significant differences from baseline. This study indicated that brexpiprazole at dose of 2 and 4 mg/d has statistically significant efficacy compared with placebo and good tolerability for patient with an acute schizophrenia exacerbation.[16]

Cariprazine (Vrylar)

In September 2015, the FDA approved the use of Cariprazine in the United States for the treatment of schizophrenia and bipolar disorder in adults. Cariprazine is a new antipsychotic with D2 and D3 receptors antagonist–partial agonist properties, and an almost 10-fold greater affinity for the D3 receptor in vitro, with high occupancy for D2 and D3 receptors in vivo. It also demonstrated pure antagonism for 5-HT1B receptor with high, moderate, and low affinities for 5-HTB1, 5-HT1A, and 5-HT2A receptors respectively.[17–19]

The efficacy of cariprazine for treatment of schizophrenia was established in three 6-week clinical trials; all the trials were multinational, multicenter, double-blind studies. The 6-week double-blind trials done by Kane and colleagues[19] and Durgam and colleagues[20] demonstrated that the total PANSS score significantly improved among patient receiving cariprazine compared with placebo. Similar improvements were noted in Clinical Global Impressions—Severity scores at the end of the study. The most common treatment adverse effects were insomnia, nausea, akathisia and extrapyramidal symptoms, and most of these side effects were mild to moderate in severity. The results of the 3 studies supported the FDA's decision that cariprazine is a safe, efficacious, and well-tolerated agent in the treatment of acute exacerbation of schizophrenia in adults.

Aripiprazole lauroxil long-acting injectable (Aristada)

A new long-acting formulation of aripiprazole (ALLAI) was recently approved by the FDA to treat adults with schizophrenia.[21] ALLAI can be administered every 4 to 6 weeks either in the gluteal or deltoid region. ALLAI is a linker lipid ester of aripiprazole and its conversion to aripiprazole in vivo is governed by slow dissolution of the aripiprazole lauroxil particles followed by hydrolysis, resulting in a steady increase in plasma concentration and an extended blood level of aripiprazole.[22] The FDA approval is based on an international, multicenter, randomized, double-blind, placebo-controlled trial.[23] The study evaluated the efficacy, safety, and tolerability of ALLAI among 623 patients aged 18 to 70 years experiencing an acute exacerbation. Patients were randomized in a 1:1:1 ratio to receive gluteal intramuscular injection of ALLAI 441 mg, ALLAI 882 mg, or matching placebo once monthly for 12 weeks. The change in PANSS total score from baseline to day 85 was the primary efficacy outcome with change in Clinical Global Impressions—Improvement score being the secondary measure. The PANSS total score (mean ± standard error) improved significantly from baseline to day 85 in the ALLAI 441 mg (-10.9 ± 1.8; $P<.001$) and 882 (-11.9 ± 1.8; $P<.001$) mg groups compared with placebo. A significant ($P\leq.004$) improvement was noted in both active treatment arms as early as day 8 and continued throughout the treatment period. ALLAI was well-tolerated with insomnia, akathisia, headache, and anxiety being the common side effects. The incidence of severe treatment-emergent adverse events were similar between the 3 groups. At the time of writing this article, it is not clear if ALLI (Aristada) offers any advantages over Abilify Maintena or suffers any shortcomings in comparison. The use of oral aripiprazole for overlap for 3 weeks in the pivotal study makes it likely that ALLAI will also have an oral overlap requirement. Using the every 6 week regimen can decrease the number of injections over a year compared with patients using every 4 week injections, but it is also not clear about the number of patients who can potentially use the 6 weekly injections. The package insert will likely allow some comparisons in the absence of head-to-head trials.

Novel Treatments in Schizophrenia

The dopaminergic hypothesis has been the predominant explanation of the pathophysiology of schizophrenia for the last half century.[24] The hypothesis not only postulates the cause of the pathognomonic symptoms, but also the pharmacologic actions and side effects of antipsychotic medications. Hyperdopaminergic activity in the mesolimbic system is implicated in the cause of the positive symptoms (ie, hallucinations and delusions) of schizophrenia. In contrast, hypodopaminergic drive in the mesocortical system may be attributed to the negative symptoms of schizophrenia, such as anhedonia, flat affect, and social isolation. Mesolimbic antipsychotic dopaminergic blockade reduces positive psychotic symptoms but at the expense of inhibition in the hypothalamo–pituitary axis and nigrostriatal pathways leading to high prolactin levels and extrapyramidal symptoms, respectively.

Dopaminergic dysfunction, however, has not been able to account for all of the symptoms observed in schizophrenia, particularly the negative symptoms.[25] New hypotheses have been suggested that may replace or complement the dopamine hypotheses. Also, a new emphasis on improving cognition in patients with schizophrenia led to the National Institute of Mental Health funded Measurement and Treatment Research to Improve Cognition in Schizophrenia (MATRICS) and Treatment Units for Research on Neurocognition and Schizophrenia (TURNS) projects to promote the development of new cognitive enhancing drugs. The MATRICS project identified 9 potential target molecules belonging to 3 neurotransmitter systems: dopaminergic, cholinergic, and glutamatergic.[26]

Glutamate System

The glutamate system has been a recent target for pharmacologic interventions in schizophrenia based on the proposed model of schizophrenia where dysfunction of the N-methyl-D-aspartate (NMDA) receptors is considered the primary convergence point in the pathology of schizophrenia (**Table 2**).[27] NMDA receptor antagonists such as phencyclidine and ketamine have shown to produce psychoticlike symptoms in healthy individuals that are similar to those seen in patients with schizophrenia.[28,29] Glutamate receptors are classified into metabotropic (mGluR) and ionotropic receptors. The metabotropic receptors are subclassified into 3 groups: group I (mGluR1 and mGluR5), group II (mGluR2 and mGluR3), and group III (mGluR4-8). Similarly, the ionotropic receptors are subclassified into alpha-amino-3-hydroxy-5-methyl-4-isoxazolepropionic acid (AMPA), Kainate, and NMDA receptors.[30] Glutamate has a direct excitatory influence on dopaminergic neurons in addition to indirect (through γ-aminobutyric acid interneuron) inhibitory action on the release of dopamine in some circuits.[31] This leads to increase in the mesolimbic dopaminergic activity and a decreased activity in the mesocortical circuit. Hypofunction of NMDA receptors is implicated in the causation of schizophrenia symptomatology, particularly the negative symptoms.

Metabotropic glutamate receptor 2/3 agonists

Pomaglumetad methionil (LY2140023) is a potent and highly selective agonist for the metabotropic glutamate mGluR2 and mGluR3 receptors. After initial promising phase II studies showing efficacy comparable with olanzapine,[32] a series of failed phase III studies by Eli Lilly with the compound LY2140023 resulted in the discontinuation of development of this molecule for treatment of schizophrenia.[33,34] A recent exploratory analysis, which included the most recent phase III study and other integrated studies, indicated that pomaglumetad shows greater improvement among patients with early in disease or paradoxically previously treated with D2 blocking drugs compared with those receiving placebo.[35] This has raised some interesting perspectives among experts about the molecular pathology among patients diagnosed with schizophrenia.[34] Previous exposure to antipsychotics could have modified the brain structure and neuroplasticity, leading to poor response to a new medication, such as the pomaglumetad. It has also been hypothesized that there may be cohorts of patients with distinct neurochemical profiles in early stages of schizophrenia who might benefit from mGluR2/3 agonists.[34]

Positive allosteric modulators of mGlu2

The available mGlu2 agonists have demonstrated a lack of subtype specificity and pose a challenge for development of tolerance with chronic use.[36] This has led to the development of positive allosteric modulators (PAMs) at mGlu2/3 receptors, such as LY487379, JNJ-42153605, JNJ-40068782, and biphenylindanone A. PAMs have shown receptor selectivity, act only in the presence of endogenous ligands, and are considered to overcome the rapid desensitization of the receptors.[37] These molecules have been tested in various preclinical trials.[38,39] ADX71149/JNJ4041183 has been the most successful PAM thus far after passing a phase IIa clinical study demonstrating safety, tolerability, and efficacy on negative symptoms in schizophrenia.[37]

Ampakines

Ampakines are PAMs of the synaptic AMPA glutamate receptors that facilitate glutamate neurotransmission.[40] CX516, a prototype of the ampakines, was compared with placebo in 4-week, double-blind study and failed to demonstrate the efficacy as a single agent.[41] Despite an earlier study suggesting positive effects on measures of attention and memory,[42] CX516 did not separate from the placebo arm with regard to PANSS total score and was not effective for cognition among 105 patients with schizophrenia when added to clozapine, olanzapine, or risperidone.[43]

Glycine System

Glycine is a coagonist and essential neurotransmitter for the activation of NMDA receptor (see **Table 2**).[31] Multiple small clinical trials, with limited power, tested a high dose of glycine and gylcine site agonists such as D-cycloserine, as an adjunct to existing treatments.[44–50] Some of these studies showed improvements in various domains in schizophrenia symptomatology among patients using the adjunctive glycine and glycine agonists compared with treatment as usual supporting the hypoglutaminergic hypothesis of schizophrenia. Sarcosine is a naturally occurring, nonselective glycine reuptake inhibitor. Sarcosine also demonstrated positive results as an adjunctive treatment to antipsychotics in multiple short-term studies.[51–53]

Table 2
Medications acting on the glutamate and glycine system

Agent	Mechanism of Action	Significant Results from Research	Phase of Development
Glutamate system			
Metabotropic glutamate receptor (mGluR) 2/3 agonists (Pomaglumetad methionil)	Highly selective agonist for the metabotropic glutamate mGluR2 and mGluR3 receptors	Initial promising phase II studies showing efficacy comparable with olanzapine followed by a series of failed phase III studies	Discontinuation of development
Positive allosteric modulators of mGlu2	Modulators of the mGlu receptors	Tested in various preclinical trials; ADX71149/JNJ4041183 has been the most successful PAM thus far after passing a phase IIa clinical study	Results awaited on further studies by Addex
Ampakines (CX516)	Positive allosteric modulators of the synaptic AMPA glutamate receptors that facilitate glutamate neurotransmission	Compared with placebo in 4-week double blind study failed to demonstrate the efficacy as a single agent. Despite an earlier study suggesting improvement of attention and memory, CX516 did not separate from the placebo arm in regards to PANSS total score and was not effective for cognition when added to clozapine, olanzapine, or risperidone	Discontinuation of development
Glycine system			
Glycine, D-cycloserine, D-serine	Coagonist and essential neurotransmitter for the activation of NMDA receptor	A metaanalysis of all available double-blind, placebo controlled trials showed that glycine, D-serine and sarcosine improved psychopathology overall, whereas D-cycloserine had no effect. Despite showing benefit when added to risperidone or olanzapine, none of these drugs add therapeutic advantage over placebo when added to clozapine	No further development
Sarcosine	Naturally occurring, nonselective GRI		

Bitopertin	GRI		An 8-week phase II study showed significantly reduced negative symptoms among the patients taking bitopertin compared with placebo. Followed by 2 failed phase III trials. A combined phase II/III trial (the CandleLyte study) compared bitopertin with placebo and zyprexa and failed to demonstrate efficacy on PANSS total score.	Removal of the drug from the pipeline of Roche in 2014
Sodium benzoate		Inhibitor of the D-amino acid oxidase increasing levels of D-serine in the synapse improving NMDA functioning	Antipsychotic effects from sodium benzoate noted in the PCP model of schizophrenia in mice. A randomized, double blind, placebo controlled study in Taiwan showed improved a variety of positive, negative, and neurocognitive symptoms.	Further studies required

Abbreviations: AMPA, alpha-amino-3-hydroxy-5-methyl-4- isoxazolepropionic acid; GRI, glycine reuptake inhibitor; mGluR, metabotropic glutamate receptor; NMDA, N-methyl-D-aspartate; PANSS, Positive and Negative Syndrome Scale; PCP, phencyclidine.

A metaanalysis of all available double-blind, placebo-controlled trials evaluating the efficacy of NMDA-enhancing molecules on schizophrenia showed that glycine, D-serine, and sarcosine improved psychopathology overall, and D-cycloserine had no effect.[54] Despite showing benefit when added to risperidone or olanzapine, none of these drugs have shown to add therapeutic advantage over placebo when added to clozapine.[54,55]

One of the avenues to enhance the NMDA receptor functioning is to increase the availability of glycine at modulatory sites on the NMDA receptors through the inhibition of glycine transporter-1 on glial cells.[56] This propelled the development and testing of glycine transporter-1 inhibitors as a potential treatment of schizophrenia. We review 2 important molecules in the glycine system that increase the synaptic glycine or D-serine concentration.

Bitopertin

Bitopertin is a glycine reuptake inhibitor that has demonstrated enhanced NMDAR signaling.[57] An 8-week, double-blind, randomized, placebo-controlled, proof-of-concept, multicenter, phase II study was conducted with 323 patients with schizophrenia who were stable on antipsychotic treatment but had significant negative symptoms. Bitopertin significantly reduced the negative symptoms among the patients taking either 10 mg/d or 30 mg/d dosing compared with placebo.[58] Unfortunately, this was followed by 2 failed phase III trials, resulting in the removal of the drug from the pipeline of Roche in 2014.[59] A combined phase II/III trial (the CandleLyte study) compared bitopertin to placebo and Zyprexa with 301 patients over 4 weeks. This study failed to demonstrate statistically significant separation between the 3 arms on the primary endpoint of change from baseline in mean PANSS total score.[60]

Sodium benzoate

NMDA receptor functioning can be enhanced by increasing the levels of D-serine in the synapse by inhibiting the D-amino acid oxidase, which metabolizes D-serine.[61] Sodium benzoate, a common food preservative, is one such D-amino acid oxidase inhibitor. An animal study examined the effects of sodium benzoate on behavioral abnormalities in mice after administration of phencyclidine. The study suggested that antipsychotic effects were noted from sodium benzoate in the phencyclidine model of schizophrenia in mice without increasing D-serine levels in the brain.[62] A randomized, double-blind, placebo-controlled study in Taiwan compared the efficacy of sodium benzoate as an adjunct to antipsychotics in subjects with schizophrenia. Sodium benzoate improved a variety of positive, negative, and neurocognitive symptoms, including a 21% improvement in PANSS total score compared with placebo.[63]

Phosphodiesterase System

Phosphodiesterases (PDEs) are a family of enzymes regulating signal transduction of neuronal membranes by maintaining the homeostasis of intracellular cyclic nucleotides by degrading cyclic adenosine monophosphate (cAMP) and cyclic guanosine monophosphate.[64] PDE10A is 1 member of the PDE family that is highly expressed in the bodies and the dendrites of medium spiny projection neurons in the striatum with minimal distribution outside the brain.[65] Parallels with D2 receptor functioning makes the PDE10A inhibitors a potential candidate for intervention in schizophrenia.[34] Also, the role of cAMP responsive element binding protein and the cAMP signaling has been demonstrated in neurodevelopment and neuroprotection.[66,67] Multiple PDE10A inhibitors are in development by various pharmaceutical companies with many of the patents directed toward improving negative and cognitive symptoms in schizophrenia

(**Table 3**).[68] Based on preclinical trials, and despite moderate adverse events, the use of PDE10A inhibitors like MP-10 and papaverine was expected to yield an antipsychotic effect along with beneficial effects on negative and cognitive symptoms.[69] However, a 4-week placebo and positive controlled randomized double-blind multicenter trial investigating fixed doses of MP-10/PF-02545920 at 5 and 15 mg failed to demonstrate the efficacy of MP-10 compared with placebo, whereas risperidone showed clear benefit.[70] This has led to further examination of the rationale and mechanism of action of this group of molecules. The discovery of PET ligands has led to assess a clinical trial studying the occupancy of PDE10A receptors by MP-10, which is completed and the results are awaited.[71]

Other PDE inhibitors are also being tested for use in treatment of negative and cognitive symptoms of schizophrenia (see **Table 3**). PDE5 inhibitors like sildenafil, a popular erectile dysfunction drug, have been hypothesized to improve the negative and cognitive symptoms.[72] Goff and colleagues[73] studied the cognitive effects of sildenafil on 15 clinically stable patients treated with various antipsychotics compared with placebo. After the administration of sildanefil 50 mg, 100 mg, and placebo in randomized order, cognitive functioning was tested 3 postbaseline sessions and another assessment for delayed recall after 48 hours. The study failed to demonstrate the cognitive enhancing effects of sildenafil among patients compared with placebo.[73] Another 8-week trial in Iran comparing sildenafil with placebo as an adjunctive therapy to risperidone demonstrated superiority of sildenafil in improving negative and PANSS total scores.[74] Intra-Cellular Therapies, Inc, is developing PDE1 inhibitors to improve cognition among patients with schizophrenia.[75]

Nicotinic Cholinergic System

Nicotinic acetylcholinergic receptors (nAChRs) mediate multiple modulatory functions in diverse synaptic and nonsynaptic locations throughout the human brain with roles in development and neuronal plasticity, contributing to learning, memory, and attention.[76] One of the subtypes of these receptors, α-7 nAChR, has been associated with P50 sensory gating found to be impaired in patients with schizophrenia. The impairment is implicated in the attention deficits and lack of attention sustainment seen in patients with schizophrenia and their unaffected relatives.[77–83]

Nicotine receptor agonists that selectively target the α-7 subtype are being tested by various pharmaceutical companies for efficacy in improving the cognitive impairment associated with schizophrenia (see **Table 3**). DMXB-A, a partial α-7 nicotinic cholinergic agonist showed promising results in improving neurocognition in a proof-of-concept study.[84] This has not been replicated in subsequent larger studies, but instead showed improvement of negative symptoms in patients with schizophrenia.[85] Another 4-week placebo-controlled study was recently completed with sustained release DXMB-A; the results are pending.[86,87] The beneficial effect on negative symptoms was replicated with other α-7 partial agonists including TC-5619 in an exploratory trial with 185 outpatients in the United States and India.[88] However, a 24-week randomized trial with 477 outpatients from 64 sites in the United States, Russia, Ukraine, Hungary, Romania, and Serbia comparing TC-5619 with placebo showed no benefit in negative or cognitive symptoms of schizophrenia.[89]

Tropisetron is a[90] 5-HT3 antagonist with high-affinity partial agonism at α-7 nAChR.[91] A short-term double-blind placebo-controlled trial with 40 patients demonstrated that tropisetron improved auditory sensory gating P50 deficits in nonsmoking individuals and cognitive functioning.[92] Subsequent studies evaluating tropisetron as an adjunctive treatment to oral antipsychotics showed that tropisetron significantly improved the overall cognitive along with P50 deficits[93] and negative symptoms

Table 3
Medications acting on the PDE system and nicotinergic system

Agent	Mechanism of Action	Significant Results from Research	Phase of Development
PDE system			
PDE10A inhibitors (eg, MP-10 and papaverine)	Regulates signal transduction of neuronal membranes by maintaining the homeostasis of intracellular cyclic nucleotides by degrading cAMP and cGMP	Preclinical trials suggested an antipsychotic effect along with beneficial effects on negative and cognitive symptoms with. A 4-week placebo- and positive-controlled randomized double-blind multicenter trial of MP-10 failed to demonstrate the efficacy compared with placebo while risperidone showed clear benefit.	Multiple PDE10A inhibitors in pharmaceutical pipeline with many of the patents directed toward improving negative and cognitive symptoms in schizophrenia
PDE5 inhibitors (eg, sildenafil)		A study of 15 clinically stable failed to demonstrate the cognitive enhancing effects of sildenafil among patients compared with placebo.	Discontinuation of development
PDE1 inhibitors		—	Intra-Cellular Therapies, Inc. is developing PDE1 inhibitors
Nicotinic cholinergic system			
DMXB-A	α-7 nAChR agonists improve the deficits with P50 sensory gating	Promising results in the proof of concept study not replicated in larger studies.	Discontinuation of development
TC-519		A 24-week multicenter trial comparing TC-5619 to placebo showed with benefit in negative or cognitive symptoms	

Tropisetron	5-HT3 antagonist with high-affinity partial agonism at α-7 nAChR	Metaanalysis of double-blinded, randomized, placebo-control trials showed that 5HT-3 receptor antagonists improved psychopathology	Results of a large randomized controlled trial awaited
EVP-6124 (Encenicline)	Highly selective partial agonist of α-7 nAChR	Phase II study showed Encenicline was well-tolerated at single doses of $\leq$180 mg	Phase III trials are under way
ABT-126	Partial agonist of α-7 nAChR	Completion of 3 phase II studies and terminating another phase II trial in 2014	Removed from the pipeline
PAM of nicotinergic system (eg, JNJ-3939406, AVL-3288)	Increase the potency and efficacy of the agonist-induced responses	JNJ-3939406 showed positive results on cognition and improved sensory gating deficits in animal studies but failed to demonstrate its effect on P50 deficits in a multicenter, randomized, double blind, placebo controlled study	AVL-3288 is currently being tested for safety, tolerability and pharmacokinetics in a phase I study

Abbreviations: cAMP, cyclic adenosine monophosphate; cGMP, cyclic guanosine monophosphate; 5HT-3, 5-hydroxytryptamine 3; nAChR, neuronal nicotinic acetylcholine receptor; PDE, phosphodiesterase.

compared with patients taking placebo.[94] A recent metaanalysis of double-blinded, randomized, placebo-controlled trials showed that 5HT-3 receptor antagonists improved psychopathology (especially negative symptoms) in patients with schizophrenia compared with placebo.[95] A large randomized controlled trial comparing tropisetron with placebo as an adjunctive treatment has been completed and the results are pending.[90]

EVP-6124 (Encenicline) is a highly selective partial agonist of α-7 nAChR with good penetrability across the blood–brain barrier.[96] In a proof-of-concept study, encenicline was compared with placebo as an adjunctive treatment to oral antipsychotics. Encenicline was well-tolerated among patients and showed positive results in various measures.[97] Based on this study, a phase II single ascending dose study was conducted to evaluate the safety, tolerability, pharmacokinetic, and pharmacodynamic profiles in healthy male volunteers. Encenicline was well-tolerated at single doses of up to 180 mg with dose-dependent pharmacodynamic effects on the central nervous system.[98] Phase III trials are under way by Forum pharmaceuticals for this drug currently.

ABT-126 is a partial agonist developed by Abbvie at α-7 nAChR that has been studied for improving cognition in Alzheimer's disease and schizophrenia.[87] After completing 3 phase II studies[99–101] and terminating another phase II trial in 2014,[102] the drug is not listed in Abbvie's pipeline. AQW051, a Novartis product, is highly selective agonist with high affinity toward α-7 nAChR.[103] Two double-blind randomized placebo-controlled phase II studies have been completed so far, but the results have not been published.[104,105] Similar to ABT-126, Novartis Pharmaceuticals does not list AQW051 in their pipeline.

PAMs are also being developed in the nicotinergic system not only to increase the potency and efficacy of the agonist induced responses, but also to alter the desensitization properties of the agonist. JNJ-39393406 showed positive results on cognition and improved sensory gating deficits in animal studies but failed to demonstrate its effect on P50 deficits in a multicenter, randomized, double-blind, placebo-controlled study.[106] AVL-3288 another PAM is currently being tested for safety, tolerability, and pharmacokinetics in a single-center, randomized, double-blind, placebo-controlled, dose-escalating phase I study.[107]

Other Compounds

Blonanserin

Blonanserin is an SGA with 5HT-2A, D2, and D3 antagonistic activity with minimal effect on histaminic and muscarinic receptors (**Table 4**).[108] It has been approved for schizophrenia and has been used in Japan since 2008 and in Korea since 2009. A systemic review in 2012 showed that blonanserin had a lower risk of hyperprolactinemia than the other pooled antipsychotics. Although blonanserin was better tolerated with respect to dizziness and akathisia, it had a higher risk of akathisia compared with risperidone. Recently, an 8-week study comparing risperidone and blonanserin showed that blonanserin was similar to risperidone in efficacy but improved quality of life compared with risperidone.[109] The Japan Useful Medication Program for Schizophrenia (JUMPS) is a 104 week, open-label, multicenter, randomized, comparative study underway in Japan, comparing treatment with either aripiprazole, blonanserin, or paliperidone in patients with schizophrenia aged 20 years or older. The primary endpoint is treatment discontinuation rate for any causes.

Minocycline

Antioxidant aberration has been implicated in the pathophysiology of schizophrenia. Microglia are key sources of free radicals leading to brain injury in various areas.[110]

Table 4 Other drugs			
Agent	Mechanism of Action	Significant Results from Research	Phase of Development
Blonanserin	5HT-2A, D2, and D3 antagonistic activity	Similar to risperidone in efficacy but improved quality of life. A large 104-week study is under way.	Approved for schizophrenia in Japan since 2008 and in Korea since 2009
Minocycline	Inhibitor of microglial activation and rescue neurogenesis	Two randomized, double-blind, placebo-controlled studies showed efficacy of minocycline as an adjunctive treatment in early phase of schizophrenia.	Further studies required

Abbreviation: 5HT-2A, 5-hydroxytryptamine 2A.

Microglia are also the intrinsic immune competent cells of the brain implicated in cytokine-induced impairment of adult neurogenesis in key areas like hippocampus.[111] The minocycline is a known inhibitor of microglial activation and rescue neurogenesis (see **Table 4**).[111,112] An open-label study of 22 patients by Miyaoka and colleagues[113] demonstrated significant clinical improvements on PANSS among patient using adjunctive minocycline. The effects were sustained at 4 weeks after the completion of the study without adverse events.[113] Two randomized, double-blind, placebo-controlled studies showed efficacy of minocycline as an adjunctive treatment in early phase of schizophrenia with respect to negative symptoms albeit their methodology had some limitations.[114,115]

Pharmaceutical Pipeline

According to a report by America's Biopharmaceutical Research Companies published in 2014, there are about 36 developing medications among various pharmaceutical companies.[116] Eight of them are in the spectrum of being in phase III studies or being currently marketed. As noted, there have been a number of drugs that have been dropped from the pipeline owing to disappointing results in clinical trials in various phases.

PDE10A inhibitors and α-7 nAChR modulators constitute the majority of these molecules in the pipeline. Some 5-HT2A antagonists, similar to lurasidone and iloperidone, which are already in the market, are also noted in the pipeline.

SUMMARY

Schizophrenia has posed a substantial challenge not only for patients and their families, but also the medical profession for many centuries. The last century has witnessed significant strides in development of treatments for schizophrenia and outcomes of these patients. But there are a large number of patients still struggling from with ongoing symptoms and for some progressively worsening course illness, necessitating the pursuit of better treatments.

The paradigm shift of focusing on specific symptom domains of schizophrenia like cognition and negative symptoms has been reflected in the research and also by the drugs in the pipeline of several of pharmaceutical companies. The marketing of these medications eventually may result in change about how schizophrenia is treated in the future.

REFERENCES

1. Lopez-Munoz F, Alamo C, Cuenca E, et al. History of the discovery and clinical introduction of chlorpromazine. Ann Clin Psychiatry 2005;17(3):113–35.
2. Shen WW. A history of antipsychotic drug development. Compr Psychiatry 1999; 40(6):407–14.
3. Leucht S, Corves C, Arbter D, et al. Second-generation versus first-generation antipsychotic drugs for schizophrenia: a meta-analysis. Lancet 2009; 373(9657):31–41.
4. AlAqeel B, Margolese HC. Remission in schizophrenia: critical and systematic review. Harv Rev Psychiatry 2012;20(6):281–97.
5. Meltzer HY. Treatment-resistant schizophrenia–the role of clozapine. Curr Med Res Opin 1997;14(1):1–20.
6. Janssen, D.o.O.-M.-J.P., Inc, Invega® Sustenna® (paliperidone palmitate) extended-release injectable suspension. United States prescribing information. 2010. Available at: http://www.invegasustenna.com/invegasustenna/shared/pi/invegasustenna.pdf. Accessed August 9, 2015.
7. Gilday E, Nasrallah HA. Clinical pharmacology of paliperidone palmitate a parenteral long-acting formulation for the treatment of schizophrenia. Rev Recent Clin Trials 2012;7(1):2–9.
8. Janssen, D.o.O.-M.-J.P., Inc. U.S FDA approves supplemental new drug applications for once monthly long-acting therapy Invega Sustenna (paliperidone palmitate) for the treatment of schizoaffective disorder. 2014.
9. Hough D, Gopal S, Vijapurkar U, et al. Paliperidone palmitate maintenance treatment in delaying the time-to-relapse in patients with schizophrenia: a randomized, double-blind, placebo-controlled study. Schizophr Res 2010;116(2–3): 107–17.
10. Kramer M, Litman R, Hough D, et al. Paliperidone palmitate, a potential long-acting treatment for patients with schizophrenia. Results of a randomized, double-blind, placebo-controlled efficacy and safety study. Int J Neuropsychopharmacol 2010;13(5):635–47.
11. Johnson&Johnson. U.S. FDA approves Invega Trinza™, first and only four-times-a-year treatment for schizophrenia. 2015. Available at: http://www.jnj.com/news/all/US-FDA-Approves-INVEGA-TRINZA-First-and-Only-Four-Times-A-Year-Treatment-for-Schizophrenia. Accessed August 9, 2015.
12. Berwaerts J, Liu Y, Gopal S, et al. Efficacy and safety of the 3-month formulation of paliperidone palmitate vs placebo for relapse prevention of schizophrenia: a randomized clinical trial. JAMA Psychiatry 2015;72(8):830–9.
13. FDA new release. Rexulti was approved by the U.S Food and drug administration as a mono-therapy for adult schizophrenia treatment, in addition as an adjunctive to an antidepressant medication to treat adults with major depressive disorder (MDD) on July 10th 2015. 2015.
14. Maeda K, Sugino H, Akazawa H, et al. Brexpiprazole I: in vitro and in vivo characterization of a novel serotonin-dopamine activity modulator. J Pharmacol Exp Ther 2014;350(3):589–604.

15. Kane JM, Skuban A, Ouyang J, et al. A multicenter, randomized, double-blind, controlled phase 3 trial of fixed-dose brexpiprazole for the treatment of adults with acute schizophrenia. Schizophr Res 2015;164(1–3):127–35.
16. Correll CU, Skuban A, Ouyang J, et al. Efficacy and safety of brexpiprazole for the treatment of acute schizophrenia: a 6-week randomized, double-blind, placebo-controlled trial. Am J Psychiatry 2015;172(9):870–80.
17. Altinbas K, Guloksuz S, Oral ET. Clinical potential of cariprazine in the treatment of acute mania. Psychiatr Danub 2013;25(3):207–13.
18. Gyertyan I, Kiss B, Sághy K, et al. Cariprazine (RGH-188), a potent D3/D2 dopamine receptor partial agonist, binds to dopamine D3 receptors in vivo and shows antipsychotic-like and procognitive effects in rodents. Neurochem Int 2011;59(6):925–35.
19. Kane JM, Zukin S, Wang Y, et al. Efficacy and safety of cariprazine in acute exacerbation of schizophrenia: results from an international, phase III clinical trial. J Clin Psychopharmacol 2015;35(4):367–73.
20. Durgam S, Starace A, Li D, et al. An evaluation of the safety and efficacy of cariprazine in patients with acute exacerbation of schizophrenia: a phase II, randomized clinical trial. Schizophr Res 2014;152(2–3):450–7.
21. FDA new release. FDA approves new injectable drug to treat schizophrenia. 2015. Available at: http://www.fda.gov/NewsEvents/Newsroom/Press Announcements/ucm465801.htm. Accessed October 7, 2015.
22. Turncliff R, Hard M, Du Y, et al. Relative bioavailability and safety of aripiprazole lauroxil, a novel once-monthly, long-acting injectable atypical antipsychotic, following deltoid and gluteal administration in adult subjects with schizophrenia. Schizophr Res 2014;159(2–3):404–10.
23. Meltzer HY, Risinger R, Nasrallah HA, et al. A randomized, double-blind, placebo-controlled trial of aripiprazole lauroxil in acute exacerbation of schizophrenia. J Clin Psychiatry 2015;76(8):1085–90.
24. Howes OD, Kapur S. The dopamine hypothesis of schizophrenia: version III–the final common pathway. Schizophr Bull 2009;35(3):549–62.
25. Laruelle M, Risinger R, Nasrallah HA, et al. Increased dopamine transmission in schizophrenia: relationship to illness phases. Biol Psychiatry 1999;46(1):56–72.
26. Marder SR. The NIMH-MATRICS project for developing cognition-enhancing agents for schizophrenia. Dialogues Clin Neurosci 2006;8(1):109–13.
27. Kantrowitz JT, Javitt DC. N-methyl-d-aspartate (NMDA) receptor dysfunction or dysregulation: the final common pathway on the road to schizophrenia? Brain Res Bull 2010;83(3–4):108–21.
28. Javitt DC, Zukin SR. Recent advances in the phencyclidine model of schizophrenia. Am J Psychiatry 1991;148(10):1301–8.
29. Lahti AC, Holcomb HH, Medoff DR, et al. Ketamine activates psychosis and alters limbic blood flow in schizophrenia. Neuroreport 1995;6(6):869–72.
30. Gibert-Rahola J, Villena-Rodriguez A. Glutamatergic drugs for schizophrenia treatment. Actas Esp Psiquiatr 2014;42(5):234–41.
31. Citrome L. Unmet needs in the treatment of schizophrenia: new targets to help different symptom domains. J Clin Psychiatry 2014;75(Suppl 1):21–6.
32. Patil ST, Zhang L, Martenyi F, et al. Activation of mGlu2/3 receptors as a new approach to treat schizophrenia: a randomized phase 2 clinical trial. Nat Med 2007;13(9):1102–7.
33. Downing AM, Kinon BJ, Millen BA, et al. A double-blind, placebo-controlled comparator study of LY2140023 monohydrate in patients with schizophrenia. BMC Psychiatry 2014;14:351.

34. Dunlop J, Brandon NJ. Schizophrenia drug discovery and development in an evolving era: are new drug targets fulfilling expectations? J Psychopharmacol 2015;29(2):230–8.

35. Kinon BJ, Millen BA, Zhang L, et al. Exploratory analysis for a targeted patient population responsive to the metabotropic glutamate 2/3 receptor agonist pomaglumetad methionil in schizophrenia. Biol Psychiatry 2015;78(11):754–62.

36. Lavreysen H, Ahnaou A, Drinkenburg W, et al. Pharmacological and pharmacokinetic properties of JNJ-40411813, a positive allosteric modulator of the mGlu2 receptor. Pharmacol Res Perspect 2015;3(1):e00096.

37. Hopkins CR. Is there a path forward for mGlu2 positive allosteric modulators for the treatment of schizophrenia? ACS Chem Neurosci 2013;4(2):211–3.

38. Cid JM, Tresadern G, Vega JA, et al. Discovery of 3-cyclopropylmethyl-7-(4-phenylpiperidin-1-yl)-8-trifluoromethyl[1,2,4]triazolo[4,3-a]pyridine   (JNJ-42153605): a positive allosteric modulator of the metabotropic glutamate 2 receptor. J Med Chem 2012;55(20):8770–89.

39. Galici R, Echemendia NG, Rodriguez AL, et al. A selective allosteric potentiator of metabotropic glutamate (mGlu) 2 receptors has effects similar to an orthosteric mGlu2/3 receptor agonist in mouse models predictive of antipsychotic activity. J Pharmacol Exp Ther 2005;315(3):1181–7.

40. Wezenberg E, Verkes RJ, Ruigt GS, et al. Acute effects of the ampakine farampator on memory and information processing in healthy elderly volunteers. Neuropsychopharmacology 2007;32(6):1272–83.

41. Marenco S, Egan MF, Goldberg TE, et al. Preliminary experience with an ampakine (CX516) as a single agent for the treatment of schizophrenia: a case series. Schizophr Res 2002;57(2–3):221–6.

42. Goff DC, Leahy L, Berman I, et al. A placebo-controlled pilot study of the ampakine CX516 added to clozapine in schizophrenia. J Clin Psychopharmacol 2001; 21(5):484–7.

43. Goff DC, Lamberti JS, Leon AC, et al. A placebo-controlled add-on trial of the Ampakine, CX516, for cognitive deficits in schizophrenia. Neuropsychopharmacology 2008;33(3):465–72.

44. Evins AE, Amico E, Posever TA, et al. D-Cycloserine added to risperidone in patients with primary negative symptoms of schizophrenia. Schizophr Res 2002; 56(1–2):19–23.

45. Goff DC, Tsai G, Manoach DS, et al. D-cycloserine added to clozapine for patients with schizophrenia. Am J Psychiatry 1996;153(12):1628–30.

46. Goff DC, Tsai G, Levitt J, et al. A placebo-controlled trial of D-cycloserine added to conventional neuroleptics in patients with schizophrenia. Arch Gen Psychiatry 1999;56(1):21–7.

47. Duncan EJ, Szilagyi S, Schwartz MP, et al. Effects of D-cycloserine on negative symptoms in schizophrenia. Schizophr Res 2004;71(2–3):239–48.

48. Heresco-Levy U, Javitt DC, Ermilov M, et al. Double-blind, placebo-controlled, crossover trial of glycine adjuvant therapy for treatment-resistant schizophrenia. Br J Psychiatry 1996;169(5):610–7.

49. Heresco-Levy U, Javitt DC, Ermilov M, et al. Efficacy of high-dose glycine in the treatment of enduring negative symptoms of schizophrenia. Arch Gen Psychiatry 1999;56(1):29–36.

50. Heresco-Levy U, Ermilov M, Lichtenberg P, et al. High-dose glycine added to olanzapine and risperidone for the treatment of schizophrenia. Biol Psychiatry 2004;55(2):165–71.

51. Lane HY, Lin CH, Huang YJ, et al. A randomized, double-blind, placebo-controlled comparison study of sarcosine (N-methylglycine) and D-serine add-on treatment for schizophrenia. Int J Neuropsychopharmacol 2010;13(4): 451–60.

52. Lane HY, Chang YC, Liu YC, et al. Sarcosine or D-serine add-on treatment for acute exacerbation of schizophrenia: a randomized, double-blind, placebo-controlled study. Arch Gen Psychiatry 2005;62(11):1196–204.

53. Tsai G, Lane HY, Yang P, et al. Glycine transporter I inhibitor, N-methylglycine (sarcosine), added to antipsychotics for the treatment of schizophrenia. Biol Psychiatry 2004;55(5):452–6.

54. Tsai GE, Lin PY. Strategies to enhance N-methyl-D-aspartate receptor-mediated neurotransmission in schizophrenia, a critical review and meta-analysis. Curr Pharm Des 2010;16(5):522–37.

55. Singh SP, Singh V. Meta-analysis of the efficacy of adjunctive NMDA receptor modulators in chronic schizophrenia. CNS Drugs 2011;25(10):859–85.

56. Hashimoto K. Glycine transporter-1: a new potential therapeutic target for schizophrenia. Curr Pharm Des 2011;17(2):112–20.

57. Pinard E, Alanine A, Alberati D, et al. Selective GlyT1 inhibitors: discovery of [4-(3-fluoro-5-trifluoromethylpyridin-2-yl)piperazin-1-yl][5-methanesulfonyl-2-((S)-2,2,2-trifluoro-1-methylethoxy)phenyl]methanone (RG1678), a promising novel medicine to treat schizophrenia. J Med Chem 2010;53(12):4603–14.

58. Umbricht D, Alberati D, Martin-Facklam M, et al. Effect of bitopertin, a glycine reuptake inhibitor, on negative symptoms of schizophrenia: a randomized, double-blind, proof-of-concept study. JAMA Psychiatry 2014;71(6):637–46.

59. Kingwell K. Schizophrenia drug gets negative results for negative symptoms. Nat Rev Drug Discov 2014;13(4):244–5.

60. Bugarski-Kirola D, Wang A, Abi-Saab D, et al. A phase II/III trial of bitopertin monotherapy compared with placebo in patients with an acute exacerbation of schizophrenia - results from the candlelyte study. Eur Neuropsychopharmacol 2014;24(7):1024–36.

61. Betts JF, Schweimer JV, Burnham KE, et al. D-amino acid oxidase is expressed in the ventral tegmental area and modulates cortical dopamine. Front Synaptic Neurosci 2014;6:11.

62. Matsuura A, Fujita Y, Iyo M, et al. Effects of sodium benzoate on pre-pulse inhibition deficits and hyperlocomotion in mice after administration of phencyclidine. Acta Neuropsychiatr 2015;27(3):159–67.

63. Lane HY, Lin CH, Green MF, et al. Add-on treatment of benzoate for schizophrenia: a randomized, double-blind, placebo-controlled trial of D-amino acid oxidase inhibitor. JAMA Psychiatry 2013;70(12):1267–75.

64. Siuciak JA. The role of phosphodiesterases in schizophrenia: therapeutic implications. CNS Drugs 2008;22(12):983–93.

65. Coskran TM, Morton D, Menniti FS, et al. Immunohistochemical localization of phosphodiesterase 10A in multiple mammalian species. J Histochem Cytochem 2006;54(11):1205–13.

66. Sakamoto K, Karelina K, Obrietan K. CREB: a multifaceted regulator of neuronal plasticity and protection. J Neurochem 2011;116(1):1–9.

67. Mantamadiotis T, Lemberger T, Bleckmann SC, et al. Disruption of CREB function in brain leads to neurodegeneration. Nat Genet 2002;31(1):47–54.

68. Kehler J. Phosphodiesterase 10A inhibitors: a 2009-2012 patent update. Expert Opin Ther Pat 2013;23(1):31–45.

69. Grauer SM, Pulito VL, Navarra RL, et al. Phosphodiesterase 10A inhibitor activity in preclinical models of the positive, cognitive, and negative symptoms of schizophrenia. J Pharmacol Exp Ther 2009;331(2):574–90.

70. DeMartinis N, Banerjee A, Kumar V, et al. Poster #212 results of a phase 2A proof-of-concept trial with a PDE10A inhibitor in the treatment of acute exacerbation of schizophrenia. Schizophr Res 2012;136(Suppl 1):S262.

71. ClinicalTrials.gov, N. A study to evaluate the PDE10 enzyme occupancy following a single dose of PF-02545920 In healthy male volunteers (PET). 2014.

72. Rodefer JS, Saland SK, Eckrich SJ. Selective phosphodiesterase inhibitors improve performance on the ED/ID cognitive task in rats. Neuropharmacology 2012;62(3):1182–90.

73. Goff DC, Cather C, Freudenreich O, et al. A placebo-controlled study of sildenafil effects on cognition in schizophrenia. Psychopharmacology (Berl) 2009; 202(1–3):411–7.

74. Akhondzadeh S, Ghayyoumi R, Rezaei F, et al. Sildenafil adjunctive therapy to risperidone in the treatment of the negative symptoms of schizophrenia: a double-blind randomized placebo-controlled trial. Psychopharmacology (Berl) 2011;213(4):809–15.

75. Deal watch: intra-cellular therapies and Takeda to develop PDE1 inhibitors for schizophrenia. Nat Rev Drug Discov 2011;10(5):329.

76. Dani JA, Bertrand D. Nicotinic acetylcholine receptors and nicotinic cholinergic mechanisms of the central nervous system. Annu Rev Pharmacol Toxicol 2007; 47:699–729.

77. Freedman R, Adler LE, Gerhardt GA, et al. Neurobiological studies of sensory gating in schizophrenia. Schizophr Bull 1987;13(4):669–78.

78. Judd LL, McAdams L, Budnick B, et al. Sensory gating deficits in schizophrenia: new results. Am J Psychiatry 1992;149(4):488–93.

79. Clementz BA, Geyer MA, Braff DL. P50 suppression among schizophrenia and normal comparison subjects: a methodological analysis. Biol Psychiatry 1997; 41(10):1035–44.

80. Siegel C, Waldo M, Mizner G, et al. Deficits in sensory gating in schizophrenic patients and their relatives. Evidence obtained with auditory evoked responses. Arch Gen Psychiatry 1984;41(6):607–12.

81. Waldo MC, Adler LE, Freedman R. Defects in auditory sensory gating and their apparent compensation in relatives of schizophrenics. Schizophr Res 1988;1(1): 19–24.

82. Potter D, Summerfelt A, Gold J, et al. Review of clinical correlates of P50 sensory gating abnormalities in patients with schizophrenia. Schizophr Bull 2006;32(4): 692–700.

83. Patterson JV, Hetrick WP, Boutros NN, et al. P50 sensory gating ratios in schizophrenics and controls: a review and data analysis. Psychiatry Res 2008;158(2): 226–47.

84. Olincy A, Harris JG, Johnson LL, et al. Proof-of-concept trial of an alpha7 nicotinic agonist in schizophrenia. Arch Gen Psychiatry 2006;63(6):630–8.

85. Freedman R, Olincy A, Buchanan RW, et al. Initial phase 2 trial of a nicotinic agonist in schizophrenia. Am J Psychiatry 2008;165(8):1040–7.

86. ClinicalTrials.gov. Nicotinic receptors and schizophrenia. 2015.

87. Hashimoto K. Targeting of alpha7 nicotinic acetylcholine receptors in the treatment of schizophrenia and the use of auditory sensory gating as a translational biomarker. Curr Pharm Des 2015;21(26):3797–806.

88. Lieberman JA, Dunbar G, Segreti AC, et al. A randomized exploratory trial of an alpha-7 nicotinic receptor agonist (TC-5619) for cognitive enhancement in schizophrenia. Neuropsychopharmacology 2013;38(6):968–75.
89. Walling D, Marder SR, Kane J, et al. Phase 2 trial of an alpha-7 nicotinic receptor agonist (tc-5619) in negative and cognitive symptoms of schizophrenia. Schizophr Bull 2016;42(2):335–43.
90. ClinicalTrials.gov. NCT00435370. Effectiveness of tropisetron plus risperidone for improving cognitive and perceptual disturbances in schizophrenia. 2014.
91. Macor JE, Gurley D, Lanthorn T, et al. The 5-HT3 antagonist tropisetron (ICS 205-930) is a potent and selective alpha7 nicotinic receptor partial agonist. Bioorg Med Chem Lett 2001;11(3):319–21.
92. Shiina A, Shirayama Y, Niitsu T, et al. A randomised, double-blind, placebo-controlled trial of tropisetron in patients with schizophrenia. Ann Gen Psychiatry 2010;9:27.
93. Zhang XY, Liu L, Liu S, et al. Short-term tropisetron treatment and cognitive and P50 auditory gating deficits in schizophrenia. Am J Psychiatry 2012;169(9): 974–81.
94. Noroozian M, Ghasemi S, Hosseini SM, et al. A placebo-controlled study of tropisetron added to risperidone for the treatment of negative symptoms in chronic and stable schizophrenia. Psychopharmacology (Berl) 2013;228(4):595–602.
95. Kishi T, Mukai T, Matsuda Y, et al. Selective serotonin 3 receptor antagonist treatment for schizophrenia: meta-analysis and systematic review. Neuromolecular Med 2014;16(1):61–9.
96. Prickaerts J, van Goethem NP, Chesworth R, et al. EVP-6124, a novel and selective alpha7 nicotinic acetylcholine receptor partial agonist, improves memory performance by potentiating the acetylcholine response of alpha7 nicotinic acetylcholine receptors. Neuropharmacology 2012;62(2):1099–110.
97. Preskorn SH, Gawryl M, Dgetluck N, et al. Normalizing effects of EVP-6124, an alpha-7 nicotinic partial agonist, on event-related potentials and cognition: a proof of concept, randomized trial in patients with schizophrenia. J Psychiatr Pract 2014;20(1):12–24.
98. Barbier AJ, Hilhorst M, van Vliet A, et al. Pharmacodynamics, pharmacokinetics, safety, and tolerability of encenicline, a selective alpha7 nicotinic receptor partial agonist, in single ascending-dose and bioavailability studies. Clin Ther 2015; 37(2):311–24.
99. ClinicalTrials.gov. NCT01678755. A phase 2 study to evaluate ABT-126 for the treatment of cognitive deficits in schizophrenia. 2015.
100. ClinicalTrials.gov. NCT01655680. A study to evaluate ABT-126 for the treatment of cognitive deficits in schizophrenia. 2015.
101. ClinicalTrials.gov. NCT01095562. Safety and efficacy study for cognitive deficits in adult subjects with schizophrenia. 2013.
102. ClinicalTrials.gov. NCT01834638. Long-term safety and efficacy of ABT-126 in subjects with schizophrenia: an extension study for subjects completing study M10–855 (NCT01655680). 2014.
103. Feuerbach D, Pezous N, Weiss M, et al. AQW051, a novel, potent and selective alpha7 nicotinic ACh receptor partial agonist: pharmacological characterization and phase I evaluation. Br J Pharmacol 2015;172(5):1292–304.
104. ClinicalTrials.gov. NCT01730768. A study to evaluate the effects of once daily doses of AQW051 on cognition, in stable schizophrenia patients. 2015.
105. NCT01163227. Effect of AQW051 on cognitive function in patients with chronic stable schizophrenia. 2013.

106. Winterer G, Gallinat J, Brinkmeyer J, et al. Allosteric alpha-7 nicotinic receptor modulation and P50 sensory gating in schizophrenia: a proof-of-mechanism study. Neuropharmacology 2013;64:197–204.
107. NCT01851603. Phase I study to evaluate the safety and pharmacokinetics of oral doses of anvylic-3288 in healthy subjects (AVL3288). 2015.
108. Tenjin T, Miyamoto S, Ninomiya Y, et al. Profile of blonanserin for the treatment of schizophrenia. Neuropsychiatr Dis Treat 2013;9:587–94.
109. Hori H, Yamada K, Kamada D, et al. Effect of blonanserin on cognitive and social function in acute phase Japanese schizophrenia compared with risperidone. Neuropsychiatr Dis Treat 2014;10:527–33.
110. Kato TA, Hyodo F, Yamato M, et al. Redox and microglia in the pathophysiology of schizophrenia. Yakugaku Zasshi 2015;135(5):739–43 [in Japanese].
111. Mattei D, Djodari-Irani A, Hadar R, et al. Minocycline rescues decrease in neurogenesis, increase in microglia cytokines and deficits in sensorimotor gating in an animal model of schizophrenia. Brain Behav Immun 2014;38:175–84.
112. Zhu F, Liu Y, Zhao J, et al. Minocycline alleviates behavioral deficits and inhibits microglial activation induced by intrahippocampal administration of granulocyte-macrophage colony-stimulating factor in adult rats. Neuroscience 2014;266:275–81.
113. Miyaoka T, Yasukawa R, Yasuda H, et al. Minocycline as adjunctive therapy for schizophrenia: an open-label study. Clin Neuropharmacol 2008;31(5):287–92.
114. Chaudhry IB, Hallak J, Husain N, et al. Minocycline benefits negative symptoms in early schizophrenia: a randomised double-blind placebo-controlled clinical trial in patients on standard treatment. J Psychopharmacol 2012;26(9):1185–93.
115. Levkovitz Y, Mendlovich S, Riwkes S, et al. A double-blind, randomized study of minocycline for the treatment of negative and cognitive symptoms in early-phase schizophrenia. J Clin Psychiatry 2010;71(2):138–49.
116. America's Biopharmaceutical Research Companies. Medicines in development for mental health. Washington DC: Pharmaceutical Research and Manufacturers of America; 2014.

Treatment-Resistant Schizophrenia

Helio Elkis, MD, PhD[a],*, Peter F. Buckley, MD[b]

KEYWORDS

- Schizophrenia • Treatment • Resistance

KEY POINTS

- Despite considerable progress in the therapeutics of schizophrenia with the advent of second-generation antipsychotics (SGAs) and particularly the use of clozapine, treatment-resistant schizophrenia (TRS) continues to be challenge.
- Many efforts have been made toward the achievement of a common definition of TRS.
- In terms of the underlying mechanisms of the development of TRS, progress has been made in terms of the elucidation of the neurochemical mechanisms, particularly in terms of dopaminergic and glutamatergic neurotransmission. Structural neuroimaging studies have shown that patients with TRS show a higher reduction of the prefrontal cortex volume when compared with non-TRS.
- Clozapine continues to be the gold standard for the treatment for TRS although various SGAs have been tested but showed no superiority.
- Various clozapine augmentation strategies with antipsychotic and other psychopharmacological drugs have been tested but unfortunately persons with partial response to clozapine remain the most difficult to treat. Nonpharmacologic strategies, such as transcranial magnetic stimulation or electroconvulsive therapy, may represent some hope for the future of these cases.

INTRODUCTION

Although treatment-resistant schizophrenia (TRS) was described 50 years ago[1] and has a gold standard treatment with clozapine based on well-defined criteria,[2] there is still a matter of great interest as well as controversy. In fact, since we published a review in this journal some years ago,[3] more than 100 articles have been published, as well as

Disclosure: Dr H. Elkis has received research grants from FAPESP (Sao Paulo Research Support Foundation), Roche, and Janssen; he has also received honoraria for travel support or board participation from Roche, Janssen, and Cristalia. Dr P.F. Buckley has nothing to disclose.
[a] Instituto de Psiquiatria HC- FMUSP, Rua Ovidio Pires de Campos 785-São Paulo, SP-05403-010, Brazil; [b] Medical College of Georgia, Augusta, GA, USA
* Corresponding author.
E-mail address: helkis@usp.br

2 books[4,5] on the subject. Therefore, the aim of the present article was to update and enhance our previous review with new evidence mainly derived from new studies, clinical trials, systematic reviews, and meta-analyses published in this period.

RESISTANCE, RESPONSE, AND REMISSION

Schizophrenia it is a chronic disorder and patients exhibit a wide range manifestations in several psychopathological dimensions, such as psychotic, negative, disorganized, cognitive, and affective symptoms.[6] Impairments in certain areas such as negative symptoms[7] and cognition[8] compromise functionality and consequently patients with chronic schizophrenia generally show disabilities in such important areas as academic, work, or social relationships.[9]

However, chronicity cannot be confused with resistance to treatment, as epidemiologic studies such as the International Study on Schizophrenia have shown that approximately 50% of the patients with chronic schizophrenia do respond to treatment and have a favorable outcome in terms of functionality measures.[10] Therefore, despite having a chronic disorder that is considered disabling, patients with schizophrenia frequently respond to antipsychotic treatment in terms of reduction of symptoms and improvement of functionality, at least in some levels.

In a meta-analysis of the outcome literature of treatment of schizophrenia encompassing the twentieth century, Hegarty and colleagues[11] observed that, after the introduction of neuroleptic therapy, only 48% of patients with chronic schizophrenia had a favorable outcome; that is, responded to treatment.

Conversely, comparing the outcome studies published before and after the neuroleptic era, Perkins and colleagues[12] observed that after the introduction of antipsychotics in the armamentarium of treatment of psychosis, two-thirds of patients achieved good and intermediate outcomes, whereas one-third had a poor outcome; that is, did not respond to treatment.

Therefore, it is well known that 30% to 40% of patients with schizophrenia do not respond adequately to treatment, but only in 1980 did poor response to treatment begin to be systematically described. In fact, early definitions of TRS included scales that were developed ad hoc by investigators,[13–15] in which resistance was generally defined as a continuum varying from the lowest to the highest levels.[3]

Two concepts play a key role for understanding the notion of TRS: response and remission.[16] Treatment response (TR) is a key concept for the understanding of TRS and is defined as a clinically significant improvement of psychopathology, which is measured according to scales such as the Brief Psychiatric Rating Scale (BPRS)[17] or the Positive and Negative Syndrome Scale (PANSS),[18] which are used to quantify response and establish thresholds.[16] For example, in the initial clozapine study, a BPRS reduction of 20% from baseline was chosen for defining treatment response[2] but, as pointed out by Correll and colleagues,[16] the choice of the cutoff point is arbitrary and various levels were used, ranging from 20% to 60% from the initial score, but the clinical significance of the reduction of each level is unclear.[19]

To illustrate this aspect, Leucht and colleagues[20] investigated the correlation between reduction in the PANSS scale and its clinical significance as measured by the Clinical Global Impression (CGI) scale and observed that 50% reduction from baseline correlated with the "much improved" level of the CGI. However the investigators noticed that in patients with TRS, even small reductions on the PANSS (eg, 25%) were clinically significant.

Using multiple instruments for the evaluation of not only psychopathological severity but also improvement in terms of functionality may represent a solution for measuring response. For this, Suzuki and colleagues[19] reviewed 33 studies that used various criteria to define TRS treatment response and treatment resistance and the investigators verified that such definitions vary widely in terms of number of trials with antipsychotics, types and doses of antipsychotic used, duration of trials, and psychopathological as well as functional outcome measures to adequately evaluate response.[21] Based on a synthesis of these studies, the investigators suggested broadening the definition of TRS and introducing measures of functionality, such as the Functional Assessment for Comprehensive Treatment of Schizophrenia (FACT-SCZ),[22] which is more specific for schizophrenia than the Global Assessment of Functions (GAF),[23] thus proposing the following criteria.[24]

Treatment Response

Response: A score of 2 or 1 in the CGI-Change OR $\geq$20 points on FACT-SCZ or $\geq$20% decrease on BPRS or PANSS.

Partial Response: A score of 3 on CGI-Change OR 10 to 20 points increase on FACT-SCZ or GAF OR $\geq$10% reduction on the BPRS or PANSS.

Treatment Resistance

A. Well-documented failure to respond to $\geq$2 antipsychotics
B. Clearly documented history of treatment failure of $\geq$1 antipsychotic plus prospective validation of treatment failure with another antipsychotic (different from the one that previously failed)
C. Dose and duration: each treatment with $\geq$600 chlorpromazine equivalents (CPZE) per day for $\geq$6 weeks
D. Lack of improvement in reducing CGI[22] $\geq$4 AND a score of $\leq$49 on FACT-SCZ or $\leq$50 on the GAF.

Otherwise, the concept of TRS is sometimes associated with remission, which would imply almost absence of symptoms, but is also related to response; that is, reduction in symptom as compared with a previously established baseline level of severity.

Remission is also an important concept to take into consideration in terms of TRS because it is considered a clinical marker between response and full recovery.[23] It is defined as the reduction of symptoms to a level that does not interfere in a patient's psychosocial function[16] and is quantified by using 8 symptoms of the PANSS, which may reach a maximum level of 3 (mild).[25]

OPERATIONAL DEFINITIONS OF TREATMENT RESISTANCE

The first operational definition of treatment resistance was proposed by Kane and colleagues[2] in the study that introduced clozapine for TRS in comparison with chlorpromazine. This definition was very important for the development of the notion of TRS and subsequent definitions used later were inspired by this seminal work[2] (**Table 1**).

Various guidelines and algorithms, such the American Psychiatric Association,[26] the Texas Medication Algorithm Project,[24] the Schizophrenia Patient Outcome Research Team (PORT),[28] the World Federation of Societies of Biological Psychiatry Guidelines,[29] and International Psychopharmacological Guidelines (IPAP),[27] have proposed definitions of TRS as presented in **Table 1**.

Such various definitions were revised by some investigators[16,30] who proposed that a patient can be considered as having TRS according to the following criteria:

1. A history of failure of at least 2 antipsychotic trials (one of them with an atypical antipsychotic) with adequate doses, with 4 to 6 weeks' duration,

Table 1
Criteria for treatment resistance

Author	Definitions and Outcome Measures
Clozapine seminal trial, Kane et al,[2] 1988	Historical: A: No period of good function within the preceding 5 y; B: At least 3 treatments with antipsychotics of at least 2 different chemical classes with dose equivalents of 1000 mg chlorpromazine for a period of 6 wk, without significant relief. Actual or cross sectional: A: BPRS (1–7° of severity) ≥45 with at least 2 of the following 4 items: conceptual disorganization, suspiciousness, hallucinatory behavior, or unusual thought content; B: CGI ≥4 (moderately ill). Prospective: No improvement after 6 wk on haloperidol (up to 60 mg/d) defined as 20% reduction of BPRS as compared with the level of severity defined by the actual criteria and/or failure to reduce CGI of ≤3 or BPRS ≤35.
Lehman et al,[26] 2004, American Psychiatric Association Guidelines	Little or no symptomatic response to at least 2 antipsychotic trials of at least 6-wk duration within the adequate dose range.
Texas Medication Algorithm Project,[24] 2006	Failure to respond to 2 trials with a single SGA, with the possibility of use of FGA in the second trial (No SGA tried in the Stage 1). Clozapine should be considered in patients with recurrent suicidality, violence, or comorbid substance abuse. Persistence of positive symptoms for >2 y warrants and >5 y requires a clozapine trial, independent of number of preceding trials.
International Psychopharmacology Algorithm Project,[27] 2006	(1) No period of good functioning in previous 5 y; (2) prior nonresponse to at least 2 antipsychotic drugs of 2 different chemical classes for at least 4–6 wk each at doses ≥400 mg equivalents of chlorpromazine or 5 mg/d risperidone; (3) moderate to severe psychopathology, especially positive symptoms: conceptual disorganization, suspiciousness, delusions, or hallucinatory behavior; (4) in keeping with our view that TRS refers to more than persistent positive symptoms, we recommend considering patients to have TRS if they exhibit any of the following after 2 trials of 4–6 wk duration each, with 2 different antipsychotics at adequate doses: persistent psychotic symptoms, recurrent mood symptoms, repeated suicide attempts or suicidal ideation, uncontrolled aggressive behavior, moderate-severe negative symptoms, or moderate-severe cognitive impairment.
Schizophrenia Patient Outcomes Research Team (PORT) Guideline,[28] 2009	Clozapine should be offered to people with schizophrenia who continue to experience persistent and clinically significant positive symptoms after 2 adequate trials of other antipsychotic agents.
Hasan et al,[29] 2012, World Federation of Societies of Biological Psychiatry (WFSBP)	TRS can be defined as a situation in which significant improvement of psychopathology and/or other target symptoms has not been demonstrated despite treatment with 2 different antipsychotics from at least 2 different chemical classes (at least 1 should be an atypical antipsychotic) in the previous 5 y at the recommended antipsychotic dosages for a treatment period of at least 2–8 wk.

Abbreviations: BPRS, Brief Psychiatric Rating Scale; CGI, Clinical Global Impression scale; FGA, first-generation antipsychotic; SGA, second-generation antipsychotic; TRS, treatment-resistant schizophrenia.
Data from Refs.[2,24,26–29]

without satisfactory response, particularly in terms of persistence of psychotic symptoms.
2. High levels of psychopathology, particularly presence of psychotic symptoms that have an impact on the patient's conduct and functionality.
3. Presence of suicidality, violence, and substance abuse.

In terms of the duration of the trials, it is important to mention that recently Samara and colleagues[31] meta-analytically reviewed the duration of a series of trials in patients with schizophrenia and found that those who do not respond in the first 2 weeks are unlikely to respond later,[31] a finding that may in the future modify the definition of TRS.

CONFOUNDING AND COMORBID CONDITIONS

Sometimes the term TRS is mistaken as lack of compliance, embedding the notion that the patient is resisting the treatment rather than the illness itself being resistant to treatment.[3,16] In fact, poor or partial adherence may represent an important factor that must be ruled out, and some investigators propose a trial with a long-acting injectable (LAI) antipsychotic to verify whether the patient is truly resistant before the introduction of clozapine.[32–34] In fact, some investigators have proposed the term "pseudo-refractoriness" for such condition.

Comorbid conditions also represent another obstacle for the correct diagnosis of TRS. For example, as happens frequently with patients with schizophrenia, patients with TRS may show higher degrees of substance abuse[35] or obsessive-compulsive symptoms or disorder,[36,37] which may contribute for the apparent inefficacy of antipsychotics. Other additional aspects are higher levels of violence as well as a higher risk for suicide when compared with non-TRS.[35]

CLINICAL FEATURES OF TREATMENT-RESISTANT SCHIZOPHRENIA

Patients with TRS differ from non-TRS or nonresponsive aspects in many respects, such as described in the following sections.

Demographic Variables

Comparing patients with TRS versus patients without TRS, some investigators found a significant mean difference in the disease onset, together with predominance of the male gender and a higher number of hospitalizations in patients with TRS.[38–41]

Other correlates are duration of illness, poor premorbid functioning, family history of schizophrenia, an absence of precipitating factors, and a history of substance abuse.[35] Duration of untreated psychosis, however, showed not to be associated with TRS, whereas poor premorbid adjustment was associated.[42]

Psychopathological Dimensions

It well established that schizophrenia is a heterogeneous disorder with various types of symptoms that can be classified according to, at least, 5 dimensions: positive or psychotic, negative, disorganization, cognitive, and anxiety-depression. Various factor analyses of the PANSS confirmed the presence of these dimensions with some small variations in terms of the name of the factors.[43] In terms of patients with TRS, Lindenmayer and colleagues[44] evaluated the effect of atypical antipsychotics on syndromal profile of 157 patients with TRS and found a factor structure similar to their original factor analysis study with patients with non-TRS; that is, positive, negative, excitement, cognitive, and depressive.

The findings of Lindenmayer and colleagues[44] were not replicated, but recently Freitas and colleagues,[45] in a preliminary study, compared 150 patients with TRS with 141 non-TRS and found that the former showed the highest loadings in the positive factor, accounting for 28% of the variance, whereas the latter showed the highest loadings in the negative factor, which accounted for 37.5% of the variance. Additionally, factors such as disorganization/cognition and depression occurred only in patients with TRS.[45]

Using the BPRS,[17] McMahon and colleagues[46] analyzed a large dataset of 1074 patients, and by using exploratory and confirmatory factor analytical methods found that 13 of the 18 items of the scale loaded into 4 factors: reality distortion (grandiosity, suspiciousness, hallucinatory behavior, unusual thought content), disorganization (conceptual disorganization, mannerism and posturing, disorientation), negative symptoms (emotional withdrawal, motor retardation, blunted affect), and anxiety/depression (anxiety, guilty feelings, depression), proposing that such factors should be used for the analysis of data of clinical trials involving patients with TRS.

Also, using a BPRS-Anchored version[47] and translated into Portuguese,[48] we analyzed a homogeneous population of 96 patients narrowly defined as having TRS based on the criteria of Kane and colleagues.[2] We found that 16 of the 18 items of the scale clustered into 4 dimensions: negative/disorganization (emotional withdrawal, disorientation, blunted affect, mannerisms and posturing, conceptual disorganization), excitement (excitement, hostility, tension, grandiosity, uncooperativeness), positive (unusual thought content, suspiciousness, hallucinatory behavior), and depression (depression, guilt feelings, motor retardation).[49]

Cognition

Patients with schizophrenia exhibit cognitive impairment that is 1 to 2 SDs below normal population scores.[50] Woodward and Meltzer,[51] who extensively reviewed various cognition studies that compared patients with TRS with those with non-TRS, arrived at the conclusion that there is relatively little evidence that cognitive impairment is more severe in patients with TRS.

Recently, however, De Bartolomeis and colleagues[52] compared 19 patients with TRS with 22 patients with non-TRS by using the Brief Assessment of Cognition in Schizophrenia.[53] They found that patients with TRS performed significantly worse in terms of verbal memory as well more severe levels of psychopathology as measured by the PANSS.

Assessment

Thus the assessment of TRS could be summarized through some items, as previously suggested by other reviewers,[23,34,35] and adapted for the present review:

- Define inadequate response using the psychopathological dimensions of schizophrenia, particularly persistence of psychotic symptoms
- Use scales such as the BPRS or the PANSS to quantify severity of symptoms
- Define what is an adequate trial in terms of duration and dose of antipsychotics
- Determine how many trials can be documented and types of antipsychotics previously used
- Use patient charts
- Use treatment response timelines
- Consider the use of LAI antipsychotic if partial or inadequate adherence to treatment

- Consider treatment response after 2 trials with adequate antipsychotic doses and duration of 4 to 6 weeks of treatment
- Consider TRS if patient has failed to reduce the baseline BPRS/PANSS score by 20% or had an increase of severity of psychopathology by $\geq 30\%$
- Check if collateral symptoms (akathisia, hypokinesia) may worsen the clinical picture
- Check comorbidities that worsen the clinical picture: obsessive-compulsive symptoms or disorder, depression, or substance abuse or dependence

ETIOLOGIC AND PATHOGENIC CORRELATES OF TREATMENT-RESISTANT SCHIZOPHRENIA

Which are the main underlying processes associated with the development of TRS?

It is has been hypothesized that schizophrenia is the result of abnormal developmental processes that began years before the onset of illness,[54] with neurodevelopmental abnormalities giving rise to the symptoms of schizophrenia during adolescence or early adulthood through the interaction of genetic and socio-cognitive factors.[55,56]

Neurodegenerative processes, in contrast, represent progressive brain diseases of the nervous system that are initiated by specific biochemical changes and that have a genetic basis. Schizophrenia was primarily regarded as a dementia, a neurodegenerative process with a deteriorating course ("dementia praecox")[57]; however, such processes are considered limited, leading to the concept of neuroprogression, which is defined as the pathologic reorganization of the central nervous system as part of the course of several mental disorders.[58]

It has been proposed that TRS could be regarded as the result of both neurodevelopmental and neurodegenerative processes through the life span and resistance to antipsychotic drugs would develop at a certain time point in the evolution of schizophrenia. The investigators of this theory propose the following stages for the development of TRS: (1) cortical pathology and deficient neuromodulatory capacity due to genetic/epigenetic etiologic factors occurring during childhood, (2) neurochemical sensitization leading to dopamine release and development of psychotic episodes occurring during adolescence, and (3) neurotoxicity with consequent development of structural neuronal changes in adulthood.[55]

According to this model, cortical neuropathology and deficient neuromodulatory capacity would be the result of genetic and/or epigenetic factors and would occur during fetal gestation and early perinatal development. Neurochemical sensitization would be the expression of a deficiency in neuromodulatory capacity that occurs in adolescence or early adulthood, triggered by environmental factors such as stress or substance abuse, whereas neurotoxicity occurs in the residual phase of the development of schizophrenia and is associated with neuronal changes or neuronal loss.[54,55]

Therefore, it is conceivable that neurodevelopmental or neurodegenerative/neuroprogessive factors may underlie the development of resistance to treatment in schizophrenia and are expressed in terms of structural or functional brain abnormalities, neurochemical abnormalities, or gene expressions. We present studies on these aspects, which compared patients with TRS with patients with non-TRS or healthy controls.

Structural Brain Abnormalities

Historically, early studies that used pneumoencephalography[59] and computed tomography (CT) scans[60] showed an inverse relationship between the degree of ventricular enlargement and treatment outcome. Some subsequent CT studies that used morphometric techniques, such as ventricular brain ratio, replicated these findings, but a meta-analysis[61] as well as conventional systematic reviews of these early studies relating brain abnormalities to clinical outcome found little evidence that ventricular enlargement is related to treatment response.[62–64]

Early MRI studies that used some descriptive definitions of treatment resistance and visual examining of imaging as well as region of interest (ROI) morphometry found no correlation between brain abnormalities in patients with TRS as compared with non-TRS.[65,66] However, using an operational definition of TRS based on PANSS scores as well as ROI morphometry, Molina and colleagues[67] found that patients with TRS had significantly less gray matter (GM) in frontal and occipital regions and significantly more white matter in frontal, parietal, and occipital regions than healthy controls but no differences were found between patients with non-TRS and controls.

Voxel-based morphometry (VBM) is a modern brain imaging technique that normalizes all the subject images to a template to compare patients with controls, taking into account each voxel.[64] A meta-analysis of this technique showed that patients with schizophrenia in general exhibit a large variety of brain abnormalities as compared with controls, particularly in areas such as superior temporal gyrus and left temporal lobe.[68]

The use of VBM in combination with selection of patients based on adequate operational definitions of TRS brought new perspectives in the investigation of the relationship between brain abnormalities and response to treatment in patients with schizophrenia. Recent work using this technique found significant differences comparing patients with TRS versus non-TRS.

Thus, Zugman and colleagues,[69] using the IPAP[27] to define treatment resistance, compared 61 patients with TRS with 67 patients with non-TRS and 80 healthy controls, and found that when compared with controls, patients with TRS showed a widespread reduction in cortical thickness in all brain regions, but when compared with non-TRS, patients with TRS showed more pronounced decreased thickness in the dorsolateral prefrontal cortex (DLPFC).

Quarantelli and colleagues,[70] using the National Institute of Clinical Excellence guidelines[71] to define treatment resistance, compared 20 patients with TRS versus 15 non-TRS and 16 controls and found that patients with TRS have more pronounced degrees of atrophy in terms of reductions of GM in the middle frontal gyrus bilaterally, into the dorsolateral superior frontal gyrus extending into the postcentral gyrus and the right medial temporal cortex.

Recently, Anderson and colleagues[72] used the APA (American Psychiatric Association) criteria[26] for defining TRS and, using an MRI device with 3 T, compared 19 patients with TRS with 18 patients with non-TRS and 20 controls. Additionally, they also did comparisons with 15 patients with clozapine-resistant schizophrenia or "ultra-TRS" (discussed later in this category as an independent item). They found a GM reduction in patients with TRS as compared with non-TRS in several cortical regions, such as superior, middle, and temporal gyri; precentral and postcentral gyri; middle and superior frontal gyri; right supramarginal gyrus; and right occipital cortex. Patients with ultra-TRS showed some differences from those with non-TRS but no differences from patients with TRS.

All these three studies are cross sectional and not longitudinal and therefore it is difficult to establish a direct relationship between the use of antipsychotics and more pronounced abnormalities in frontal and prefrontal cortex (PFC) found in patients with TRS as compared with non-TRS.

A recent systematic review by Nakajima and colleagues[73] investigated structural neuroimaging studies in patients with TRS as compared with (1) healthy controls, (2) patients with non-TRS, and (3) as predictors of clozapine response (a topic to be discussed later). In terms of structural neuroimaging, the investigators included 5 studies,[69,74–77] but except for the study by Zugman and colleagues,[69] which compared patients with TRS versus non-TRS based on clear operational definition, the other studies investigated resistant hallucinations,[74,77] compared with patients with TRS with other disorders,[75] or included chronic patients, not selected according to particular TRS operational criteria.[76] Due to the heterogeneity of studies, not surprisingly the investigators found no evidence of a correlation between TRS and structural neuroimaging parameters.[73]

Functional and Molecular Neuroimaging

Functional neuroimaging techniques provide indirect ways of investigating the brain activity in vivo, whereas molecular neuroimaging provides a direct way of investigating these activities. Borgio and colleagues[64] reviewed these studies extensively in a previous review.

As previously mentioned, recently Nakajima and colleagues[73] also published an extensive review on functional neuroimaging studies in patients with TRS and found a few studies that compared these patients with healthy controls or patients with non-TRS, whereas most studies were related to clozapine response in this field. Nakajima and colleagues[73] point out that a series of studies suggest that, when patients with TRS are compared with healthy controls, they exhibit hypo metabolism in the PFC and hyper metabolism in the basal ganglia.[78,79]

Based on functional and neurochemical data, it has been proposed that patients with schizophrenia have an increased dopamine (DA) synthesis.[80–83] In relation to treatment resistance, various studies on this issue were reviewed by Demjaha and Howes[84] showing that the results are contradictory. Thus, to test the role of DA synthesis in relation to treatment resistance, Demjaha and Howes[84] compared 12 patients defined as TRS by the criteria of Kane and colleagues[2] with 12 patients with non-TRS (responders) as well as 12 controls in terms of their striatal dopamine synthesis capacity using 18F-DOPA PET. All patients were treated with nonclozapine antipsychotics. Patients with TRS showed similar levels of DA synthesis as compared with healthy controls, whereas patients with non-TRS showed a higher DA synthesis capacity, leading one to speculate that DA may not be the key aberrant neurotransmitter in TRS.[85]

To investigate the role of other neurotransmitters in TRS, Demjaha and colleagues[86] in another study used DOPA PET and proton magnetic resonance spectroscopy to evaluate DA as well as glutamate (GLU) functions. They compared 6 patients with TRS with 8 treatment responders and 10 healthy volunteers and found the same pattern as their previous study, with responders showing elevated striatal DA synthesis when compared with patients with TRS or healthy controls. However, they found the opposite pattern across groups in terms of GLU activity in the cingulate cortex because, when compared with controls or responders, patients with TRS showed a significant elevation of GLU activity, albeit the comparison between responders and TRS was shown to be nonsignificant.[86]

Genetics

The issue of the influence of genetic factors in TRS was extensively reviewed by De Luca and colleagues.[87] In this review, the investigators sought to review the pharmacokinetic but mainly pharmacodynamic factors of TRS, particularly in terms of clozapine response in relation to serotonin (5HT) system genes and DA system genes as well as other genes.

In terms of the influence of the 5HT system, most studies compared patients with TRS versus non-TRS using the criteria of Kane and colleagues.[2] These studies found some association between some genes of the 5HT system (eg, *HTR2A: His452Tyr, T102c*) but not in others (*5HT2C: Cys23Ser*).[88–91]

The COMT (catechol-ortho-methyltransferase) is a key enzyme in the metabolism of dopamine, which is known to be dysregulated in schizophrenia. It is located in the cytogenetic band of 22q11.2 on chromosome 22. In terms of its polymorphisms, a G-A transition in *codon 158* of the *COMT* gene results in the substitution of valine to methionine.[92]

This *COMT Val158Met* polymorphism has been extensively studied in association with aggressive behavior, violence, suicide, and the use of cannabis in patients with schizophrenia.[87] Using a very restrictive definition of TRS (patients hospitalized for 1 year and receiving daily the equivalent of 1000 mg chlorpromazine during this period), Inada and colleagues[92] compared 100 patients with schizophrenia with 201 healthy controls and observed no association between *COMT* polymorphism or alleles (H and L) with a diagnosis of schizophrenia, although the rate of TRS tended to be higher in patients with *COMT L/L* genotype than in those without TRS.

Among these genes was *DISC-1* (Disrupted-In-Schizophrenia), which, along with *Neuregulin-1–ErbB4*, plays a key role in neurodevelopment, and is considered a candidate gene for schizophrenia.[31] This was further investigated through 4 single nucleotide polymorphisms (SNPs) in 32 patients with TRS as compared with 95 patients with non-TRS, but no association was found between *DISC 1* and TRS.[93]

The association between 384 markers (SNPs) from candidate genes was investigated in 85 patients defined as having TRS according to the APA definition of treatment resistance[26] and compared with 115 patients with non-TRS. The investigators found a significant trend with the *SNP rs2152324* in the *NALCN* gene but after false discovery rate correction, the *P* value was not significant.[94]

The role of inflammation in TRS has been studied for a long time,[95,96] and recently the gene *FAS*, which plays a key role in this association, was investigated in 96 patients defined as having TRS by the criteria of Kane and colleagues,[2] in comparison with 77 patients with non-TRS. The researchers found a significant association between the *SNP rs7085850* and 2 haplotypes that were significantly associated with TRS in this sample.[94]

More recently, various publications have reported evidence of the association of TRS with the dopaminergic system in terms of *DRD1* polymorphysms[97] and DA transporter,[98] as well as other genes such as *BDNF*[99] or *rs2237457* located on chromosome 7p12.2 and tested as a possible biomarker.[100] However, in pharmacokinetic terms, the cytochrome P450 system (*CYP2D6*) was found not to be associated with TRS.[101]

Other Biological and Clinical Correlates of Treatment-Resistant Schizophrenia

Several studies sought to investigate the relationship between TRS and various pharmacologic or clinical correlates. For example, it was found that these patients have altered T-cell functions as well as alterations of inflammatory process mediated by interleukins.[102] Body temperature is increased in drug-naïve schizophrenia, whereas antipsychotics may decrease body temperature. Shiloh and colleagues[103] confirmed the hypothesis that psychopathology as measured by the PANSS is correlated with corneal body temperature.

TREATMENT OF TREATMENT-RESISTANT SCHIZOPHRENIA
Pharmacologic Treatments

Clozapine
The advent of antipsychotics represented a turning point for treatment of schizophrenia and chlorpromazine in 1950 and proved to be efficacious in replacing previous treatments, such as psychosurgery or insulin therapy.[11] However, cases of resistance to neuroleptics were described in 1960[1] and then a series of strategies were proposed until 1990, such as augmentation with lithium addition,[104] high-dose antipsychotics,[105,106] electroconvulsive therapy (ECT),[107] and even psychosurgery for extreme cases.[108,109]

Clozapine emerged as a drug for TRS in a trial in comparison with chlorpromazine in patients operationally defined as treatment resistant[2] and then started to be used worldwide in 1990.[110] Since then, evidence of efficacy and effectiveness of clozapine in patients with TRS comes from many sources.

First, in terms of *efficacy*, clozapine was shown to be more efficacious when compared with first-generation antipsychotics (FGAs) or second-generation antipsychotics (SGAs) in a series of early randomized controlled trials that were included in various meta-analyses,[111–114] although some systematic reviews questioned the superiority of clozapine in comparison with conventional antipsychotics.[115]

Geddes and colleagues,[116] using meta-regression, found that depending on the comparator dose, SGAs were not superior to conventional antipsychotics; however, clozapine exhibited the highest effect sizes. In contrast, Davis and colleagues[117] meta-analyzed 124 randomized controlled trials that compared various SGAs (clozapine, amisulpride, risperidone, olanzapine, zotepine, sertindole, quetiapine, ziprasidone, remoxipride) with haloperidol and found that only clozapine, amisulpride, risperidone, and olanzapine were superior to haloperidol. However, clozapine showed almost twice the effect size (0.49) in comparison with some other SGAs (amisulpride = 0.29, risperidone = 0.25, olanzapine = 0.21).

This study was replicated by Leucht and colleagues[118] in a meta-analysis that included 150 trials and 21,533 participants, and again clozapine, amisulpride, risperidone, and olanzapine proved to be superior to haloperidol, a standard antipsychotic for the treatment of schizophrenia, with clozapine showing the highest efficacy in terms of improvement of positive, negative, depressive, and total symptoms (**Fig. 1**).

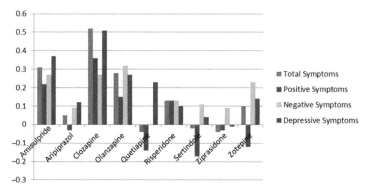

Fig. 1. Efficacy of clozapine in comparison with other SGAs for the treatment of schizophrenia. (*Data from* Leucht S, Corves C, Arbter D, et al. Second-generation versus first-generation antipsychotic drugs for schizophrenia: a meta-analysis. Lancet 2009;373(9657):31–41.)

Leucht and colleagues compared each SGA versus conventional antipsychotics in these 3 meta-analyses, as well as a meta-analysis performed by the Cochrane Schizophrenia Group,[119] and found that clozapine showed the highest effect size in comparison with all other SGAs in measures of the improvement of positive, negative, and total psychopathology.[118]

Therefore, these meta-analyses have shown that, when compared with FGAs, clozapine was superior in terms of improvement of psychopathology, particularly positive, negative, and depressive and total psychopathology.

However, again Leucht and colleagues,[120] in a meta-analysis comparing head to head all SGAs, found clozapine to be superior only to zotepine and to risperidone in doses higher than 400 mg per day, a finding replicated by a Cochrane meta-analysis comparing clozapine with every SGA.[121]

In terms of effectiveness, in the phase 2 Clinical Antipsychotic Trials of Intervention Effectiveness (CATIE) study, 99 patients who had not responded to atypical antipsychotics in the previous phase were assigned to clozapine (n = 49), olanzapine (n = 19), quetiapine (n = 15), or risperidone (n = 16). Patients assigned to clozapine had greater reductions in the PANSS total score as well as the lowest discontinuation.[122]

In the CutLass study, 136 patients with schizophrenia who showed a poor response to 2 or more antipsychotics were randomly assigned to clozapine (n = 67) or to another SGA (n = 69) (risperidone, olanzapine, quetiapine, or amisulpride). Clozapine proved to be superior in terms of reduction of the PANSS but not in quality of life, an important effectiveness outcome.[123]

Rehospitalization is another important effectiveness outcome, and we evaluated 262 patients discharged from the Institute of Psychiatry of the University of São Paulo during a 3-year follow-up of use of clozapine, FGAs, or SGAs. Overall, patients with clozapine had remained free of readmission for a longer period, particularly when compared with patients with SGAs.[41] Large population studies in Sweden involving more than 25,000 patients also found that the use of clozapine was associated with reduction of risk of rehospitalizations.[124]

Therefore, there is no dispute about the efficacy of clozapine in TRS and it is the drug of choice for such condition, being recommended by all guidelines for the treatment of schizophrenia when patients do not respond to a certain number of trials with nonclozapine antipsychotics.[24,26,28,29,71]

Alternatives to clozapine

Because clozapine may be intolerable for some patients,[125] various clinical trials tried other nonclozapine drugs as alternatives for TRS, such as an FGA, levomepromazine,[126] and various SGAs, such as aripiprazole,[127,128] sertindole,[129] ziprasidone,[130] quetiapine,[131] and/or combinations with amisulpride,[132] as well as LAIs, such as risperidone.[133]

Clozapine was also compared to other SGA in terms of efficacy and effectiveness in patients with TRS, particularly with Risperidone.[134,135] Various clinical trials tested the efficacy of high dose olanzapine (equal or higher than 30 mg/day) in comparison with standard doses of clozapine[136–143] and most of them were included in a meta-analysis which found no differences between clozapine and high dose olanzapine in terms of frequency of relapses. However clozapine showed superiority over high dose olanzapine in terms of improvement of psychotic, negative as well as overall symptoms.[144]

Suicide

Since the InterSePT study, which showed clozapine was superior to olanzapine in the reduction of attempts or suicide risk in patients with schizophrenia, clozapine became also the drug of choice for the reduction of the risk of recurrent suicidal behavior in patients with schizophrenia or schizoaffective disorder who are judged to be at chronic risk for reexperiencing suicidal behavior.[145]

A meta-analysis that included 6 studies confirmed that the use of clozapine was associated with threefold overall reduction of risk of suicidal behaviors,[146] whereas large mortality population studies developed in Finland[147] and Sweden[124] found that clozapine significantly reduced the risk of suicide.

Response and incomplete response to clozapine
Predictors of clozapine treatment response

Plasma clozapine levels Plasma systematic reviews previously published showed a series of clinical aspects that are predictors of treatment response to clozapine, such as higher baseline levels of psychopathology and functioning in the previous year,[148] and among them adequate dosing and plasma levels represent important aspects. Doses of 300 to 600 mg correlate with plasma threshold response.[149] Previous studies of plasma clozapine levels have shown that levels equal to or higher than 350 ng/mL predict good response, although this can be influenced by factors such as smoking.[150,151] An excellent systematic review provided by Remington and colleagues[152] involving 24 studies among 69 articles, established useful guidelines for such issue, as follows:

a. Plasma levels higher than 250 to 400 ng/mL are associated with increased chance of clinical response.
b. Doses exceeding 500 to 600 mg per day carry an increased risk of seizures.
c. Increasing plasma levels (600–838 ng/mL) does not improve clinical response.
d. There is not a clear relationship between levels and serious side effects such as agranulocytosis and seizures.
e. Plasma levels are more closely related to oral doses than either clinical response or side effects.

Pharmacogenetics The pharmacogenetics of clozapine was extensively reviewed by Foster and Buckley.[153] This review showed that various neurotransmitter systems are involved in clozapine response such as the D1 receptor gene *DRD1* as well as the D2 receptor gene (*DRD2*) promotor region -141Ins/Del polymorphism. Additionally the reviewers provided evidence regarding clozapine response in different ethnicities showing that in Caucasian populations 3 haplotypes located in the 5–8 region are involved in clozapine response, whereas in the African American populations the SNPs *Taq(-) 1A* and *Taq 1B* and *r1125394* were strongly associated with treatment response to clozapine.

Others polymorphisms have been studied involving clozapine response such as the *5HT3* receptor (*r1062613*) as well as *GSK3* gene,[154] the *5HT* transporter gene,[155] the *neurorexin 1*[156,157] and *D4/ D5* variants.[158] Another important review on the pharmacogenetics of clozapine response was published by Kohlrausch.[159]

Structural neuroimaging Pioneer work of Friedman and colleagues[160] using CT Scans showed that the degree of prefrontal atrophy was inversely related to response to clozapine and this finding was replicated by other CT or MRI studies.[161–163] Subsequent studies were unable to replicate these findings[164,165]; however, as previously mentioned, recent work of Zugman and colleagues[69] using VBM showed that patients with TRS showed more pronounced decreased thickness in the DLPFC when compared with non-TRS. Therefore, future studies with new neuroimaging technics are needed to address the issue of the relationship between the degree of cortical thickness of the DLPFC and clozapine response.

Only one study showed that patients treated with clozapine showed a correlation between improvement of psychotic symptoms and temporal gray volume, whereas improvement of disorganization symptoms were inversely related to baseline intracranial volume and hippocampal volume.[166]

Functional neuroimaging Previous work of Molina and colleagues[166–168] using Single Photon Emission Tomography (SPECT) or Positron Emission Tomography (PET) have shown an association between clozapine treatment and reduction of metabolic activity in pre-frontal regions and thalamus[166–168] although it is unclear whether this parameter is related to clinical efficacy.[73] However some authors propose that treatment with clozapine may alleviate hyperactivity in the limbic system in schizophrenia better than other antipsychotics and thus may facilitate activation of the regions involved in cognitive tasks.[169] Nakajima and colleagues[73] reviewed extensively these studies and found no evidence of a correlation between brain modifications associated with the use of clozapine and treatment response.

Partial response to clozapine

It is estimated that 30% of patients receiving clozapine treatment remain symptomatic, particularly in terms of the persistence of psychotic symptoms.[3,170] These patients are termed "clozapine unresponsives," "clozapine partial responders," "clozapine-resistant," or having "ultraresistant schizophrenia" or "super-refractory schizophrenia."[39,171–174] For the sake of clarity we call these TRS subtypes super-refractory schizophrenia (SRS).[39]

There is a general agreement that patients with SRS have persistence of psychotic symptoms after adequate treatment with adequate doses at least for 6 months.[3] However, to our knowledge, only Mouaffak and colleagues[173] have proposed an operationalized definition, using the following multidimensional criteria:

1. At least 8 weeks of treatment with clozapine with plasma levels of >350 µg/L and failure to improve by at least 20% in total BPRS score.
2. Persistent psychotic symptoms, defined as ≥ 4 (moderate) on at least 2 to 4 positive symptom items of the BPRS (18 items, graded 1–7).[17]
3. Current presence of at least moderately severe illness on the BPRS (score ≥ 45) and a score of ≥ 4 (moderate) on the CGI scale.[22]
4. Persistence of illness as defined as no stable period of good social and/or occupational functioning within the past 5 years (inability to maintain work and relationships) and GAF ≤ 40.

In recent years, various excellent reviews[171,173–178] have shed some light on the various aspects of the treatment of this complex condition. We summarize the major aspects of pharmacological treatment, providing the best evidence of efficacy based on the most recent systematic reviews or meta-analyses. Additionally, we discuss evidence for other nonpharmacologic interventions of SRS.

Clozapine antipsychotic augmentation

Various antipsychotics, such as loxapine, olanzapine, pimozide, and ziprasidone, were initially used for clozapine augmentation in patients with SRS. Subsequently, sulpiride, amisulpride, aripiprazole, and risperidone were tested in a series of randomized controlled trials but none of them proved to be effective in terms of improvement of clozapine efficacy when compared with controls[3]

Barbui and colleagues,[179] in a systematic review of 21 studies involving FGAs and SGAs, found an effect favoring the use of a second antipsychotic in open-label studies. However, in terms of a randomized controlled trial, the addition of amisulpride, risperidone, or sulpiride showed no benefit in terms of improving clozapine efficacy.

Other Pharmacologic Agents

Various pharmacologic agents, such as antiepileptics/mood stabilizers (lamotrigine, topiramate), antidepressants (citalopram, fluoxetine, fluvoxamine, mirtazapine), glutamatergic agents (CX 516, D-cycloserine, D-serine, glycine, sarcosine), allopurinol, memantine, and tetrabenazine have been tested in various clinical trials.[180–182] Among them, the use of lamotrigine showed some evidence of efficacy,[183] but as demonstrated by Sommer and colleagues,[180] the positive effect disappeared after the removal of an outlier. In fact, these investigators showed that pharmacologic augmentation of clozapine has not yet been demonstrated to be superior to placebo.

Nonpharmacologic Augmentation Strategies

Transcranial magnetic stimulation and transcranial direct current stimulation
The use of transcranial magnetic stimulation (TMS) particularly for resistant auditory hallucinations, as well as persistent negative symptoms, has been extensively reviewed[184,185] with some promising results but it is not formally indicated to be used in daily routine clinical practice for patients with TRS or SRS.

Electroconvulsive therapy
ECT is recommended for the treatment of schizophrenia in various guidelines and algorithms for treatment of schizophrenia.[24,26–29] The use of ECT in TRS was extensively reviewed by Champattana,[186] who included 9 uncontrolled studies. Other reviews have shown the ECT is used as an augmentation strategy, particularly for incomplete responders to clozapine and the number of controlled studies is scarce.[187,188]

However, recently, Petrides and colleagues[189] published results of a randomized controlled trial in which patients with partial response to clozapine were assigned to ECT plus clozapine or treatment as usual (TAU). Patients who were considered nonresponders of the clozapine group received an 8-week open trial of ECT (crossover phase). ECT was performed 3 times per week for the first 4 weeks and twice weekly for the last 4 weeks. Response was defined as 40% reduction in symptoms on BPRS and CGI. Fifty percent of patients of the ECT group responded to treatment, whereas none of the patients of the TAU showed any improvement.[189]

Cognitive behavior therapy
Cognitive behavioral therapy (CBT) has been extensively used in patients with schizophrenia, particularly for the improvement of symptoms such as hallucinations and delusions.[190] A meta-analysis of 12 randomized controlled trials showed that, when compared with controls, patients with medication-resistant psychosis who have received CBT improved significantly in terms of psychotic symptoms as well as general symptoms.[191]

Among these studies, 2 used CBT in patients with partial response to clozapine. Results have shown that patients who received CBT improved in terms of general psychopathology[192] as well as psychotic symptoms[193] in comparison with controls (befriending).

SUMMARY

Despite considerable progress in the therapeutics of schizophrenia with the advent of SGAs and particularly the use of clozapine, TRS continues to be challenge.

Many efforts have been made toward the achievement of a common definition of TRS.

In terms of the underlying mechanisms of the development of TRS, progress has been made in terms of the elucidation of the neurochemical mechanisms, particularly in terms of dopaminergic and glutamatergic neurotransmission. Structural neuroimaging studies have shown that patients with TRS show a higher reduction of the PFC volume when compared with non-TRS.

Clozapine continues to be the gold standard for the treatment of TRS, although various SGAs have been tested but have shown no superiority.

Various clozapine augmentation strategies with antipsychotic and other psychopharmacological drugs have been tested, but unfortunately persons with partial response to clozapine remain the most difficult to treat patients. Nonpharmacologic strategies, such as TMS or ECT, may represent some hope for the future of these cases.

NOTE TO READERS

In the time this article was being published, Samara and colleagues[194] published an impressive Network Metanalysis (NMA) which integrated 40 blinded Randomized Controlled Trials (RCTs) involving antipsychotics such as Clozapine as well as Chlorpromazine, Haloperidol, Fluphenazine, Risperidone, Olanzapine and Quetiapine in patients with TRS. They found that there is insufficient evidence to affirm that any antipsychotic is more efficacious for patients with TRS and, in contrast with unblinded effectiveness studies, such as the CATIE[122] or CutLass[123], the RCTs included in study provided little evidence of the superiority of Clozapine compared with other SGA.

However the authors showed to be cautious about their own findings which they considered not definitive, particularly regarding methodological aspects of NMA, as well as particularities of the RCTs included in the study, such as the definition of TRS, mean Clozapine doses-which were significantly below as compared with studies of Clozapine vs FGA- as well the degree of severity of cases. They remarked that the superiority of Clozapine over the FGAs has been demonstrated repeatedly, establishing this antipsychotic as the gold standard treatment for patients with TRS and that evidence from blinded RCTs for the comparison of Clozapine with other SGAs is still lacking and, consequently, more trials are warranted, particularly including more severe cases.[194]

Commenting the results of this study Kane and Correll[195] called the attention for the fact that, due to the complexities and methodological issues involving the studies, the results of this very well done metanalysis may eventually confuse clinicians, patients and families. They also pointed out that the results of the study by Samara and colleagues, is in contrast of another metanalysis published by Leucht[196] and colleagues, which, using similar methodology (multi-treatments metanalysis), compared 15 different antipsychotics with placebo in patients with schizophrenia and found that Clozapine showed the highest effect size as compared with other SGA such as Olanzapine or Risperidone.[195]

REFERENCES

1. Itil TM, Keskiner A, Fink M. Therapeutic studies in "therapy resistant" schizophrenic patients. Compr Psychiatry 1966;7(6):488–93.
2. Kane J, Honigfeld G, Singer J, et al. Clozapine for the treatment-resistant schizophrenic. A double-blind comparison with chlorpromazine. Arch Gen Psychiatry 1988;45(9):789–96.
3. Elkis H. Treatment-resistant schizophrenia. Psychiatr Clin North Am 2007;30(3): 511–33.
4. Elkis H, Meltzer HY, editors. Therapy-resistant schizophrenia. Basel (Switzerland): Karger; 2010.

5. Buckley PF, editor. Treatment-refractory schizophrenia—a clinical conundrum. Heildelberg (Germany): Springer; 2014.

6. American Psychiatric Association. Diagnostic and statistical manual of mental disorders, 5th edition: DSM-5. Washington, DC: American Psychiatric Press; 2013.

7. Buchanan RW. Persistent negative symptoms in schizophrenia: an overview. Schizophr Bull 2007;33(4):1013–22.

8. Green MF, Kern RS, Braff DL, et al. Neurocognitive deficits and functional outcome in schizophrenia: are we measuring the "right stuff"? Schizophr Bull 2000;26(1):119–36.

9. Reichenberg A, Feo C, Prestia D, et al. The course and correlates of everyday functioning in schizophrenia. Schizophr Res Cogn 2014;1(1):e47–52.

10. Harrison G, Hopper K, Craig T, et al. Recovery from psychotic illness: a 15- and 25-year international follow-up study. Br J Psychiatry 2001;178:506–17.

11. Hegarty JD, Baldessarini RJ, Tohen M, et al. One hundred years of schizophrenia: a meta-analysis of the outcome literature. Am J Psychiatry 1994; 151(10):1409–16.

12. Perkins DO, Miller-Andersen L, Lieberman JA. Natural history and predictors of clinical outcome. In: Lieberman JA, Scott Stroup T, Perkins DO, editors. Textbook of schizophrenia. Washington, DC: American Psychiatric Publishing; 2006. p. 289–301.

13. Csernansky JG, Yesavage JA, Maloney W, et al. The treatment response scale: a retrospective method of assessing response to neuroleptics. Am J Psychiatry 1983;140(9):1210–3.

14. Brenner HD, Dencker SJ, Goldstein MJ, et al. Defining treatment refractoriness in schizophrenia. Schizophr Bull 1990;16(4):551–61.

15. Brenner H, Merlo M. Definition of therapy-resistant schizophrenia and its assessment. Eur Psychiatry 1995;10(Suppl 1):11S–117S.

16. Correll CU, Kishimoto T, Nielsen J, et al. Quantifying clinical relevance in the treatment of schizophrenia. Clin Ther 2011;33(12):B16–39.

17. Overall J, Gorham D. The brief psychiatric rating scale. Psychol Rep 1962;10: 799–812.

18. Kay SR, Fiszbein A, Opler LA. The positive and negative syndrome scale (PANSS) for schizophrenia. Schizophr Bull 1987;13(2):261–76.

19. Suzuki T, Remington G, Mulsant BH, et al. Defining treatment-resistant schizophrenia and response to antipsychotics: a review and recommendation. Psychiatry Res 2012;197(1–2):1–6.

20. Leucht S, Kane JM, Kissling W, et al. What does the PANSS mean? Schizophr Res 2005;79(2–3):231–8.

21. Suzuki T, Remington G, Mulsant BH, et al. Treatment resistant schizophrenia and response to antipsychotics: a review. Schizophr Res 2011;133(1–3):54–62.

22. Guy W. ECDEU assessment manual for psychopharmacology. Rockville (MD): US Department of Health, Education and Welfare; 1976.

23. Tracy DK, Shergill S. Treatment-refractory schizophrenia: definition and assessment. In: Buckley PF, Gaughran F, editors. Treatment-refractory schizophrenia—a clinical conundrum. Heildelberg (Germany): Springer; 2014. p. 1–19.

24. Moore TA, Buchanan RW, Buckley PF, et al. The Texas Medication Algorithm Project antipsychotic algorithm for schizophrenia: 2006 update. J Clin Psychiatry 2007;68(11):1751–62.

25. Andreasen NC, Carpenter WT Jr, Kane JM, et al. Remission in schizophrenia: proposed criteria and rationale for consensus. Am J Psychiatry 2005;162(3): 441–9.

26. Lehman AF, Lieberman JA, Dixon LB, et al. Practice guideline for the treatment of patients with schizophrenia, 2nd edition. Am J Psychiatry 2004;161(2 Suppl): 1–56.

27. The International Psychopharmacology Algorithm Project, 2016. Available at: http://www.ipap.org.

28. Buchanan RW, Kreyenbuhl J, Kelly DL, et al. The 2009 schizophrenia PORT psychopharmacological treatment recommendations and summary statements. Schizophr Bull 2010;36(1):71–93.

29. Hasan A, Falkai P, Wobrock T, et al. World Federation of Societies of Biological Psychiatry (WFSBP) Guidelines for Biological Treatment of Schizophrenia, part 1: update 2012 on the acute treatment of schizophrenia and the management of treatment resistance. World J Biol Psychiatry 2012;13(5):318–78.

30. Stahl SM, Morrissette DA, Citrome L, et al. "Meta-guidelines" for the management of patients with schizophrenia. CNS Spectr 2013;18(3):150–62.

31. Samara MT, Leucht C, Leeflang MM, et al. Early improvement as a predictor of later response to antipsychotics in schizophrenia: a diagnostic test review. Am J Psychiatry 2015;172(7):617–29.

32. Kane JM, Correll CU. Past and present progress in the pharmacologic treatment of schizophrenia. J Clin Psychiatry 2010;71(9):1115–24.

33. Kane JM, Kishimoto T, Correll CU. Non-adherence to medication in patients with psychotic disorders: epidemiology, contributing factors and management strategies. World Psychiatry 2013;12(3):216–26.

34. Lambert T. Disease management: multidimensional approaches to incomplete recovery in psychosis. In: Elkis H, Meltzer H, editors. Therapy-resistant schizophrenia. Basel (Switzerland): Karger; 2010. p. 87–113.

35. Lindenmayer J, Khan A. Assessment of therapy-resistant schizophrenia. In: Elkis H, Meltzer H, editors. Therapy-resistant schizophrenia. Basel (Switzerland): Karger; 2010. p. 9–32.

36. Cunill R, Castells X, Simeon D. Relationships between obsessive-compulsive symptomatology and severity of psychosis in schizophrenia: a systematic review and meta-analysis. J Clin Psychiatry 2009;70(1):70–82.

37. Sa AR, Hounie AG, Sampaio AS, et al. Obsessive-compulsive symptoms and disorder in patients with schizophrenia treated with clozapine or haloperidol. Compr Psychiatry 2009;50(5):437–42.

38. Meltzer HY, Rabinowitz J, Lee MA, et al. Age at onset and gender of schizophrenic patients in relation to neuroleptic resistance. Am J Psychiatry 1997; 154(4):475–82.

39. Henna Neto J, Elkis H. Clinical aspects of super-refractory schizophrenia: a 6-month cohort observational study. Rev Bras Psiquiatr 2007;29(3):228–32.

40. Castro AP, Elkis H. Rehospitalization rates of patients with schizophrenia discharged on haloperidol, risperidone or clozapine. Rev Bras Psiquiatr 2007; 29(3):207–12.

41. Werneck AP, Hallak JC, Nakano E, et al. Time to rehospitalization in patients with schizophrenia discharged on first generation antipsychotics, non-clozapine second generation antipsychotics, or clozapine. Psychiatry Res 2011;188(3): 315–9.

42. Bobo W, Meltzer H. Duration of untreated psychosis and premorbid function: relationship with treatment response and treatment-resistant schizophrenia.

In: Elkis H, Meltzer H, editors. Therapy- resistant schizophrenia. Basel (Switzerland): Karger; 2010. p. 74–86.

43. Lindenmayer JP, Grochowski S, Hyman RB. Five factor model of schizophrenia: replication across samples. Schizophr Res 1995;14(3):229–34.

44. Lindenmayer JP, Czobor P, Volavka J, et al. Effects of atypical antipsychotics on the syndromal profile in treatment-resistant schizophrenia. J Clin Psychiatry 2004;65(4):551–6.

45. Freitas RR, Vizzotto ADB, Avrichir B, et al. Comparison of the Positive and Negative Syndrome Scales (PANSS) factor structure in patients with refractory versus non refractory schizophrenia. Schizophr Bull 2015;41:S103.

46. McMahon RP, Kelly DL, Kreyenbuhl J, et al. Novel factor-based symptom scores in treatment resistant schizophrenia: implications for clinical trials. Neuropsychopharmacology 2002;26(4):537–45.

47. Woerner MG, Mannuzza S, Kane JM. Anchoring the BPRS: an aid to improved reliability. Psychopharmacol Bull 1988;24(1):112–7.

48. Romano F, Elkis H. Tradução e adaptação de um instrumento para avaliação psicopatológica das psicoses: a Escala Breve de Avaliação Psiquiátrica-Versão Ancorada (BPRS-A). J Bras Psiquiatr 1996;45:43–9.

49. Alves TM, Pereira JC, Elkis H. The psychopathological factors of refractory schizophrenia. Rev Bras Psiquiatr 2005;27(2):108–12.

50. Saykin AJ, Shtasel DL, Gur RE, et al. Neuropsychological deficits in neuroleptic naive patients with first-episode schizophrenia. Arch Gen Psychiatry 1994;51(2):124–31.

51. Woodward N, Meltzer H. Neuropsychology of treatment-resistant schizophrenia. In: Elkis H, Meltzer H, editors. Therapy-resistant schizophrenia. Basel (Switzerland): Karger; 2010. p. 33–51.

52. de Bartolomeis A, Balletta R, Giordano S, et al. Differential cognitive performances between schizophrenic responders and non-responders to antipsychotics: correlation with course of the illness, psychopathology, attitude to the treatment and antipsychotics doses. Psychiatry Res 2013;210(2):387–95.

53. Keefe RS, Goldberg TE, Harvey PD, et al. The Brief Assessment of Cognition in Schizophrenia: reliability, sensitivity, and comparison with a standard neurocognitive battery. Schizophr Res 2004;68(2–3):283–97.

54. Rapoport JL, Giedd JN, Gogtay N. Neurodevelopmental model of schizophrenia: update 2012. Mol Psychiatry 2012;17(12):1228–38.

55. Sheitman BB, Lieberman JA. The natural history and pathophysiology of treatment resistant schizophrenia. J Psychiatr Res 1998;32(3–4):143–50.

56. Howes OD, Murray RM. Schizophrenia: an integrated sociodevelopmental-cognitive model. Lancet 2014;383(9929):1677–87.

57. Kraepelin E. Dementia praecox and paraphrenia (From the German edition of the textbook of psychiatry). Edinburgh (Scotland): E&S Livingstone; 1919.

58. Jarskog L, Gilmore J. Neuroprogressive theories. In: Lieberman J, Stroup T, Perkins D, editors. Textbook of schizophrenia. Washington, DC: The American Psychiatric Publishing; 2006. p. 137–49.

59. Cazzullo C. Biological and clinical studies on schizophrenia related to pharmacological treatment. Recent Adv Biol Psychiatry 1963;18(9):114–43.

60. Weinberger DR, Bigelow LB, Kleinman JE, et al. Cerebral ventricular enlargement in chronic schizophrenia. An association with poor response to treatment. Arch Gen Psychiatry 1980;37(1):11–3.

61. Friedman L, Lys C, Schulz SC. The relationship between structural brain imaging parameters to antipsychotic treatment response: a review. J Psychiatry Neurosci 1992;17(2):42–54.

62. Sharma T, Kerwin R. Biological determinants of difficult to treat patients with schizophrenia. Br J Psychiatry Suppl 1996;(31):5–9.

63. Crosthwaite C, Reveley MA. Structural imaging and treatment response in schizophrenia. In: Reveley MA, Deakin W, editors. The psychopharmacology of schizophrenia. London: Arnold; 2000. p. 89–108.

64. Borgio J, Rocha D, Elkis H, et al. Neuroimaging of treatment-resistant schizophrenia. In: Elkis H, Meltzer H, editors. Therapy-resistant schizophrenia. Basel (Switzerland): Karger; 2010. p. 63–73.

65. Lawrie SM, Ingle GT, Santosh CG, et al. Magnetic resonance imaging and single photon emission tomography in treatment-responsive and treatment-resistant schizophrenia. Br J Psychiatry 1995;167(2):202–10.

66. Lawrie SM, Abukmeil SS, Chiswick A, et al. Qualitative cerebral morphology in schizophrenia: a magnetic resonance imaging study and systematic literature review. Schizophr Res 1997;25(2):155–66.

67. Molina V, Reig S, Sanz J, et al. Differential clinical, structural and P300 parameters in schizophrenia patients resistant to conventional neuroleptics. Prog Neuropsychopharmacol Biol Psychiatry 2008;32(1):257–66.

68. Honea R, Crow TJ, Passingham D, et al. Regional deficits in brain volume in schizophrenia: a meta-analysis of voxel-based morphometry studies. Am J Psychiatry 2005;162(12):2233–45.

69. Zugman A, Gadelha A, Assunção I, et al. Reduced dorso-lateral prefrontal cortex in treatment resistant schizophrenia. Schizophr Res 2013;148(1–3):81–6.

70. Quarantelli M, Palladino O, Prinster A, et al. Patients with poor response to antipsychotics have a more severe pattern of frontal atrophy: a voxel-based morphometry study of treatment resistance in schizophrenia. Biomed Res Int 2014;2014:325052.

71. National Institute of Health and Clinical Excellence. Core interventions in the treatment and management of schizophrenia in primary and secondary care. London: NICE Schizophrenia; 2002.

72. Anderson VM, Goldstein ME, Kydd RR, et al. Extensive gray matter volume reduction in treatment-resistant schizophrenia. Int J Neuropsychopharmacol 2015;18(7):pyv016.

73. Nakajima S, Takeuchi H, Plitman E, et al. Neuroimaging findings in treatment-resistant schizophrenia: a systematic review: lack of neuroimaging correlates of treatment-resistant schizophrenia. Schizophr Res 2015;164(1–3):164–75.

74. Cachia A, Paillere-Martinot ML, Galinowski A, et al. Cortical folding abnormalities in schizophrenia patients with resistant auditory hallucinations. Neuroimage 2008;39(3):927–35.

75. Sun J, Maller JJ, Daskalakis ZJ, et al. Morphology of the corpus callosum in treatment-resistant schizophrenia and major depression. Acta Psychiatr Scand 2009;120(4):265–73.

76. Holleran L, Ahmed M, Anderson-Schmidt H, et al. Altered interhemispheric and temporal lobe white matter microstructural organization in severe chronic schizophrenia. Neuropsychopharmacology 2014;39(4):944–54.

77. Kubera KM, Sambataro F, Vasic N, et al. Source-based morphometry of gray matter volume in patients with schizophrenia who have persistent auditory verbal hallucinations. Prog Neuropsychopharmacol Biol Psychiatry 2014;50:102–9.

78. Molina Rodriguez V, Montz Andree R, Perez Castejon MJ, et al. Cerebral perfusion correlates of negative symptomatology and parkinsonism in a sample of treatment-refractory schizophrenics: an exploratory 99mTc-HMPAO SPET study. Schizophr Res 1997;25(1):11–20.

79. Rodriguez VM, Andree RM, Castejon MJ, et al. Fronto-striato-thalamic perfusion and clozapine response in treatment-refractory schizophrenic patients. A 99mTc-HMPAO study. Psychiatry Res 1997;76(1):51–61.

80. Howes OD, Montgomery AJ, Asselin MC, et al. Elevated striatal dopamine function linked to prodromal signs of schizophrenia. Arch Gen Psychiatry 2009; 66(1):13–20.

81. Howes OD, Kapur S. The dopamine hypothesis of schizophrenia: version III–the final common pathway. Schizophr Bull 2009;35(3):549–62.

82. Howes OD, Bose SK, Turkheimer F, et al. Dopamine synthesis capacity before onset of psychosis: a prospective [18F]-DOPA PET imaging study. Am J Psychiatry 2011;168(12):1311–7.

83. Howes O, Bose S, Turkheimer F, et al. Progressive increase in striatal dopamine synthesis capacity as patients develop psychosis: a PET study. Mol Psychiatry 2011;16:885–6.

84. Demjaha A, Howes O. Dopamine and biology and course of treatment resistance. In: Buckley P, Gaughran F, editors. Treatment-refractory schizophrenia—a clinical conundrum. Berlin; Heildelberg (Germany): Springer-Verlag; 2014. p. 31–43.

85. Demjaha A, Murray RM, McGuire PK, et al. Dopamine synthesis capacity in patients with treatment-resistant schizophrenia. Am J Psychiatry 2012;169(11): 1203–10.

86. Demjaha A, Egerton A, Murray RM, et al. Antipsychotic treatment resistance in schizophrenia associated with elevated glutamate levels but normal dopamine function. Biol Psychiatry 2014;75(5):e11–3.

87. De Luca V, Souza R, Panariello F, et al. Genetic studies in treatment-resistant schizophrenia. In: Elkis H, Meltzer H, editors. Therapy-resistant schizophrenia. Basel (Switzerland): Karger; 2010. p. 52–62.

88. Yu YW, Tsai SJ, Lin CH, et al. Serotonin-6 receptor variant (C267T) and clinical response to clozapine. Neuroreport 1999;10(6):1231–3.

89. Arranz M, Collier D, Sodhi M, et al. Association between clozapine response and allelic variation in 5-HT2A receptor gene. Lancet 1995;346(8970):281–2.

90. Arranz MJ, Collier DA, Munro J, et al. Analysis of a structural polymorphism in the 5-HT2A receptor and clinical response to clozapine. Neurosci Lett 1996; 217(2–3):177–8.

91. Arranz MJ, Munro J, Owen MJ, et al. Evidence for association between polymorphisms in the promoter and coding regions of the 5-HT2A receptor gene and response to clozapine. Mol Psychiatry 1998;3(1):61–6.

92. Inada T, Nakamura A, Iijima Y. Relationship between catechol-O-methyltransferase polymorphism and treatment-resistant schizophrenia. Am J Med Genet B Neuropsychiatr Genet 2003;120B(1):35–9.

93. Hotta Y, Ohnuma T, Hanzawa R, et al. Association study between Disrupted-in-Schizophrenia-1 (DISC1) and Japanese patients with treatment-resistant schizophrenia (TRS). Prog Neuropsychopharmacol Biol Psychiatry 2011;35(2): 636–9.

94. Jia P, Jayathilake K, Zhao Z, et al. Association of FAS, a TNF-alpha receptor gene, with treatment resistant schizophrenia. Schizophr Res 2011;129:211–2.

95. Lin A, Kenis G, Bignotti S, et al. The inflammatory response system in treatment-resistant schizophrenia: increased serum interleukin-6. Schizophr Res 1998; 32(1):9–15.

96. Maes M, Bocchio Chiavetto L, Bignotti S, et al. Increased serum interleukin-8 and interleukin-10 in schizophrenic patients resistant to treatment with neuroleptics and the stimulatory effects of clozapine on serum leukemia inhibitory factor receptor. Schizophr Res 2002;54(3):281–91.

97. Ota VK, Spindola LN, Gadelha A, et al. DRD1 rs4532 polymorphism: a potential pharmacogenomic marker for treatment response to antipsychotic drugs. Schizophr Res 2012;142(1–3):206–8.

98. Bilic P, Jukic V, Vilibic M, et al. Treatment-resistant schizophrenia and DAT and SERT polymorphisms. Gene 2014;543(1):125–32.

99. Zhang JP, Lencz T, Geisler S, et al. Genetic variation in BDNF is associated with antipsychotic treatment resistance in patients with schizophrenia. Schizophr Res 2013;146(1–3):285–8.

100. Li J, Meltzer HY. A genetic locus in 7p12.2 associated with treatment resistant schizophrenia. Schizophr Res 2014;159(2–3):333–9.

101. van de Bilt MT, Prado CM, Ojopi EP, et al. Cytochrome P450 genotypes are not associated with refractoriness to antipsychotic treatment. Schizophr Res 2015; 168(1-2):587–8.

102. Altamura AC, Bassetti R, Cattaneo E, et al. Some biological correlates of drug resistance in schizophrenia: a multidimensional approach. World J Biol Psychiatry 2005;6(Suppl 2):23–30.

103. Shiloh R, Schapir L, Bar-Ziv D, et al. Association between corneal temperature and mental status of treatment-resistant schizophrenia in patients. Eur Neuropsychopharmacol 2009;19(9):654–8.

104. Lerner Y, Mintzer Y, Schestatzky M. Lithium combined with haloperidol in schizophrenic patients. Br J Psychiatry 1988;153:359–62.

105. Little KY, Gay TL, Vore M. Predictors of response to high dose antipsychotics in chronic schizophrenics. Psychiatry Res 1989;30(1):1–9.

106. Brotman AW, McCormick S 3rd. A role for high-dose antipsychotics. J Clin Psychiatry 1990;51(4):164–6.

107. Fink M, Sackeim HA. Convulsive therapy for schizophrenia. Schizophr Bull 1966; 22(1):27–39.

108. da Costa DA. The role of psychosurgery in the treatment of selected cases of refractory schizophrenia: a reappraisal. Schizophr Res 1997;28(2–3):223–30.

109. Soares MS, Paiva WS, Guertzenstein EZ, et al. Psychosurgery for schizophrenia: history and perspectives. Neuropsychiatr Dis Treat 2013;9:509–15.

110. Meltzer HY. Treatment-resistant schizophrenia–the role of clozapine. Curr Med Res Opin 1997;14(1):1–20.

111. Taylor DM, Duncan-McConnell D. Refractory schizophrenia and atypical antipsychotics. J Psychopharmacol 2000;14(4):409–18.

112. Chakos M, Lieberman J, Hoffman E, et al. Effectiveness of second-generation antipsychotics in patients with treatment-resistant schizophrenia: a review and meta-analysis of randomized trials. Am J Psychiatry 2001;158(4):518–26.

113. Wahlbeck K, Cheine M, Essali A, et al. Evidence of clozapine's effectiveness in schizophrenia: a systematic review and meta-analysis of randomized trials. Am J Psychiatry 1999;156(7):990–9.

114. Wahlbeck K, Cheine M, Essali MA. Clozapine versus typical neuroleptic medication for schizophrenia. Cochrane Database Syst Rev 2000;(2):CD000059.

115. Moncrieff J. Clozapine v. conventional antipsychotic drugs for treatment-resistant schizophrenia: a re-examination. Br J Psychiatry 2003;183:161–6.
116. Geddes J, Freemantle N, Harrison P, et al. Atypical antipsychotics in the treatment of schizophrenia: systematic overview and meta-regression analysis. BMJ 2000;321(7273):1371–6.
117. Davis JM, Chen N, Glick ID. A meta-analysis of the efficacy of second-generation antipsychotics. Arch Gen Psychiatry 2003;60(6):553–64.
118. Leucht S, Corves C, Arbter D, et al. Second-generation versus first-generation antipsychotic drugs for schizophrenia: a meta-analysis. Lancet 2009;373(9657):31–41.
119. Adams CE, Coutinho ES, Davis J, et al. Cochrane Schizophrenia Group. Schizophr Bull 2008;34(2):259–65.
120. Leucht S, Komossa K, Rummel-Kluge C, et al. A meta-analysis of head-to-head comparisons of second-generation antipsychotics in the treatment of schizophrenia. Am J Psychiatry 2009;166(2):152–63.
121. Asenjo Lobos C, Komossa K, Rummel-Kluge C, et al. Clozapine versus other atypical antipsychotics for schizophrenia. Cochrane Database Syst Rev 2010;(11):CD006633.
122. McEvoy JP, Lieberman JA, Stroup TS, et al. Effectiveness of clozapine versus olanzapine, quetiapine, and risperidone in patients with chronic schizophrenia who did not respond to prior atypical antipsychotic treatment. Am J Psychiatry 2006;163(4):600–10.
123. Lewis SW, Barnes TR, Davies L, et al. Randomized controlled trial of effect of prescription of clozapine versus other second-generation antipsychotic drugs in resistant schizophrenia. Schizophr Bull 2006;32(4):715–23.
124. Ringback Weitoft G, Berglund M, Lindstrom EA, et al. Mortality, attempted suicide, re-hospitalisation and prescription refill for clozapine and other antipsychotics in Sweden—a register-based study. Pharmacoepidemiol Drug Saf 2014;23(3):290–8.
125. Mortimer AM, Singh P, Shepherd CJ, et al. Clozapine for treatment-resistant schizophrenia: National Institute of Clinical Excellence (NICE) guidance in the real world. Clin Schizophr Relat Psychoses 2010;4(1):49–55.
126. Lal S, Thavundayil JX, Nair NP, et al. Levomepromazine versus chlorpromazine in treatment-resistant schizophrenia: a double-blind randomized trial. J Psychiatry Neurosci 2006;31(4):271–9.
127. Duggal HS, Mendhekar DN. High-dose aripiprazole in treatment-resistant schizophrenia. J Clin Psychiatry 2006;67(4):674–5.
128. Kane JM, Meltzer HY, Carson WH Jr, et al. Aripiprazole for treatment-resistant schizophrenia: results of a multicenter, randomized, double-blind, comparison study versus perphenazine. J Clin Psychiatry 2007;68(2):213–23.
129. Kane JM, Potkin SG, Daniel DG, et al. A double-blind, randomized study comparing the efficacy and safety of sertindole and risperidone in patients with treatment-resistant schizophrenia. J Clin Psychiatry 2011;72(2):194–204.
130. Kane JM, Khanna S, Rajadhyaksha S, et al. Efficacy and tolerability of ziprasidone in patients with treatment-resistant schizophrenia. Int Clin Psychopharmacol 2006;21(1):21–8.
131. Lindenmayer JP, Citrome L, Khan A, et al. A randomized, double-blind, parallel-group, fixed-dose, clinical trial of quetiapine at 600 versus 1200 mg/d for patients with treatment-resistant schizophrenia or schizoaffective disorder. J Clin Psychopharmacol 2011;31(2):160–8.

132. Quintero J, Barbudo E, Molina JD, et al. The effectiveness of the combination therapy of amisulpride and quetiapine for managing treatment-resistant schizophrenia: a naturalistic study. J Clin Psychopharmacol 2011;31:240–2.

133. Meltzer HY, Lindenmayer JP, Kwentus J, et al. A six month randomized controlled trial of long acting injectable risperidone 50 and 100mg in treatment resistant schizophrenia. Schizophr Res 2014;154(1–3):14–22.

134. Wahlbeck K, Cheine M, Tuisku K, et al. Risperidone versus clozapine in treatment-resistant schizophrenia: a randomized pilot study. Prog Neuropsychopharmacol Biol Psychiatry 2000;24(6):911–22.

135. Bondolfi G, Dufour H, Patris M, et al. Risperidone versus clozapine in treatment-resistant chronic schizophrenia: a randomized double-blind study. The Risperidone Study Group. Am J Psychiatry 1998;155(4):499–504.

136. Tollefson GD, Birkett MA, Kiesler GM, et al. Double-blind comparison of olanzapine versus clozapine in schizophrenic patients clinically eligible for treatment with clozapine. Biol Psychiatry 2001;49(1):52–63.

137. Bitter I, Dossenbach MR, Brook S, et al. Olanzapine versus clozapine in treatment-resistant or treatment-intolerant schizophrenia. Prog Neuropsychopharmacol Biol Psychiatry 2004;28(1):173–80.

138. Kumra S, Kranzler H, Gerbino-Rosen G, et al. Clozapine and "high-dose" olanzapine in refractory early-onset schizophrenia: a 12-week randomized and double-blind comparison. Biol Psychiatry 2008;63(5):524–9.

139. Meltzer HY, Bobo WV, Roy A, et al. A randomized, double-blind comparison of clozapine and high-dose olanzapine in treatment-resistant patients with schizophrenia. J Clin Psychiatry 2008;69(2):274–85.

140. Volavka J, Czobor P, Sheitman B, et al. Clozapine, olanzapine, risperidone, and haloperidol in the treatment of patients with chronic schizophrenia and schizoaffective disorder. Am J Psychiatry 2002;159(2):255–62.

141. Conley RR, Tamminga CA, Bartko JJ, et al. Olanzapine compared with chlorpromazine in treatment-resistant schizophrenia. Am J Psychiatry 1998;155(7):914–20.

142. Naber D, Riedel M, Klimke A, et al. Randomized double blind comparison of olanzapine vs. clozapine on subjective well-being and clinical outcome in patients with schizophrenia. Acta Psychiatr Scand 2005;111(2):106–15.

143. Kishi T, Suzuki T, Sekiguchi H, et al. Efficacy and tolerability of high dose olanzapine in Japanese patients with treatment-resistant schizophrenia. Asian J Psychiatr 2013;6(1):86–7.

144. Souza JS, Kayo M, Tassell I, et al. Efficacy of olanzapine in comparison with clozapine for treatment-resistant schizophrenia: evidence from a systematic review and meta-analyses. CNS Spectr 2013;18(2):82–9.

145. Meltzer HY, Alphs L, Green AI, et al. Clozapine treatment for suicidality in schizophrenia: International Suicide Prevention Trial (InterSePT). Arch Gen Psychiatry 2003;60(1):82–91.

146. Hennen J, Baldessarini RJ. Suicidal risk during treatment with clozapine: a meta-analysis. Schizophr Res 2005;73(2–3):139–45.

147. Tiihonen J, Lonnqvist J, Wahlbeck K, et al. 11-year follow-up of mortality in patients with schizophrenia: a population-based cohort study (FIN11 study). Lancet 2009;374(9690):620–7.

148. Chung C, Remington G. Predictors and markers of clozapine response. Psychopharmacology (Berl) 2005;179(2):317–35.

149. Kinon BJ, Ahl J, Stauffer VL, et al. Dose response and atypical antipsychotics in schizophrenia. CNS Drugs 2004;18(9):597–616.

150. Miller DD, Fleming F, Holman TL, et al. Plasma clozapine concentrations as a predictor of clinical response: a follow-up study. J Clin Psychiatry 1994; 55(Suppl B):117–21.

151. Potkin SG, Bera R, Gulasekaram B, et al. Plasma clozapine concentrations predict clinical response in treatment-resistant schizophrenia. J Clin Psychiatry 1994;55(Suppl B):133–6.

152. Remington G, Agid O, Foussias G, et al. Clozapine and therapeutic drug monitoring: is there sufficient evidence for an upper threshold? Psychopharmacology (Berl) 2013;225(3):505–18.

153. Foster A, Buckley P. Pharmacogenetics and treatment resistant schizophrenia. In: Buckley P, Gaughran F, editors. Treatment-refractory schizophrenia: a clinical conundrum. Heildelberg (Germany): Springer; 2014. p. 179–83.

154. Souza RP, Romano-Silva MA, Lieberman JA, et al. Association study of GSK3 gene polymorphisms with schizophrenia and clozapine response. Psychopharmacology (Berl) 2008;200(2):177–86.

155. Kohlrausch FB, Salatino-Oliveira A, Gama CS, et al. Influence of serotonin transporter gene polymorphisms on clozapine response in Brazilian schizophrenics. J Psychiatr Res 2010;44(16):1158–62.

156. Souza RP, Meltzer HY, Lieberman JA, et al. Influence of neurexin 1 (NRXN1) polymorphisms in clozapine response. Hum Psychopharmacol 2010;25(7–8): 582–5.

157. Lett TA, Tiwari AK, Meltzer HY, et al. The putative functional rs1045881 marker of neurexin-1 in schizophrenia and clozapine response. Schizophr Res 2011; 132(2–3):121–4.

158. Hwang R, Tiwari AK, Zai CC, et al. Dopamine D4 and D5 receptor gene variant effects on clozapine response in schizophrenia: replication and exploration. Prog Neuropsychopharmacol Biol Psychiatry 2012;37(1):62–75.

159. Kohlrausch FB. Pharmacogenetics in schizophrenia: a review of clozapine studies. Rev Bras Psiquiatr 2013;35(3):305–17.

160. Friedman L, Knutson L, Shurell M, et al. Prefrontal sulcal prominence is inversely related to response to clozapine in schizophrenia. Biol Psychiatry 1991;29(9): 865–77.

161. Honer WG, Smith GN, Lapointe JS, et al. Regional cortical anatomy and clozapine response in refractory schizophrenia. Neuropsychopharmacology 1995; 13(1):85–7.

162. Konicki PE, Kwon KY, Steele V, et al. Prefrontal cortical sulcal widening associated with poor treatment response to clozapine. Schizophr Res 2001;48(2–3): 173–6.

163. Arango C, Breier A, McMahon R, et al. The relationship of clozapine and haloperidol treatment response to prefrontal, hippocampal, and caudate brain volumes. Am J Psychiatry 2003;160(8):1421–7.

164. Bilder RM, Wu H, Chakos MH, et al. Cerebral morphometry and clozapine treatment in schizophrenia. J Clin Psychiatry 1994;55(Suppl B):53–6.

165. Lauriello J, Mathalon DH, Rosenbloom M, et al. Association between regional brain volumes and clozapine response in schizophrenia. Biol Psychiatry 1998; 43(12):879–86.

166. Molina V, Reig S, Sarramea F, et al. Anatomical and functional brain variables associated with clozapine response in treatment-resistant schizophrenia. Psychiatry Res 2003;124(3):153–61.

167. Molina Rodriguez V, Montz Andree R, Perez Castejon MJ, et al. SPECT study of regional cerebral perfusion in neuroleptic-resistant schizophrenic patients who

responded or did not respond to clozapine. Am J Psychiatry 1996;153(10): 1343–6.

168. Molina V, Gispert JD, Reig S, et al. Cerebral metabolic changes induced by clozapine in schizophrenia and related to clinical improvement. Psychopharmacology (Berl) 2005;178(1):17–26.

169. Molina V, Tamayo P, Montes C, et al. Clozapine may partially compensate for task-related brain perfusion abnormalities in risperidone-resistant schizophrenia patients. Prog Neuropsychopharmacol Biol Psychiatry 2008;32(4):948–54.

170. Elkis H, Meltzer HY. Refractory schizophrenia. Rev Bras Psiquiatr 2007;29(Suppl 2):S41–7 [in Portuguese].

171. Buckley P, Miller A, Olsen J, et al. When symptoms persist: clozapine augmentation strategies. Schizophr Bull 2001;27(4):615–28.

172. Anil Yagcioglu AE, Kivircik Akdede BB, Turgut TI, et al. A double-blind controlled study of adjunctive treatment with risperidone in schizophrenic patients partially responsive to clozapine: efficacy and safety. J Clin Psychiatry 2005;66(1): 63–72.

173. Mouaffak F, Tranulis C, Gourevitch R, et al. Augmentation strategies of clozapine with antipsychotics in the treatment of ultraresistant schizophrenia. Clin Neuropharmacol 2006;29(1):28–33.

174. Barnes TR, McEvedy CJ, Nelson HE. Management of treatment resistant schizophrenia unresponsive to clozapine. Br J Psychiatry Suppl 1996;(31):31–40.

175. Williams L, Newton G, Roberts K, et al. Clozapine-resistant schizophrenia: a positive approach. Br J Psychiatry 2002;181:184–7.

176. Remington G. Augmenting clozapine response in treatment-resistant schizophrenia. In: Elkis H, Meltzer H, editors. Therapy-resistant schizophrenia. Basel (Switzerland): Karger; 2010. p. 129–51.

177. Souza J, Kayo M, Henna Neto J, et al. New therapeutic strategies for resistance to clozapine and treatment-resistant schizophrenia. In: Elkis H, Meltzer H, editors. Therapy-resistant schizophrenia. Basel (Switzerland): Karger; 2010. p. 152–64.

178. Castle D, Keks N. What can we do if clozapine fails? pharmacologic choices and differential outcomes. In: Buckley P, Gaughran F, editors. Treatment-refractory schizophrenia—a clinical conundrum. Heildelberg (Germany): Springer; 2014. p. 93–106.

179. Barbui C, Signoretti A, Mule S, et al. Does the addition of a second antipsychotic drug improve clozapine treatment? Schizophr Bull 2009;35(2):458–68.

180. Sommer IE, Begemann MJ, Temmerman A, et al. Pharmacological augmentation strategies for schizophrenia patients with insufficient response to clozapine: a quantitative literature review. Schizophr Bull 2012;38(5):1003–11.

181. Porcelli S, Balzarro B, Serretti A. Clozapine resistance: augmentation strategies. Eur Neuropsychopharmacol 2012;22(3):165–82.

182. Miyamoto S, Jarskog LF, Fleischhacker WW. New therapeutic approaches for treatment-resistant schizophrenia: a look to the future. J Psychiatr Res 2014; 58:1–6.

183. Tiihonen J, Wahlbeck K, Kiviniemi V. The efficacy of lamotrigine in clozapine-resistant schizophrenia: a systematic review and meta-analysis. Schizophr Res 2009;109(1–3):10–4.

184. Jandl M, Kaschka W. Treatment of therapy-resistant auditory hallucinations in schizophrenia patients by repetitive transcranial magnetic stimulation. In: Elkis H, Meltzer H, editors. Therapy-resistant schizophrenia. Basel (Switzerland): Karger; 2010. p. 177–94.

185. Rosenquist P, Ahmed A, McCall WV. Therapeutic brain stimulation in treatment resistant schizophrenia. In: Buckley P, Gaughran F, editors. Treatment-refractory schizophrenia—a clinical conundrum. Heildelberg (Germany): Springer; 2014. p. 107–20.

186. Champattana W. Electroconvulsive therapy for treatment-refractory schizophrenia. In: Elkis H, Meltzer H, editors. Therapy-resistant schizophrenia. Basel (Switzerland): Karger; 2010. p. 165–76.

187. Sinclair D, Adams CE. Treatment resistant schizophrenia: a comprehensive survey of randomised controlled trials. BMC Psychiatry 2014;14:253.

188. Pompili M, Lester D, Dominici G, et al. Indications for electroconvulsive treatment in schizophrenia: a systematic review. Schizophr Res 2013;146(1–3):1–9.

189. Petrides G, Malur C, Braga RJ, et al. Electroconvulsive therapy augmentation in clozapine-resistant schizophrenia: a prospective, randomized study. Am J Psychiatry 2015;172(1):52–8.

190. Hunter E, Johns L, Onwumere J, et al. Cognitive behavioural therapy for psychosis. In: Buckley P, Gaughran F, editors. Treatment-refractory schizophrenia—a clinical conundrum. Heildelberg (Germany): Springer; 2014.

191. Burns AM, Erickson DH, Brenner CA. Cognitive-behavioral therapy for medication-resistant psychosis: a meta-analytic review. Psychiatr Serv 2014;65(7):874–80.

192. Barretto EM, Kayo M, Avrichir BS, et al. A preliminary controlled trial of cognitive behavioral therapy in clozapine-resistant schizophrenia. J Nerv Ment Dis 2009; 197(11):865–8.

193. Pinto A, La Pia S, Mennella R, et al. Cognitive-behavioral therapy and clozapine for clients with treatment-refractory schizophrenia. Psychiatr Serv 1999;50(7): 901–4.

194. Samara MT, Dold M, Gianatsi M, et al. Efficacy, acceptability, and tolerability of antipsychotics in treatment-resistant schizophrenia: a network meta-analysis. JAMA Psychiatry 2016;73(3):199–210.

195. Kane JM, Correll CU. The role of clozapine in treatment-resistant schizophrenia. JAMA Psychiatry 2016;73(3):187–8.

196. Leucht S, Cipriani A, Spineli L, et al. Comparative efficacy and tolerability of 15 antipsychotic drugs in schizophrenia: a multiple-treatments meta-analysis. Lancet 2013;382(9896):951–62.

Transcending Psychosis
The Complexity of Comorbidity in Schizophrenia

Sun Young Yum, MD[a], Michael Y. Hwang, MD[b],*,
Henry A. Nasrallah, MD[c], Lewis A. Opler, MD, PhD[d]

KEYWORDS

- Schizophrenia • Comorbid disorder • Pathogenesis • Diagnosis • Treatment

KEY POINTS

- Conceptual issues of comorbidity in schizophrenia are discussed.
- The biological pathogenesis of comorbidity in schizophrenia is reviewed.
- Subtyping strategy of schizophrenia with comorbid disorder is discussed.
- Diagnostic and clinical issues of comorbidity in schizophrenia are discussed.
- Treatment and outcome of schizophrenias with comorbid disorder are considered.

CONCEPTUAL ISSUES OF COMORBIDITY IN SCHIZOPHRENIA

Physicists spent many years debating whether light was best conceptualized as waves or as particles, until it became apparent that it could be conceptualized simultaneously as both waves and particles. Long-standing debates in psychiatry on categorical versus dimensional conceptualizations of psychiatric disorders may someday arrive at a similar conclusion.

Mastery of diagnostic categorization has been considered a core competency of a modern-day psychiatrist. This approach suffers from inadequate attention to other coexisting conditions. Once a clinician arrives at a categorization within the hierarchical diagnostic system, all symptoms tend to be viewed as a part of that diagnostic entity.

With the recent emergence of dimensional approaches to psychiatric research, there seems to be an increasing expectation that symptoms will neatly fit to

Disclosure: Dr M.Y. Hwang is Staff Physician, Department of Veterans Administration and Former Member of FDA Advisory Board. Dr S.Y. Yum is a full time employee of Boehringer Ingelheim Pharmaceutical.

[a] Department of Clinical Medical Science, Seoul National University, Seoul, South Korea; [b] Department of Psychiatry, New York Medical College, Franklin Delano Roosevelt VA Medical Center (116), 2094 Albany Post Road, Montrose, NY 10548, USA; [c] Department of Psychiatry, St Louis University, St Louis, MO 63104, USA; [d] Predoctoral Program in Clinical Psychology, Long Island University, Brookville, NY 11548, USA
* Corresponding author.
E-mail address: Michael.hwang@va.gov

Abbreviations and acronyms	
DSM-IV	*Diagnostic and Statistical Manual of Mental Disorders*, 4th edition
DSM-V	*Diagnostic and Statistical Manual of Mental Disorders*, 5th edition
FDA	US Food and Drug Administration
OC	Obsessive–compulsive
OCD	Obsessive-compulsive disorder
OCS	Obsessive–compulsive symptoms
RDoC	Research Domain Criteria

corresponding circuits across the diagnoses. This approach fails to take into account a more macroscopic view of how symptoms do not exist in a vacuum, and often, the context of the symptom presentation can be more important than the symptom itself.

The diagnostic and treatment issues of coexisting psychiatric symptoms and/or disorders in schizophrenia remain conceptually controversial and clinically challenging. Schizophrenia is a complex, heterogeneous, and disabling psychiatric disorder that disrupts cognitive, perceptual, and emotional functioning. It has become increasingly clear over the years that there are many dimensions within the category of schizophrenic spectrum disorder.[1] However one may pause to question whether lumping all symptoms into one disorder or treating each symptom phenomena as a distinct condition can be regarded as a categorical or dimensional approach. Both concepts are compatible with either approach.

Traditional medical training encourages finding one diagnosis that can explain multiple symptoms and signs. Therefore, once a diagnosis of schizophrenia is made, symptoms beyond overt psychosis have generally been considered as byproducts or associated symptoms of schizophrenic spectrum disorder. There is an emphasis on arriving at a categorical diagnosis that can explain most of the clinical problems while recognizing the existence of different symptom dimensions within the categorization.

Proponents of the concept of comorbidity in schizophrenia have argued that symptoms such as depression,[2] dementia,[3] panic,[4] obsessive–compulsive disorder (OCD),[5] posttraumatic stress disorder,[6] and eating disorders[7] are separate disorders. In this view, the symptom dimensions are emphasized, but in the context of the categorical diagnosis.

Because both views recognize both categories and dimensions, we may already be more advanced in our phenomenological discussion than the physicists. So, why is there still a need to continue talking about comorbidities? This discussion is clinically important; in the former case, treatment of psychosis may lead to resolution of other associated symptoms, whereas in the latter case symptoms other than psychosis need separate clinical attention.

This paper discusses these conceptual aspects of comorbidities in schizophrenia, with a focus on schizophrenia and OCD comorbidity as an example to illustrate the arguments.

CLINICAL SUBTYPES

Identifying subgroups with distinct clustering of symptoms to predict longitudinal clinical course have been proposed as a foundation to systematically understanding the pathogeneses and treatment implications of schizophrenia.[1] Delineation of phenotypes has been viewed as fundamental to identifying candidate genes. Alternatively, dissecting behavioral correlates was seen as necessary for finding the responsible neural circuits. Subtyping with comorbidities has been proposed as phenomenologic groundwork for biological understanding of schizophrenia.

Despite long debates and some advances, the following questions remain:

1. What are the diagnostic criteria for defining comorbid disorders in schizophrenia?
2. What is the biopsychosocial basis for comorbidity?
3. What are the optimal pharmacologic and psychological treatments?
4. Are well-recognized comorbidity subtypes (eg, schizoaffective disorder, schizoobsessive disorder) a clinically meaningful approach?

One of the most important factors contributing to the in upsurge of research and clinical interest in comorbidities was the modifications in the *Diagnostic and Statistical Manual of Mental Disorders*, 4th edition (DSM-IV),[8] which acknowledged the possibility of distinct comorbid psychiatric disorders in patients with schizophrenia. Since its debut in the DSM-IV, recognition of OCD as a comorbidity in schizophrenia has steadily increased to an estimated rate of more than 20%[9] from less than 5% in the early 20th century.[10,11] Evidence also suggests that the prevalence rates of OCD or obsessive-compulsive symptoms (OCS) vary according to the stage of psychotic illness, as well as in patient populations at high risk for developing schizophrenia.[9,12]

Clinical and research evidence to date suggest that schizophrenia with OCS may constitute a distinct subgroup of schizophrenic illness with clinical and biological profiles that is mediated by multiple underlying psychobiological pathogenic processes. The clinical obsessive–compulsive (OC) phenomena observed in psychotic disorders are similar to those observed in individuals with traditional OCD. Frequent clinical manifestations include aggressive sexual and religious obsessions with checking compulsions, obsessions of contamination with cleaning compulsions, and hoarding.[5] OCS can also present in the form of preoccupations and rituals related to eating and body image.[7] Consequently, the old clinical and research categorization of neurotic and psychotic OC phenomena has become controversial. This dated understanding of comorbidity still remains in clinical practice, but how it will evolves in the context of the *Diagnostic and Statistical Manual of Mental Disorders*, 5th edition, remains to be seen.

The new fifth edition of the DSM has minor changes for categorizing schizophrenia, but includes some notable changes in the conceptualization of OCD.[13]

1. OCD and related disorders now have a designated new chapter separate from anxiety disorder.
2. The previous DSM-IV specifier "with poor insight" has been modified to allow for varying digress of insight: good or fair insight, poor insight, and absent insight/delusional OCD (ie, complete conviction that OCD beliefs are true). This insight specifier is intended to improve differential diagnosis by emphasizing that the presence or absent insight or delusional belief warrants a diagnosis of the relevant OC and related disorder, rather than psychotic disorder.
3. The DSM-5 includes a new category for substance-/medication-induced OC and related disorder. This reflects the recognition that substances and medications can present with symptoms similar to primary OC and related disorders.

The DSM-5 supports the diagnosis of OCD without the need for traditionally important distinction between severe neurotic obsessions and psychotic delusional preoccupations manifested in psychotic disorders. Furthermore, evidence suggests that the onset, clinical course, treatment response, and prognosis of comorbid disorders are diverse. Depression, panic, and OC phenomena may first manifest during the premorbid phase as well as in late phases of schizophrenic illness. A recent metaanalysis of the temporal sequence of schizophrenia and OCD, however, showed that OCD symptoms precede the onset of schizophrenia.[14]

Based on the recent research evidence we have previously suggested a subtyping strategy for OC schizophrenia based on the chronology of symptom emergence[5]:

1. OCS occurring during prodromal phase of psychotic illness. OC symptoms in this group may worsen during the course of the illness accompanied by functional deterioration.
2. In some patients, the OCS may resolve independent of the progression of psychotic illness.
3. The OCS or OCD may emerge or persist during course of the schizophrenic illness:
   a. OCS may develop as a part of acute psychotic exacerbation of preoccupation, with or without ritualistic behaviors. The psychotic preoccupations or ruminations that emerge along with the acute phase of psychotic illness, may resolve with overall improvement of psychosis.
   b. OCS may develop or exacerbate after treatment with atypical antipsychotics that possess a potent antiserotonergic receptor profile. Recent reports found that such drugs may induce OC manifestations that respond to the anti-OC pharmacologic regimen.

Alternatively, subtyping could be based on longitudinal functional outcome. Although evidence of its long-term clinical impact needs further study, current evidence suggests that comorbid OCD in schizophrenia is associated with greater psychosis, worse cognitive and psychosocial functioning, and increased suicide risk.[15–17]

Advances in neurobiological and pharmacological science have provided important feedback on behavioral phenomenology. Although discovered by chance, it was found that lithium, tricyclics, antipsychotics, barbiturates, and benzodiazepines validated categorical diagnoses of bipolar disorder, major depression, schizophrenia, and anxiety. Pharmacologic assays of these drugs led to hypotheses about pathogenesis of psychiatric illnesses within categorical diagnoses. There are also hopes that advances in molecular biology will allow syndromic illnesses to be subcategorized based on their etiopathogenesis.

NEUROBIOLOGICAL EVIDENCE OF OBSESSIVE–COMPULSIVE PHENOMENA IN SCHIZOPHRENIA
Preclinical Studies

For many years, animals with spontaneous stereotypies have been explored as models of OCD. Many of the behaviors such as induced polydipsia, food restriction–induced hyperactivity, repetitive pacing, and self-injurious behaviors are induced by stressful environments. It is difficult to tease apart the effect of stress and anxiety, and whether the manifest repetitive behaviors are consequent. These animals show variable responses to anti-OCD pharmacotherapy. Non–anxiety-related stereotypic behaviors in the mouse model such as the marble burying test (which is a nonaversive stimulus) are reduced by traditional anti-OCD drugs as well as antiserotonergic antipsychotics.[18,19] Interestingly, this behavior is also extinguished by aripiprazole via 5-HT1A receptor-independent mechanisms and a selective dopamine D2 receptor antagonist, L-741,626.[20]

Animal assays in schizophrenia have made notable progress over the years, relying previously only on those with face validity (ie, symptoms look alike in animal and human) to assays developed from bottom-up reverse translation with a priori hypothesis (eg, risk genes), which provide better construct validity. Of the latter, the candidate gene approach is one of the most promising in terms of informing us of the neurodevelopmental aspects underlying the disorders. One example is the NR1 hypomorphic mice. Of the glutamate N-methyl-$_D$-aspartate receptors, NR1 subunit is consistently associated with schizophrenia. The Nr1neo$^{-/-}$ mice exhibit the specific behavioral phenotypes including increased locomotor activity, deficits in prepulse inhibition, repetitive behavior, and excessive grooming.[21,22] These are emerging as animal assays for schizophrenia and have been shown to have some predictive validity for pharmacologic effects. However, more accurately, Nr1neo/mice are models of glutamate hypofunction. This glutamate theory may support our previous hypotheses about dopamine and serotonin signaling convergence, as well as circuits for OCD and schizophrenia. In addition to genetic studies, the interface between these 2 disorders may be sought through the neuroendocrine and neuroimmune systems.

In summary, animal models of OCD respond to traditional anti-OCD as well as antipsychotic medications. In addition, a candidate gene identified in schizophrenia leads to behavioral phenotypes consistent with OCS.

Clinical Evidence

Previous biomarker studies have demonstrated possibilities for both distinct as well as overlapping neurobiological pathogenesis of OCD and schizophrenia. Neuroimaging studies have shown volumetric as well as functional differences between OCD and schizophrenia.[23,24] The challenge in interpreting these findings is determining whether the differences shown in regions of interest are casual or reactive. In contrast, neuropsychological testing in OCD has demonstrated deficits in the orbitofrontostriatal circuit, which is also implicated in schizophrenia. Much of the manifest OCS resemble childhood behaviors that resolve with age. It has been suggested that maturation of the prefrontal cortex and its subcortical connections are critical to inhibiting ritualistic, repetitive behaviors and replace them with more goal-directed behaviors.[25] One of the electrophysiologic markers often denoted as an endophenotype of schizophrenia, the P300, was shown to have significantly smaller amplitudes in both schizophrenia and OCD, although this deficit was correlated with differential cognitive deficits on neuropsychological testing.[26]

For atypical, antipsychotic-induced de novo emergence of OCS, there may be a genetic risk factor. In a pharmacogenetic case control association study of schizophrenia outpatients, patients with and without atypical antipsychotic-induced OCS showed sequence variations in the glutamate transporter gene *SLC1A1* that were associated with susceptibility to atypical antipsychotic–induced OCS.[27]

Finally, the comorbidity in schizophrenia may have a genetic basis. Recent genetic advances have recognized the phenomenon of pleiotropy in schizophrenia, where 1 gene can influence multiple clinical phenotypic traits. For example, a large genome-wide association study of 33,332 psychiatric patients and 27,888 healthy controls found a genetic link (the calcium channel gene *CACNA1C*) across 5 major psychiatric disorders: schizophrenia, autism spectrum disorders, major depression, attention deficit hyperactivity disorder, and bipolar disorder.[28] The *CACNA1C* gene has been associated with neurocognitive deficits[29] as well as schizotypal personality,[30] both of which are linked to schizophrenia. Pleiotropy may explain why some comorbidities such as anxiety are observed very commonly in patients with bipolar disorder or why OCD is often seen in patients with schizophrenia.

FUTURE PROSPECTS

For now, schizophrenia with comorbid conditions needs to be looked at both from a categorical and from a dimensional perspective. The debates over the validity of the DSM-5 categories and the call to complement them with a dimensional approach, such as the Research Domain Criteria (RDoC)[31] are not new. The publication of the DSM-5 in 2013 is a welcome development. It offers the best way of describing psychiatric disorders and like the DSM-IV, it allows room for flexible thinking, including recognition of comorbid conditions in clinical practice.

The simultaneous announcement of the National Institutes of Mental Health RDoC Project need not be seen as an attack on the DSM-5, but rather as a call to find meaningful system that is, relevant in clinical practice and for future research as we move on from the DSM-5 toward "precision psychiatry."[32]

Like physicists learning to think of light as both waves and particles, we need to be able to work with categorical systems like the DSM-5 and *International Classification of Diseases,* 11th edition, while ensuring that all dimensions of psychopathology are attended to in individual patients.

New drugs in development addressing dimensional aspects of schizophrenia may also pave the way for better phenomenological and biological understanding of the illness. The US Food and Drug Administration (FDA) has traditionally held the view that symptoms or symptom clusters of a defined DSM syndrome as well as comorbid conditions cannot be recognized as separate indications due to concerns over pseudospecificity. Fortunately, the FDA's position has evolved in recent years to accommodate the "real world" of clinical practice. For example, negative symptoms in schizophrenia are now recognized by the FDA as a legitimate target for drug development. But the FDA has asked several questions along the way: (1) Are negative symptoms phenomenologically distinct with independent clinical course from other symptoms of schizophrenia? (2) Is there evidence that negative symptoms respond differently to drug treatment than do other schizophrenic symptoms? and (3) Is the pathophysiology of negative symptoms understood to be different from that of other schizophrenic symptoms?[33,34]

The FDA has also recognized cognitive impairment in schizophrenia as a possible target indication, and progress has been made in discussions about cognitive impairment in depression. While these may be considered exceptions that will not be applicable to all comorbidities, they are nonetheless a big leap forward towards a systematic and individualized management of schizophrenic patients with comorbid disorders.

REFERENCES

1. Opler LA, Hwang MY. Schizophrenia: a multidimensional disorder. Psychiatr Ann 1994;24(9):491–5.
2. Siris SG, Addington D, Azorin JM, et al. Depression in schizophrenia: recognition and management in the USA. Schizophr Res 2001;47(2–3):185–97.
3. Jeste DV, Symonds LL, Harris MJ, et al. Nondementia nonpraecox dementia praecox? Late-onset schizophrenia. Am J Geriatr Psychiatry 1997;5(4): 302–17.
4. Sandberg L, Siris SG. "Panic disorder" in schizophrenia. J Nerv Ment Dis 1987; 175(10):627–8.
5. Hwang MY, Kim SW, Yum SY, et al. Management of schizophrenia with obsessive-compulsive features. Psychiatr Clin North Am 2009;32(4):835–51.
6. Vogel M, Spitzer C, Barnow S, et al. The role of trauma and PTSD-related symptoms for dissociation and psychopathological distress in inpatients with schizophrenia. Psychopathology 2006;39(5):236–42.
7. Yum SY, Caracci G, Hwang MY. Schizophrenia and eating disorders. Psychiatr Clin North Am 2009;32(4):809–19.

8. American Psychiatric Association (APA). Task Force on DSM-IV. Diagnostic and statistical manual of mental disorders: DSM-IV. 4th edition. Washington, DC: American Psychiatric Association; 1994.

9. Craig T, Hwang MY, Bromet EJ. Obsessive-compulsive and panic symptoms in patients with first-admission psychosis. Am J Psychiatry 2002;159(4):592–8.

10. Jahrreis W. Obsessions during schizophrenia. Arch Psychiatr Nervenkr 1926;77: 740–88.

11. Rosen I. The clinical significance of obsessions in schizophrenia. J Ment Sci 1957;103:773–85.

12. Poyurovsky M, Fuchs C, Weizman A. Obsessive-compulsive disorder in patients with first-episode schizophrenia. Am J Psychiatry 1999;156(12):1998–2000.

13. American Psychiatric Association (APA). DSM-5 Task Force. Diagnostic and statistical manual of mental disorders: DSM-5. 5th edition. Washington, DC: American Psychiatric Association; 2013.

14. Devulapalli KK, Welge JA, Nasrallah HA. Temporal sequence of clinical manifestation in schizophrenia with co-morbid OCD: review and meta-analysis. Psychiatry Res 2008;161(1):105–8.

15. Hwang MY, Morgan JE, Losconzcy MF. Clinical and neuropsychological profiles of obsessive-compulsive schizophrenia: a pilot study. J Neuropsychiatry Clin Neurosci 2000;12(1):91–4.

16. Ucok A, Ceylan ME, Tihan AK, et al. Obsessive compulsive disorder and symptoms may have different effects on schizophrenia. Prog Neuropsychopharmacol Biol Psychiatry 2011;35(2):429–33.

17. de Haan L, Sterk B, Wouters L, et al. The 5-year course of obsessive-compulsive symptoms and obsessive-compulsive disorder in first-episode schizophrenia and related disorders. Schizophr Bull 2013;39(1):151–60.

18. Matsushita M, Egashira N, Harada S, et al. Perospirone, a novel antipsychotic drug, inhibits marble-burying behavior via 5-HT1A receptor in mice: implications for obsessive-compulsive disorder. J Pharmacol Sci 2005;99(2):154–9.

19. Harasawa T, Ago Y, Itoh S, et al. Role of serotonin type 1A receptors in fluvoxamine-induced inhibition of marble-burying behavior in mice. Behav Pharmacol 2006;17(7):637–40.

20. Egashira N, Okuno R, Matsushita M, et al. Aripiprazole inhibits marble-burying behavior via 5-hydroxytryptamine (5-HT)1A receptor-independent mechanisms. Eur J Pharmacol 2008;592(1–3):103–8.

21. Mohn AR, Gainetdinov RR, Caron MG, et al. Mice with reduced NMDA receptor expression display behaviors related to schizophrenia. Cell 1999;98(4):427–36.

22. Gandal MJ, Anderson RL, Billingslea EN, et al. Mice with reduced NMDA receptor expression: more consistent with autism than schizophrenia? Genes Brain Behav 2012;11(6):740–50.

23. Kwon JS, Shin YW, Kim CW, et al. Similarity and disparity of obsessive-compulsive disorder and schizophrenia in MR volumetric abnormalities of the hippocampus-amygdala complex. J Neurol Neurosurg Psychiatr 2003;74(7): 962–4.

24. Kim JJ, Youn T, Lee JM, et al. Morphometric abnormality of the insula in schizophrenia: a comparison with obsessive-compulsive disorder and normal control using MRI. Schizophr Res 2003;60(2–3):191–8.

25. Gillan CM, Papmeyer M, Morein-Zamir S, et al. Disruption in the balance between goal-directed behavior and habit learning in obsessive-compulsive disorder. Am J Psychiatry 2011;168(7):718–26.

26. Kim MS, Kang SS, Youn T, et al. Neuropsychological correlates of P300 abnormalities in patients with schizophrenia and obsessive-compulsive disorder. Psychiatry Res 2003;123(2):109–23.

27. Kwon JS, Joo YH, Nam HJ, et al. Association of the glutamate transporter gene SLC1A1 with atypical antipsychotics-induced obsessive-compulsive symptoms. Arch Gen Psychiatry 2009;66(11):1233–41.

28. Cross-Disorder Group of the Psychiatric Genomics Consortium. Identification of risk loci with shared effects on five major psychiatric disorders: a genome-wide analysis. Lancet 2013;381(9875):1371–9.

29. Hori H, Yamamoto N, Fujii T, et al. Effects of the CACNA1C risk allele on neurocognition in patients with schizophrenia and healthy individuals. Sci Rep 2012; 2:634.

30. Roussos P, Bitsios P, Giakoumaki SG, et al. CACNA1C as a risk factor for schizotypal personality disorder and schizotypy in healthy individuals. Psychiatry Res 2013;206(1):122–3.

31. Cuthbert BN. The RDoC framework: facilitating transition from ICD/DSM to dimensional approaches that integrate neuroscience and psychopathology. World Psychiatry 2014;13(1):28–35.

32. Insel TR. The NIMH Research Domain Criteria (RDoC) Project: precision medicine for psychiatry. Am J Psychiatry 2014;171(4):395–7.

33. Laughren T, Levin R. Food and Drug Administration perspective on negative symptoms in schizophrenia as a target for a drug treatment claim. Schizophr Bull 2006;32(2):220–2.

34. Laughren T, Levin R. Food and Drug Administration commentary on methodological issues in negative symptom trials. Schizophr Bull 2011;37(2):255–6.

Detecting and Managing Adverse Effects of Antipsychotic Medications
Current State of Play

Donna Ames, MD[a,b,*], Sian M. Carr-Lopez, PharmD[c,d],
Mary A. Gutierrez, PharmD, BCPP[e], Joseph M. Pierre, MD[f,g],
Jennifer A. Rosen, PharmD, BCPP[h,i,j], Susan Shakib, PharmD, BCPS[k,l],
Lynn M. Yudofsky, MD[m]

KEYWORDS

- Antipsychotic medication • Adverse effects • First-generation antipsychotics
- Second-generation antipsychotics • Weight gain • Hyperlipidemia • QT prolongation
- Hyperprolactinemia

KEY POINTS

- This review provides a summary of the most recent evidence of the adverse effects profiles of each of the currently available antipsychotic medications.
- This article reviews the relative propensity for certain antipsychotics to induce weight gain, diabetes, hyperlipidemia (HLP), cardiac side effects, sudden death, sexual side effects, and osteoporosis.

Continued

---

[a] Department of Psychiatry, Psychosocial Rehabilitation and Recovery Center, West Los Angeles Veterans Affairs Medical Center, 11301 Wilshire Boulevard, Los Angeles, CA 90073, USA; [b] David Geffen School of Medicine at UCLA, 10833 Le Conte Avenue, Los Angeles, CA 90095, USA; [c] Pharmacy Service, Veterans Affairs Northern California Health Care System, 10535 Hospital Way, Mather, CA 95655, USA; [d] Department of Pharmacy Practice, University of the Pacific, 3601 Pacific Avenue, Stockton, CA 95211, USA; [e] Chapman University School of Pharmacy, 9401 Jeronimo Road, Irvine, CA 92618, USA; [f] Schizophrenia Treatment Unit, West Los Angeles VA Medical Center, Los Angeles, CA 90073, USA; [g] Department of Psychiatry & Biobehavioral Sciences, David Geffen School of Medicine at UCLA, 10833 Le Conte Avenue, Los Angeles, CA 90095, USA; [h] Department of Pharmacy, Veterans Affairs Northern California Healthcare System, 150 Muir Road, Martinez, CA 94553, USA; [i] University of the Pacific School of Pharmacy, 3601 Pacific Avenue, Stockton, CA 95211, USA; [j] University of Southern California School of Pharmacy, 1985 Zonal Avenue, Los Angeles, CA 90089, USA; [k] Thomas J. Long School of Pharmacy & Health Sciences, University of the Pacific 3601 Pacific Avenue, Stockton, CA 95211, USA; [l] Department of Pharmacy, Veterans Affairs Long Beach Healthcare System, 5901 East 7th Street, Long Beach, CA 90822, USA; [m] Semel Institute for Neuroscience & Human Behavior, UCLA, 760 Westwood Plaza, Suite C8-193, Los Angeles, CA 90024, USA
* Corresponding author.
E-mail address: Donna.ames@va.gov

Psychiatr Clin N Am 39 (2016) 275–311
http://dx.doi.org/10.1016/j.psc.2016.01.008
0193-953X/16/$ – see front matter Published by Elsevier Inc.

Continued

- Readers will learn about appropriate clinical approaches to recognizing, monitoring and mitigating adverse effects.
- Guidelines for appropriate monitoring of these medications' adverse effects are presented.

INTRODUCTION

Antipsychotic drugs (APDs) are some of the most frequently prescribed medications, not only for psychotic disorders and symptoms but also for a wide range of both on-label and off-label indications, including affective disorders, anxiety disorders, behavioral disturbances, and insomnia. Because second-generation APDs (SGAs) have largely replaced first-generation APDs (FGAs) as first-line options due to their substantially decreased risk of extrapyramidal side effects, attention has shifted to other clinically concerning adverse events associated with APD therapy. The focus of this article is to update the authors' previous review[1] of the nonextrapyramidal side effects associated with SGAs, including weight gain, diabetes, HLP, cardiac side effects, mortality risk, hyperprolactinemia (hPRL), sexual side effects, and osteoporosis. Issues surrounding diagnosis and monitoring as well as clinical management are addressed.

WEIGHT GAIN

Relative to the general population, treatment-naïve patients with schizophrenia and bipolar disorder have a higher prevalence of obesity and being overweight.[2,3] Nonetheless, controlled clinical trials have consistently demonstrated greater degrees of weight gain during treatment with APDs compared with placebo, although individual differences in relative weight gain exist between medications. Weight gain and obesity are concerning due to an associated decrease in medication adherence and an increase in the risk of cardiovascular disease.[2,4] This is especially concerning among those with severe mental illnesses (SMIs), who seem at significantly higher risk for cardiovascular morbidity and mortality, which is the most common cause of death in this population.[2,4]

Mechanisms

The precise mechanism underlying APD-induced weight gain is not fully understood. Several theoretic mechanisms have been postulated involving neurochemical mechanisms that result in imbalances between energy intake and expenditure.[5,6] It has been speculated that APD-induced weight gain may involve antagonism of histamine H_1 and serotonin 2C receptors[5,7,8] inasmuch as brain serotonin seems to play a role in influencing satiety and hunger, whereas the histaminergic system affects food intake and energy regulation.[9] It has been speculated that APD-induced weight gain may involve antagonism of histaminergic H1 and serotonin 2C receptors.[10]

Available clinical evidence suggests that APD-induced weight gain may arise from an increase in appetite and food intake, in conjunction with delayed signaling of satiety.[11,12] A 6-week double-blind randomized controlled trial (RCT) comparing the eating behavior of patients taking CLZ and OLZ revealed an increase in food cravings and binge eating over time for both medications.[13] Between the 2 treatment groups, food cravings and binge eating were more frequent with OLZ (48.9% and 16.7%, respectively) relative to CLZ (23.3% and 8.9%, respectively). These results suggest that APDs influence feeding behaviors that contribute to weight gain.

First-Generation Antipsychotics

Contrary to popular belief, FGAs can be associated with clinically significant weight gain (defined by the US Food and Drug Administration [FDA] as a greater than 7% increase in total body weight relative to baseline), with lower potency APDs, such as chlorpromazine (CPM) and thioridazine, having a greater risk than higher potency agents.[14] In the European First Episode Schizophrenia Trial (EUFEST),[15] which evaluated treatment with haloperidol (HAL), OLZ, quetiapine (QTP), ziprasidone (ZIP), or amisulpride (AMI) over 12 months in first-episode schizophrenia, HAL was associated with significant weight in 53% of patients, with an average weight gain of 7.3 kg. In another study, drug-naïve patients with first-episode psychosis treated with HAL for 12 months gained an average of 9.56 kg.[5] The Clinical Antipsychotic Trials of Intervention Effectiveness (CATIE) compared several different SGAs to perphenazine over 18 months among subjects with schizophrenia who were previously treated with APDs for an average of 14 years.[16] Although an average weight loss of 0.9 kg weight loss per month was reported among perphenazine-treated subjects, 12% of subjects experienced significant weight gain. FGAs do carry a weight gain liability and switching from an SGA to an FGA does not guarantee weight loss.

Second-Generation Antipsychotics

Evidence suggests that different SGAs are associated with varying magnitudes of weight gain.[17] The CATIE study[16] demonstrated that significant weight gain was much more frequent among those treated with OLZ (30% of treated subjects) relative to QTP (16%), risperidone (RIS) (14%), or ZIP (7%). Likewise, OLZ was associated with the greatest amount of weight gain (4.3 kg) followed by QTP (0.50 kg) and RIS (0.36 kg), whereas ZIP was associated with weight loss (−0.73 kg). Although the CATIE study included patients with a long history of previous APD treatment, the Comparison of Atypicals for First Episode (CAFE) and EUFEST studies included first-episode psychosis patients with minimal or no prior APD exposure. The CAFE study evaluated the metabolic profiles of OLZ, QTP, and RIS over 52 weeks.[18] After just 12 weeks, significant weight gain was observed in 59.8% of subjects treated with OLZ, 32.5% with RIS, and 29.2% with QTP. At 52 weeks, 80% of OLZ-treated subjects had significant weight gain compared with 57.6% with RIS and 50% with QTP. Similarly, in the EUFEST study, significant weight gain occurred with 86% of OLZ-treated subjects compared with 65% on QTP, 63% on AMI, and 37% on ZIP. A third study evaluating the effects of HAL, OLZ, and RIS in drug-naïve patients with first-episode psychosis found mean weight gain of 12.02 kg on OLZ, 8.99 kg on RIS, and 9.56 kg on HAL over 1 year.[19]

At this time, few head-to-head trials are available to accurately determine comparable differences in weight gain between all SGAs inclusive of the more recently approved agents, such as paliperidone (PAL), asenapine (ASE), iloperidone (ILP), and lurasidone (LUR). Based on the manufacturers' package inserts, weight gain during short-term clinical trials with these medications seems modest but variable. In a 6-week trial of PAL, significant weight gain was observed in 6% to 9% of subjects treated with doses of 3 mg/d to 12 mg/d compared with 5% on placebo.[20] Short-term 4-week and 6-week trials of ILP were associated with significant weight gain in 12% to 18% of subjects, with a mean gain of 2 kg.[20] For LUR, 4.8% of subjects with schizophrenia and 2.4% with bipolar depression experienced significant weight gain over 6 weeks, with mean weight gains of 0.43 kg and 0.29 kg, respectively.[21] Finally, in a longer 52-week trial of ASE, 14.7% of subjects had significant weight gain, with an average gain of 0.9 kg.[22]

Leucht and colleagues[23] conducted a meta-analysis that compared the efficacy and side-effect profile of 15 oral APDs for acute treatment of schizophrenia. The magnitude of weight gain for individual medications compared with placebo, from greatest to least, was OLZ, zotepine, CLZ, ILP, CPM, sertindole, QTP, RIS, PAL, ASE, AMI, aripiprazole (ARI), LUR, ZIP, and HAL. All APDs except HAL, ZIP, and LUR yielded more weight gain than placebo. Looking at between-medication differences, CLZ, ILP, CPM, sertindole, QTP, RIS, and PAL were associated with significantly greater weight gain than HAL, ZIP, LUR, ARI, AMI, and ASE (except for PAL vs ASE).

Time Course of Weight Gain

When weight gain occurs in the context of APD therapy, it tends to occur in 3 stages, with a rapid increase in body weight within the first 3 months of starting treatment (stage 1), followed by a continued steady increase in weight for at least 1 year or longer (stage 2) and finally a plateau of weight with continued therapy (stage 3).[24] Zipursky and colleagues[25] studied the time course of weight gain in patients with first-episode psychosis treated with OLZ and HAL. During the first 12 weeks of treatment, patients rapidly gained weight on OLZ (mean 9.2 kg) and HAL (mean 3.7 kg), and weight gain continued until it reached plateaus of 15.5 kg and 7.1 kg, respectively, after a year. After the first year of treatment, weight was maintained with minimal change.

A 10-year naturalistic study followed weight change in patients with schizophrenia or schizoaffective disorder who had received treatment with CLZ for up to 10 years.[26] Using a random slopes model to analyze weight change over time, the investigators found a linear coefficient of 0.095 kg weight gain per month, with a mean gain of approximately 13.6 kg at endpoint. In this study, weight gain resumed after an initial period of stability, suggesting that weight gain may sometimes continue for a prolonged period before showing a ceiling effect for certain medications like CLZ.[27]

Kinon and colleagues[28] retrospectively investigated the relationship between early rapid weight gain and the course of weight change in patients treated with OLZ over 1 year. Within 2 weeks of treatment, approximately 15% of patients rapidly gained an average of 4% of their body weight. A weight plateau was reached at 38 weeks, with those patients having rapid initial weight gain gaining more weight and reaching a significantly higher plateau at endpoint. Rapid initial weight gain with APD treatment may, therefore, be predictive of greater cumulative weight gain in the long run.

Risk Factors

Aside from individual medication differences, it is important for clinicians to know which other factors might affect weight gain in a particular patient. For example, Simon and colleagues[29] performed a review to investigate a possible correlation between SGA dose and the magnitude of weight gain. They found that for OLZ and CLZ, weight gain was proportional to both dose and plasma drug concentrations. In another retrospective analysis, serum OLZ concentrations greater than 20.6 ng/mL were associated with clinically significant weight gain.[30] An 8-week RCT examining 3 different doses of OLZ (10 mg, 20 mg, and 40 mg daily) found that mean weight gain was significantly greater at 40 mg/d compared with the 10 mg/d.[31] Weight change and OLZ plasma levels were not, however, significantly correlated. In another study evaluating long-acting injectable OLZ over 24 weeks, subjects were randomly assigned to receive high (300 mg every 2 weeks), medium (405 mg every 4 weeks), and low (150 mg every 2 weeks) doses.[32] The incidence of significant weight gain was greatest in the high-dose group (21%) compared with the medium-dose (15%) and low-dose (16%) groups.

The evidence for a relationship between RIS dosing and weight gain is less clear. Some studies have supported a relationship whereas others have not.[29] No studies to date have explored correlations between plasma concentrations of RIS and weight change. Looking at the limited number of studies involving ARI, AMI, QTP, sertindole, and ZIP, Simon and colleagues[29] found scant evidence to support a dose-relationship with weight gain for these medications and no studies examining plasma concentrations.

Beyond medication dose, APD-induced weight gain varies from individual to individual, raising the question of whether there are patient-related predictors of weight gain. Most studies to date have identified an inverse relationship between pretreatment body mass index (BMI) and subsequent APD-associated weight gain.[33–35] Low baseline BMI may predict a more rapid weight gain compared with heavier counterparts, who may ultimately gain more weight and reach a higher plateau.[36] Other potential risk factors for weight gain include younger age, lack of previous APD therapy, higher parental BMI, and nonsmoking status.[36] In a 3-year prospective cohort study involving drug-naïve patients, poor social functioning and lack of response for negative symptoms were correlated with weight gain.[37] Some studies have suggested that women are at higher risk for APD-associated weight gain,[33,36] but others have not identified any a gender difference.[25]

Monitoring and Management

Clinicians should educate patients so that they are aware of the weight gain propensity of APDs and ask patients if they are noticing any changes in weight and clothing or belt size. A consensus statement from the American Diabetes Association, American Psychiatric Association, and American Association of Clinical Endocrinologists recommended monitoring of weight, BMI, and waist circumference on initial APD therapy as well as every 4 weeks for 3 months and quarterly thereafter.[38] Individual and family histories of obesity, diabetes, dyslipidemia, hypertension, and cardiovascular disease should be elicited to identify risks of weight gain and other metabolic concerns.

Switch strategies

If APD treatment is associated with a subsequent gain of greater than or equal to 5% baseline weight, clinicians should consider switching from an APD associated with more weight gain to one that is more weight neutral, although such switches carry the risk that APD response might be lost.[38] Over the course of a year-long study, subjects who had gained weight on OLZ, RIS, or QTP were switched to either ARI or ZIP.[39] Those who switched to ZIP lost an average of 6.3 kg with a BMI reduction of 2.3, whereas those who switched to ARI lost an average of only 0.7 kg with BMI reduction of 0.2. The proportion of patients who lost greater than or equal to 7% of their body weight or were no longer considered obese likewise favored ZIP over ARI as a switch agent. These data are consistent not only with the notion that ZIP is among least likely SGAs to cause weight gain but also that beyond weight neutrality, actual weight loss can be achieved when switching from an APD associated with weight gain to one that is more weight neutral.

Behavioral interventions

Patients taking APDs, particularly those who are or who become overweight or obese, should be provided with education on proper nutrition and exercise.[38] There are several vital elements of successful psychosocial weight-loss programs, including a low-calorie, low-fat diet and increased physical activity, in combination with behavioral therapy.[40–43] A meta-analysis that evaluated behavioral and pharmacologic interventions for weight loss found that nutritional counseling in combination with exercise demonstrated maximal benefit.[44]

Pharmacologic interventions

Several pharmacologic interventions for weight loss have been studied in patients with schizophrenia who are taking APDs. Beyond its use in the management of diabetes, metformin has been studied for its efficacy in the prevention and reversal of

APD-induced weight gain.[45–47] A 12-week trial examined weight change among patients with first-episode psychosis taking SGAs, who were randomized to receive metformin alone, lifestyle intervention with metformin, lifestyle intervention, or placebo.[47] Lifestyle intervention in combination with metformin was most effective for weight loss (−4.7 kg), followed by metformin alone (−3.2 kg) and lifestyle intervention alone (−1.4 kg). Placebo-treated subjects gained 3.1 kg at endpoint. This finding, along with other positive studies,[48] supports the use of metformin in addition to behavioral weight-loss strategies. The efficacy of several other medications for APD-induced weight gain has also been explored. A 12-week trial randomized overweight patients treated with SGAs to placebo or topiramate (100 mg/d or 200 mg/d).[49] Weight loss was greatest with topiramate (200 mg/d; −6.8%), relative to topiramate (100 mg/d; −2.2%) and placebo (−0.4%). Orlistat has been studied in patients with OLZ-induced and CLZ-induced weight gain, with weight loss observed in men but not women.[50] Sibutramine has been evaluated for its potential in APD-induced weight gain with mixed results[51–53] but was removed from the market in 2010 due to cardiac concerns. Clinicians should be mindful that the addition of medications for weight loss may be associated with additional adverse effects.

DIABETES

Patients with schizophrenia and bipolar disorder have a 2 to 3 times greater risk of diabetes and obesity than the general population, with an estimated prevalence of 10% to 15%.[54,55] Although the observation that diabetes is overrepresented among those with schizophrenia dates back to before the introduction and widespread use of APDs,[56,57] subsequent research clearly indicates a strong association between treatment with APDs and insulin resistance, glucose dysregulation, and the development of type 2 diabetes mellitus.[58,59] In 2004, the FDA required that the package labeling of all SGAs include warnings about an increased risk of hyperglycemia, diabetes mellitus, and severe hyperglycemia associated with ketoacidosis.[38]

Mechanisms

Type 2 diabetes mellitus evolves from abnormalities in insulin action and secretion in combination with genetic, environmental, and lifestyle factors. In patients with SMI, insulin resistance and glucose dysregulation may be further influenced by psychiatric disease itself or its associated pharmacotherapy.[14,55,60] Although the underlying mechanism of APD influenced glucose dysregulation is not fully understood, APDs may increase the risk of diabetes by fostering insulin resistance, reducing insulin secretion, or increasing weight.[55,61]

The weight gain liabilities of APDs suggest that obesity plays a significant role in the development of APD-associated insulin resistance and diabetes. In addition, abdominal adiposity in particular seems associated with a greater risk of type 2 diabetes mellitus and cardiovascular disease.[62] Such abdominal or omental adiposity is typical of APD-associated weight gain.[63]

APD-associated insulin resistance has been reported without concomitant weight gain in short-term studies.[55] To evaluate the metabolic effects of APDs independent of weight gain, healthy subjects were administered OLZ, ARI, or placebo for 9 days.[64] In the absence of weight gain, OLZ resulted in significant increases in postprandial insulin, glucagon-like peptide 1, and insulin resistance, whereas ARI resulted in insulin resistance but did not affect postprandial hormones compared with placebo. Increased insulin resistance has been demonstrated using the homeostatic model assessment for patients receiving OLZ, CLZ, and RIS.[65,66]

The affinity of APDs for the muscarinic M3 receptor has been suggested as playing a role in their diabetic liability. The M3 receptor is present on the pancreatic ß-cells that maintain proper glucose homeostasis and insulin release.[67,68] Of the SGAs, CLZ and OLZ have been consistently associated with a high risk of insulin resistance and glucose dysregulation and also have among the highest binding affinities for M3 receptors.[69]

Differential Effects of Antipsychotic Drugs

Both FGAs and SGAs have been associated with an increased risk for new-onset diabetes.[67] Similar to the risk of weight gain, however, the incidence of insulin resistance is not equivalent among all APDs.[38] In the CATIE study,[16] after 18 months of treatment, mean blood glucose increased most with OLZ (15.0 ± 2.8 mg/dL), followed by QTP (6.8 ± 2.5 mg/dL), RIS (6.7 ± 2.0 mg/dL), perphenazine (5.2 ± 2.0 mg/dL), and ZIP (2.3 ± 3.9 mg/dL). Likewise, increases in mean glycosylated hemoglobin A_{1c} (HbA_{1c}) were greatest with OLZ (0.41 ± 0.09%) compared with perphenazine (0.10 ± 0.06%), RIS (0.08 ± 0.04%), and QTP (0.05 ± 0.05%). Patients treated with ZIP had a mean reduction in HbA_{1c} ($-0.10 ± 0.14\%$). After 1 year of APD treatment among previously medication-naïve patients in the EUFEST study, emergent hyperglycemia (defined as blood glucose $\geq$100 mg/dL) occurred in 30% of OLZ-treated subjects, 22% of QTP-treated subjects or ZIP-treated subjects, 21% of AMI-treated subjects, and 18% of HAL-treated subjects.[15] Mean fasting insulin levels also increased for all APDs (AMI 8.6 ± 3.1 mU/L, OLZ 2.5 ± 3.9 mU/L, QTP 2.1 ± 1.2 mU/L, HAL 2.0 ± 1.4 mU/L, and ZIP 0.1 ± 2.0 mU/L).

In a retrospective chart review of 590 patients, glucose levels were followed for 2.5 years preinitiation and postinitiation of CLZ, OLZ, RIS, QTP, HAL or fluphenazine.[70] There were significant increases in glucose from baseline for CLZ, OLZ, and HAL of 14%, 21%, and 17%, respectively. Furthermore, significant increases in maximum glucose levels were noted for CLZ (31%) and OLZ (37%). After initiation of CLZ, 13% of patients required initiation of a glucose-lowering agent and 6% of OLZ-treated patients required adjustment of their glucose-lowering medications. Patients on other APDs did not require pharmacologic intervention. Wani and colleagues[71] evaluated the prevalence of glucose dysregulation in treatment-naïve patients with schizophrenia using fasting blood glucose (FBG) and oral glucose tolerance test at baseline and after 14 weeks of APD treatment. After 14 weeks of randomized treatment with ARI, RIS, HAL, and OLZ, there was a significant increase in mean FBG (ARI 7.2 mg/dL, RIS 11.5 mg/dL, HAL 11.9 mg/dL, OLZ 26.8 mg/dL), and oral glucose tolerance test (ARI 12.3 mg/dL, RIS 15.3 mg/dL, HAL 18.37, OLZ 44.5 mg/dL) for all medication groups. OLZ-treated patients had significant plasma glucose elevation compared with RIS, ARI, and HAL. In a 6-week, double-blind RCT involving treatment-naïve patients with schizophrenia, FBG and 2-hour postprandial blood sugar (PPBS) levels were monitored in subjects treated with OLZ, RIS, and HAL.[34] Mean FBG and PPBS increases were observed in patients on OLZ (FBG 6.6 ± 12.7 mg/dL, PPBS 21.5 ± 32.2 mg/dL), HAL (FBG 6.8 ± 14.1 mg/dL, PPBS 6.7 ± 12.6 mg/dL), and RIS (FBG 4.3 ± 12.5 mg/dL, PPBS 21.0 ± 23.4 mg/dL). Treatment-emergent diabetes was noted in the HAL (3.2%) and OLZ (2.9%) groups but not in the RIS group. Another RCT of subjects with schizophrenia and schizoaffective disorders examined glucose changes during treatment with CLZ, OLZ, RIS, or HAL.[58] After 8 weeks, mean blood glucose significantly increased by 17.1 mg/dL from baseline in the CLZ group and by 8.4 mg/dL in the HAL group. Subjects receiving OLZ had a clinically significant increase blood glucose from baseline after 14 weeks (14.3 mg/dL), although only 14% developed glucose levels greater than 125 mg/dL. RIS was not associated with statistically significant changes in glucose.

For simplicity's sake, hyperglycemia and diabetes among SGAs can be stratified into 3 tiers of risk, with CLZ and OLZ having the highest liability, QTP and RIS having moderate risk, and ARI and ZIP having the lowest risk.[2,14] There is currently a lack of adequate head-to-head studies evaluating the newer SGAs, such as PAL, ASE, ILP, and LUR, for risk stratification. Based on short-term studies of less than 12 weeks' duration, manufacturer-reported incidence of FBG greater than or equal to 126 mL/dL were 3.2% to 4.8% for PAL, 4.9% to 7.4% for ASE, 10.7% for ILP, and 5.6% to 12.7% for LUR. Mean changes in FBG were −0.6 to 3.2 mg/dL for ASE, 6.6 mg/dL for ILP, −0.4 to 2.6 mg/dL for LUR, and −0.7 to 4.3 mg/dL for PAL. Based on longer-term studies (≥24 weeks), the reported mean changes in FBG were 2.4 mg/dL for ASE, −1.8 to 5.4 mg/dL for ILP, 0.8 to 2.3 mg/dL for LUR, and 3.3 to 4.6 mg/dL for PAL.

Monitoring and Management

When monitoring patients taking APDs, clinicians should ask patients about any symptoms of diabetes, such as increase in thirst or frequency of urination. In addition to monitoring weight, waist circumference, and blood pressure, consensus guidelines recommend baseline laboratory testing for FBG and lipids. FBG should be reassessed at 12 weeks and annually thereafter, with HbA_{1c} testing used as a supplementary measure of chronic glycemia. Additional metabolic monitoring is recommended, including assessing personal or family history of diabetes and measurement of blood pressure at baseline, at 12 weeks, and yearly thereafter.[38]

On initiation of APD therapy, education and lifestyle recommendations, including proper nutrition and physical activity, are recommended to mitigate diabetes risk.[38] Because diabetes is a chronic and progressive disease, patients should be educated about maintaining a long-term, balanced diet with restrictions of carbohydrate intake. Additionally, increased physical activity should be recommended to promote calorie expenditure and weight loss and to improve cardiovascular outcomes.[41–43] Education regarding the microvascular and macrovascular risks associated with diabetes is especially important for patients with SMI who are less likely to be evaluated for retinopathy or diabetic foot complications compared with the general population.[72] Once diabetes is present, the management and treatment goals for those with SMI should follow the same guidelines and algorithms as for the general population, including the initiation of appropriate diabetic pharmacotherapy for glycemic control.[73] As with weight gain, switching APDs in the interest of decreasing blood glucose is an option; however, risk of relapse may occur if the medication switched to is less effective. A multidisciplinary approach, including collaboration between psychiatrists, primary care clinicians, endocrinologists, nutritionists, and pharmacists, may improve patient outcomes.

HYPERLIPIDEMIA

In addition to weight gain and glucose dysregulation, SGAs have been shown to cause HLP. HLP encompasses triglycerides and cholesterol, which is composed of low-density lipoproteins (LDLs), commonly known as "bad cholesterol," and high-density lipoproteins (HDLs), commonly known as "good cholesterol." That APDs can lead to HLP is of clinical significance due to the long-term consequences on overall cardiovascular health in individuals taking this class of medications, particularly those with chronic psychotic disorders, such as schizophrenia. Moreover, it has been shown that patients with chronic psychosis are more likely to have such deleterious side effects go undetected due to limitations in access to care.[74]

Mechanisms

Although there are multiple hypotheses, the exact mechanism by which APDs induce HLP remains elusive.[75] Studies have postulated that weight gain, diet changes, and glucose intolerance lead to lipid abnormalities; however, some research has revealed that APDs increase lipids independently of these factors that normally predispose individuals to HLP.[76] Saari and colleagues[77] conducted a general population-based study of 5654 members of a birth cohort in Finland who received clinical examinations at age 31. Fasting serum total cholesterol, HDL, LDL, and triglyceride levels were measured along with assessment of HLP risk factors. The sample was divided into 4 groups: those taking FGAs, those taking SGAs, those taking both FGAs and SGAs, and those not taking any APDs. The study showed that the prevalence of hypercholesterolemia, high LDL, and hypertriglyceridemia were elevated in patients taking APDs (31.1%, 20.0%, and 22.2%, respectively) compared with those not taking them (12.2%, 10.2%, and 7.0%, respectively). The researchers adjusted for HLP risk factors (gender, waist circumference, physical exercise, diet, alcohol intake, and smoking) and demonstrated that in individuals treated with APDs, the risk of hypercholesterolemia was 2.8 (95% CI, 1.4–5.6); of hypertriglyceridemia 2.3 (95% CI, 1.0–5.4); and of high LDL 1.6 (95% CI, 0.7–3.5). This study suggests, therefore, that APDs can cause HLP apart from other predisposing factors, even in a young population. One limitation of the study, however, was the small sample of individuals (n = 45) taking APDs.

Although HLP is concerning because of its association with cardiac risk, some research has suggested that the increase in lipids associated with SGA treatment may explain their therapeutic effects. A study by Procyshyn and colleagues[78] revealed that improvement of psychotic symptoms on CLZ correlated with the changes in serum lipids. The study incorporated a subset of data from a double-blind RCT of individuals with schizophrenia who were poor CLZ responders. While controlling for weight, they examined the association between serum lipid concentrations and Positive and Negative Syndrome Scale (PANSS) scores and found that changes in serum lipid concentration predicted changes in symptoms over that of changes in weight.[78] An increase in serum triglyceride concentration was associated with a decrease in total PANSS score and an increase in either serum total cholesterol concentration, serum triglyceride concentration, or their combined effect was associated with a decrease in PANSS-negative subscale scores.[78] Spivak and colleagues[79] conducted a retrospective review of 70 patients receiving CLZ and 30 patients receiving FGAs for 6 months. Among CLZ-treated subjects, significant reductions in aggression and suicidal behavior were accompanied by increases in triglycerides, whereas those on FGAs had increased cholesterol levels but no improvements in aggression or suicidality. The investigators speculated that triglycerides might be related to clinical improvements with CLZ.[79]

Differential Effects of Antipsychotic Drugs

Overall, SGAs seem to have a greater effect on lipids than FGAs.[80] Within FGAs, low-potency phenothiazines, such as CPM, are associated with greater risk of HLP than high-potency butyrophenones, such as HAL.[76] Sasaki and colleagues[81] conducted a cross-sectional study of individuals with chronic schizophrenia to compare HLP in patients receiving phenothiazines to those receiving butyrophenones; 17 patients were receiving phenothiazines (perphenazine and trifluoperazine) and 14 received a butyrophenone (HAL). Those receiving phenothiazine treatment had higher mean triglyceride levels (163 ± 65 mg/dL) than those receiving HAL (104 ± 52 mg/dL).[76]

In 2005, Koro and Meyer[76] reviewed the literature dating back to 1970 and found that the low-potency FGA CPM and the SGAs CLZ, OLZ, and QTP have the highest risk of HLP, whereas high-potency FGAs, such as HAL, along with the SGAs ZIP, RIS, and ARI, have the lowest risk.[76] A subsequent study by de Leon and colleagues[82] examined the association of APDs and HLP in 360 participants with SMI. Patients were divided into 3 groups: 57 subjects on OLZ, 105 on QTP, and 198 on other APDs (RIS, ZIP, ARI or FGAs). After correcting for potential confounders, it was reported that patients taking OLZ had significantly higher mean total serum cholesterol levels (178 mg/dL vs 192 mg/dL) and mean triglyceride levels (172 mg/dL vs 202 mg/dL) compared with those in the "other" medication group APDs.[82] Likewise, patients taking QTP had significantly higher mean total serum cholesterol levels (178 mg/dL vs 194 mg/dL) and mean triglyceride levels (172 mg/dL vs 225 mg/dL) compared with the other medications.[82] A matched case-control study by Olfson and colleagues[83] reviewed 13,133 incident cases of HLP in individuals with psychotic disorders who were matched to 72,140 control subjects and patients who were prescribed either no APD or 1 APD. The relative risk of developing new onset HLP was highest with CLZ, followed by OLZ, RIS, QTP, ZIP FGAs, and ARI.[83] The study concluded that subjects taking CLZ, OLZ, QTP, RIS, ZIP, and FGAs had a higher risk of developing HLP compared with those not taking any APDs. Only treatment with ARI was associated with no significant risk of HLP.

As with ARI, it seems that some of the newer SGAs may have a relatively benign lipid profile. Meltzer and colleagues[84] conducted a pooled analysis of 3 different 6-week placebo-controlled studies examining the safety and efficacy of the oral extended-release formulation of PAL in 1326 subjects with schizophrenia. Changes in serum levels of total cholesterol, HLD, LDL, and triglycerides were minimal with PAL treatment.[84] Similarly, a pooled analysis of 3 different 6-week trials involving 1943 patients with schizophrenia treated with ILP reported that lipid levels remained unaffected, with decreases in triglycerides levels.[85] Kemp and colleagues[86] conducted a post hoc analysis using data from 17 ASE trials involving patients with bipolar disorder and schizophrenia who were treated with ASE, OLZ, or placebo. In placebo-controlled trials, changes in lipids did not differ significantly between ASE and placebo, except for mean triglyceride levels, which did not change substantially with ASE (+1.8 mg/dL) but decreased with placebo (−12.2 mg/dL). Within OLZ-controlled trials, ASE treatment was associated with small decreases in mean total cholesterol (−0.4 mg/dL), LDL (−0.3 mg/dL), and triglycerides (−0.9 mg/dL), whereas OLZ increased these parameters (+6.2 mg/dL, +3.1 mg/dL, and +24.3 mg/dL, respectively). The study concluded that lipid changes on ASE were comparable to placebo, whereas OLZ significantly increased lipids compared with ASE. LUR was compared with ZIP in a short-term 21-day trial of subjects with schizophrenia and schizoaffective disorder.[87] In this study, both LUR and ZIP were associated with a small endpoint reductions in median total cholesterol (−6.4 vs −4.4 mg/dL) with no endpoint change in median triglycerides (0.0 vs 0.0 mg/dL). A review of other LUR studies likewise concluded that LUR has insignificant effects on lipids.[88]

In summary, the available literature indicates that among SGAs, CLZ, OLZ, and QTP carry the greatest risk of HLP. RIS has a moderate effect on lipids, whereas ZIP and ARI seem more benign. Although the newer SGAs, including PAL, ILP, ASE, and LUR, seem lipid neutral, additional research is needed to corroborate early evidence.

Monitoring and Management

Clinicians should inquire if their patients have any family or personal history of lipid abnormalities prior to initiating treatment with APDs. As discussed previously, it is recommended that fasting lipids be monitored at the start of APD therapy, at 12 weeks, and every 5 years thereafter (or yearly in the setting of HLP).[38] Differences in lipid profiles among various APDs highlight the potential utility of switching to a more lipid neutral SGA in the setting of HPL associated with other APDs. The effectiveness of switching in this manner is supported by a retrospective study of veterans with schizophrenia or schizoaffective disorder who were switched from OLZ to other APDs.[89] This trial found that switching from OLZ to ZIP was associated with significant decreases in both mean LDL cholesterol (−16.9 mg/dL) and triglyceride levels (−62.9 mg/dL).

CARDIAC ADVERSE EFFECTS

In 2001, evidence from a large, controlled, epidemiologic study underscored concerns about the proarrhythmic effects of FGAs, including sudden cardiac death (SCD).[90] Between 2004 and 2006, case reports of drug-induced torsades de pointes (TdP) involving RIS, QTP, and ZIP were published,[91–93] followed in 2009 by epidemiologic data establishing an association between SGAs and increased risk for SCD.[94]

Detecting Patients at Risk for Serious Ventricular Dysrhythmias

Estimating the risks of serious but rare adverse events with SGAs is difficult from a methodological perspective. Recently, the Cardiac Safety Research Consortium published recommendations on when cardiovascular safety outcome trials are indicated, recognizing the intense resources required to complete such studies.[95] Without existing outcomes data from large, longitudinal clinical trials, clinicians must estimate risk based on surrogate markers, such as corrected QT (QTc) interval prolongation (QT_cIP) or in vitro and epidemiologic data, to assist with risk assessment.

Corrected QT interval prolongation

The risk for serious ventricular dysrhythmias (SVDs), specifically TdP, is estimated by a drug's propensity to prolong the QT interval. Because heart rate influences QT interval, a QTc interval is reported. Formulas to correct the QT interval include the Bazett square root, which is the most commonly used correction in clinical practice, and the Fridericia formula, which has advantages over Bazett in patients with extreme heart rates. Definitions of normal QTc interval range from less than 0.4 to less than 0.44 seconds. Women tend to have longer QTc intervals than men so that gender-specific norms have been defined at less than 450 milliseconds (ms) for men and less than 460 ms for women.[96] A QTc interval greater than 500 ms[97] or an increase of 60 ms from baseline is indicative of increased risk of TdP.[98] Prolonged QTc may or may not develop into SVDs, such that QTc is regarded as an imperfect but accepted surrogate marker for TdP. The use of a QT nomogram is reportedly better able to predict TdP than the Bazett formula.[99] Other methods, including QT dispersion, QT variability markers, and U wave analysis, may help identify patients at risk for SVDs.[96,100,101]

In vitro studies

The human ether-à-go-go-related gene (hERG) regulates production of the delayed rectifier potassium current–rapid (I_{Kr}). This rectifying current represents outward flow of potassium from cardiac conduction cells and thus ventricular repolarization. Patients with primary (hereditary) QTcIP have altered hERG expression, providing a laboratory model to examine the potential of drugs and drug concentrations to prolong

QT interval via drug effects on the I_{Kr}.[96] Most medications that prolong the QT interval block I_{Kr}. Different APDs produce variable effects on I_{Kr} with dose-dependent suppression of the I_{Kr}.[102] Recent data indicate that APDs with high potency for hERG potassium channel blockade are associated with the highest risk of SVDs and SCD, connecting in vitro findings and clinical outcomes.[103] Limitations of this laboratory-based assessment, however, exist.[97] Moreover, drug-induced blockade of the T-type calcium channels or autonomic neurocardiac function are also implicated in QTcIP.[100]

Epidemiologic data

Observational epidemiologic studies are limited in their ability to establish causality between SGAs and SCD and must control for numerous potential confounders.[97] Ray and colleagues[94] calculated the adjusted incidence for SCD in a retrospective cohort of Tennessee Medicaid enrollees, including 44,216 users of FGAs; 46,089 users of SGAs; and 186,600 matched nonuser controls. They found that both FGAs and SGAs increased risk for SCD. The risk for SCD was increased regardless of the existence of indication for use and a significant dose relationship between SGA and SCD. Limitations of this work include not controlling for smoking or disease severity and unclear diagnostic validity of SCD.

Murray-Thomas and colleagues[104] assessed mortality, including SCD, cardiac mortality, and all-cause mortality (excluding suicide), in 3 populations: APD users (n = 183,392, of whom 115,491 were prescribed FGAs and 67,901 were prescribed SGAs), matched controls from the general population (n = 544,726), and APD nonusers with psychiatric disorders (n = 193,920). Compared with controls, both APD users and nonusers had higher rates of all-cause mortality such that psychiatric disease states themselves seemed to influence mortality. APD users had a higher adjusted relative risk compared with controls and nonusers for all-cause mortality, cardiac mortality, and SCD. SGAs were associated with lower adjusted relative risk for all-cause mortality during the first year of therapy and were similar to the rate of FGAs thereafter. The investigators postulated that increased mortality over time may be related to metabolic side effects or APD polypharmacy.

Weeke and colleagues[105] examined the associated risk of APDs and out-of-hospital cardiac arrest (OHCA) using the Danish Cardiac Arrest Registry. Of the 28,947 OHCA patients evaluated, 2205 (7.6%) were receiving treatment with an APD agent at the time of the arrest, and APD use was associated with increased risk. As a class, FGAs were associated with increased risk whereas SGAs were not. Individually, OLZ, QTP, RIS, and CLZ were evaluated, but only QTP was associated with increased OHCA risk.

Using a national database, Wu and colleagues[103] examined more than 17,000 cases of ventricular arrhythmia and/or SCD and exposure to APD treatment. QTP and RIS use was associated with ventricular arrhythmia and/or SCD whereas CLZ, OLZ, ARI, AMI, and ZIP were not. The researchers noted that the small number of patients taking newer APDs may have had an impact on the results.

Reducing Risk

Patient factors

Prior to initiating therapy with an SGA, patients should be evaluated to determine their risk for SVDs (**Box 1**). A vast majority of cases of drug-induced QTcIP occur in individuals with at least 1 risk factor.[106] It is prudent to obtain each patient's family history of heart disease and sudden premature death prior to initiating treatment. For high-risk patients prescribed SGAs, clinicians should monitor electrolytes, routinely assess

---

Box 1
Risk factors that predispose individuals to corrected QT interval prolongation

Prolonged baseline QTc

Female gender

Hypokalemia

Hypomagnesemia

Diuretic use

Advanced age

Bradycardia

Congestive heart failure or cardiac hypertrophy

Cardiac ischemia

Diabetes mellitus

Hypertension

Renal or hepatic failure

Drug combinations that block ion channels (prolong QT interval) or inhibit enzymatic metabolism

Drug exposure via high doses or in individuals with genetic polymorphism in enzymatic metabolism

Data from Refs.[97,102,107]

---

the medication profile for drug-drug interactions, and conduct ECG monitoring.[97] Routine ECG monitoring is not warranted for all patients but can be used for individuals with an established risk of SVDs/SCD.[108]

Drug interactions
Drug interactions can influence adverse drug outcomes through both pharmacodynamic and pharmacokinetic mechanisms. Drugs with a pharmacodynamic propensity for SVD include loop diuretics which may result in electrolyte wasting, or agents that prolong QT interval such as the macrolide or fluoroquinolone antibiotics or imidazole antifungal agents, methadone, certain antidepressants, and antiarrhythmic agents such as sotalol. Less commonly used medications, such as antimalarials or pentamidine, are also clinically important and may be less well recognized.[100] Pharmacokinetic interactions are caused by decreased SGA elimination from the body, particularly by drugs known to be strong cytochrome P450 (CYP) enzyme inhibitors. Medications with mild to moderate risk of QTcIP may create heightened risk when prescribed with a metabolic inhibitor.[109]

Patients with major depressive disorders
Several SGAs are approved for use as adjunctive treatment of major depression disorder. Drug interactions, particularly between fluoxetine (a potent CYP2D6 and moderate CYP3A4 inhibitor) and RIS, ARI, or ILP, may result in increased serum concentration of the SGA and, therefore, an increased risk of adverse outcomes.[110,111] More pharmacokinetic and pharmacodynamic data are needed to adjust dosing when agents are combined with attention to the risk of TdP when adding an SGA to selective serotonin reuptake inhibitors.[112]

Cardiovascular factors

The risk of SCD is heightened in patients with concomitant severe cardiovascular disease.[90] SGAs are associated with a worsening of cardiovascular risk factors. A review of clinical practice found highly variable rates of screening for cardiovascular risk factors, such as obesity, hypertension, diabetes, and dyslipidemia, in patients with SMI.[113] With long-term therapy, drug-induced worsening of cardiovascular health may lead to coronary heart disease, diabetes, hypertension, or heart failure, which could in turn increase the risk for SCD associated with SGA.

Risk in children and adolescents

Clinical trials involving SGAs in children and adolescents have included ARI, OLZ, PAL, QTP, RIS, and ZIP. Compared with baseline QTc intervals, endpoint QTc intervals were significantly increased for RIS and ZIP, with ZIP producing the greatest increase. Compared with pooled placebo arms, ZIP significantly increased QTc, whereas ARI decreased QTc interval.[114]

Drug-specific factors

Comparisons of SGAs and their ability to prolong QTc interval may assist prescribers with drug selection in at-risk patients.[96–98,115–117] The FDA-approved product labeling for all SGAs includes cautionary statements about prescribing to patients with risk factors for QTcIP. The 3 newest agents approved by the FDA include ILP, ASE, and LUR. In patients given ILP, pooled ECG data using the Fridericia QTc showed QTcIP may be dose related and similar to the changes seen with HAL and ZIP. Pharmacogenomic studies have found single nucleotide polymorphisms related to QTcIP with ILP.[118] ASE is described as having modest effect on QTcIP, comparable to that of QTP.[119] LUR seems associated with a low risk of QTcIP[120,121] but is contraindicated for use with strong CYP3A4 inhibitors or inducers, and dosage reductions are recommended when prescribed concomitantly with a moderate CYP3A4 inhibitor. Further experience in clinical practice, particularly when prescribed along with interacting medications, may alter LUR's future safety rating.

A multiple-treatments meta-analysis of APDs enabled the creation of a hierarchy of comparative drug effect on QTcIP.[23] QTcIP was ranked lowest for LUR and highest with sertindole. There was no statistically significant difference compared with placebo for LUR, ARI, PAL, and ASE.

Long-acting injectables

Available data suggest that the safety profiles of oral RIS, PAL, and ARI are comparable to their long-acting injection formulations.[122,123] A meta-analysis of long-acting injectable formulations of PAL, RIS, and OLZ reported no significant QTcIP in the long-acting injection group compared with placebo or oral APD control groups.[124]

Management of Patients Who Experience Corrected QT Interval Prolongation

Patients at risk for QTcIP should be educated to seek emergency care if they experience palpitations, lightheadedness, dizziness, or syncope. High-risk patients should have a baseline ECG, then monthly ECGs for the first 6 months and every 6 to 12 months thereafter. Periodic electrolyte assessment is also recommended. In response to QTcIP, dose reduction or discontinuation of the offending drug should be instituted when the QTc interval is 470 ms to 500 ms for men, 480 ms to 500 ms for women, or when the QTc interval increases 60 ms or more from baseline. Stopping the APD is recommended if the QTc interval is greater than or equal to 500 ms and ECGs should be monitored until the QTc interval normalizes.[106]

Further Considerations

Examining baseline QTc has the potential to identify approximately 90% of individuals with long QT syndrome[96]; 5% to 10% of individuals who develop drug-induced TdP carry gene mutations related to prolonged QTc; the future availability of practical and economically viable genetic screening could influence SGA drug and dose selection. Genome-wide association studies hold promise as a source of biomarkers for efficacy and adverse effects of SGAs.[125] Guidelines for the use of SGAs that take into account concomitant conditions, such as heart failure or coronary heart disease, similar to the guidelines for use of antiarrhythmic agents in the management of atrial fibrillation could be developed.[126] Finally, risk scoring for hospitalized patients has been developed and validated.[127] Developing a predictive mathematical model to calculate a risk score for ambulatory patients, similar to the Framingham Risk Score,[128] could also have utility. Individuals with a high risk score for drug-induced dysrhythmias would be best suited to APDs with a low propensity for this adverse effect. Overall, although SVDs and SCD are rare events, risk factors originating with the patient and with the SGA should be assessed and considered as part of the drug selection process.

MORTALITY
Mortality in Schizophrenia

It is well known that individuals with schizophrenia have a greater risk of early mortality compared with the general population, with a reduced life expectancy of 10 to 25 years.[129] A systematic review of international studies found a median standard mortality ratio of 2.58 for schizophrenia, meaning that persons with the illness have between a 2-fold to 3-fold increase in death compared with age-matched controls.[130] This mortality gap for schizophrenia has been increasing since the 1970s, despite greater longevity for the general population.[130]

There are many potential explanations for greater mortality risk in schizophrenia, ranging from high rates of comorbid medical illnesses, such as obesity, diabetes, and cardiovascular disease; unhealthy lifestyles, including poor diet, lack of exercise, and tobacco dependence; limited access to and utilization of health care resources; suicide; and negative biases against persons with schizophrenia on the part of health care providers that compromise care.[129,131] With increased attention to metabolic side effects over the past several decades, APDs have themselves been implicated as an important culprit in the mortality gap of schizophrenia.

Exploring the potential contribution of APD treatment to mortality is methodologically challenging. RCTs are vital for identifying medication-specific effects but generally involve small numbers of healthy individuals with only short-term follow-up, such that death is too infrequent an event for statistical comparison. Isaac and Koch[132] performed a pooled analysis of 23 phase II and phase III RCTs of 4-week to 6-week duration involving APDs for schizophrenia and schizoaffective disorder submitted to the European Medicines Agency and the FDA for drug licensing. Among a total of 7553 patients, 7 died, with 2 of 5738 on APDs and 5 of 1815 on placebo. This study suggests an increased risk of death for patients with schizophrenia who are not taking medications.

In contrast to RCTs, observational cohort studies allow for much larger epidemiologic databases and longer follow-up periods that provide a better estimate of mortality rates. As nonrandomized and uncontrolled comparisons, however, such studies have myriad confounds and methodological limitations that hamper causal conclusions about medication effects. Such limitations include uncertainty about medication adherence, potential differences in medical comorbidities between treatment groups, and diagnostic uncertainty. Perhaps the most important confound is disease severity, whereby those persons not taking APDs in an observational study might have a more mild form of schizophrenia or might not really have schizophrenia at all, in which case they might be expected to live longer. This possibility presents an alternative explanation to claims about APDs increasing mortality.

Looking at the data, Weinmann and associates[133] published a systematic review of 12 cohort studies that tracked death rates among those with schizophrenia and schizoaffective disorder over 2-year to 17-year follow-up. With considerable heterogeneity among the included studies, meta-analysis was not possible and results were variable, with some studies finding a greater increased risk of death associated with APDs and others finding the opposite. The investigators cautiously concluded that it was possible that APDs are associated with greater mortality in schizophrenia.

More recently, a retrospective cohort study examined mortality rates over an 11-year follow-up period for all patients in Finland admitted to a hospital with a diagnosis of schizophrenia between 1996 and 2006.[134] This study found a persistent mortality gap that was larger among younger patients. In terms of medications, the overall risk of death was lower for those currently taking any APDs compared with those not taking them, with an adjusted hazard ratio (HR) of 0.68. Longer-term APD treatment was associated with a lower risk of death. De Hert and colleagues[135] have highlighted methodological critiques of this study, including the improbably large number of patients categorized as not taking any APDs and the exclusion of deaths occurring during hospitalization.

Subsequent studies have failed to provide clarity on the issue of APD-associated mortality. For example, 2 analyses from a large general practice database in the United Kingdom found an increased mortality risk for those treated with APDs compared with psychiatric nonusers, although these studies were not limited to individuals with schizophrenia and excluded suicides.[104,136] In contrast, a review of placebo-controlled FDA registration medication trials found that mortality was lower among patients with schizophrenia taking APDs compared with those on placebo.[137] Likewise, a large cohort study from Sweden prospectively followed individuals with schizophrenia over 5 years, comparing them to age-matched and gender-matched controls.[138] Among both chronic and first-episode patients, the highest mortality rates were observed for those with no APD exposure, a finding the investigators claimed was consistent with the only other 5 large prospective cohorts involving actual filled prescriptions.

The available evidence supporting a causal role of APDs as a contributor to the mortality gap in schizophrenia is, therefore, at best, equivocal. In the absence of evidence-based alternatives to APD therapy, clinicians are, therefore, left to cautiously consider risk-benefit analyses, including available information on individual medications. Although the mechanism of APD-associated mortality has been presumed related to metabolic and cardiovascular risk, studies focusing on comparisons between APDs have not supported this hypothesis. For example, several studies have found lower mortality risk with SGAs compared with FGAs, contrary to expectations.[139,140] In addition, the study by Tiihonen and colleagues[138] found that CLZ treatment was associated with the lowest mortality rate. Such findings argue against cardiometabolic and QTc-related explanations of APD-associated mortality.[138,140] They also raise the possibility that any increase in mortality with SGAs or APDs in general might be counterbalanced by other benefits affecting longevity, such as decreasing rates of suicide.[137,138]

Management of the mortality risk in schizophrenia could be enhanced by patient participation in holistic wellness programs using evidence-based psychotherapy that promotes recovery and stress management and even provides smoking cessation. The Department of Veterans Affairs has mandated the development of programs, called Psychosocial Rehabilitation and Recovery Centers, that provide wellness and holistic treatments to veterans with SMI. It has yet to be seen if such programs can reduce mortality.

Mortality in Dementia

In contrast to patients with schizophrenia, an increased mortality risk with APDs in the treatment of elderly patients with dementia is better established. Concerns about elevated mortality in this population arose starting in the late 1990s as pharmaceutical companies were pursuing FDA indications for SGAs in the management of dementia-related psychosis. Based on a review of studies involving elderly patients with dementia, the FDA issued warnings about a possible increased risk of cerebrovascular adverse events for RIS, OLZ, and ARI.[141,142] By 2005, the FDA further observed that 15 of 17 RCTs involving RIS, OLZ, QTP, and ARI in the treatment of behavioral disorders in dementia demonstrated a greater rate of death for those treated with these medications compared with placebo, with an overall 1.6-fold to 1.7-fold increased mortality risk.[143] The most frequent causes of death were cardiovascular events (eg, heart failure and sudden death) and pneumonia. These findings resulted in a black box warning for the medications studied as well as all other available SGAs at the time. This included medications for which there was minimal evidence of risk due to lack of clinical trials in the demented elderly, such as CLZ, ZIP, and Symbyax, a branded combination of OLZ and fluoxetine.

After the FDA warnings, Schneider and associates[142] published an independent meta-analysis of 15 RCTs of mostly 10-week to 12-week duration involving RIS, OLZ, QTP, and ARI for the treatment of psychosis and behavioral disturbances in dementia. This analysis included data from 3353 patients with a mean age of 81.2 years, most of whom were diagnosed with Alzheimer disease.[142] Although there was no statistically significant increase in death for any individual medications (odds ratio [OR] = 1.3–1.9), the investigators did find a significantly increased risk of death overall for all SGAs combined (OR = 1.54). They concluded that the number needed to harm (NNH) was 100, indicating that for every 100 patients treated over 10 to 12 weeks, 1 death would be expected. An updated meta-analysis likewise found an increased risk of death with SGAs, with an NNH of 87.[144] These consistent findings stand in contrast to a recent meta-analysis that failed to find any significant increase in risk of death with APD treatment (OR = 1.06), though there was a significant increase in stroke risk (OR = 2.62).[145] Because all of these meta-analyses were based mostly on the same controlled trials, it is likely that this third disparate finding was related to methodological issues, including the inclusion of redundant data sets.

A Canadian cohort of elderly demented patients found a statistically significant increase risk of death with new-use of SGAs compared with nonuse, with adjusted HRs of 1.31 and 1.55 for 30-days' and 180-days' follow-up, respectively.[146] Over a follow-up period of 8 years, a smaller cohort study from Finland determined an HR of 2.07.[147] Potential confounds within observational studies involving the elderly may be considerable, however,[148] and it is likely that more severe dementia and co-morbid medical disease among those who receive APDs is an even greater confound in such studies than among adults with schizophrenia.

Managing Mortality Risk in Dementia

Clinically, there are several issues to consider when weighing the risks and benefits of APD use among the elderly patients with dementia. First, it seems that, compared with placebo, APD treatment can be efficacious for various targets within dementia, including psychiatric symptoms (paranoia) and behavioral disturbances (eg, anger, aggression, and agitation).[144,145,149] Based on the NNH estimate of 100, however, there seems to be a heavy toll of 1 death for every 9 to 25 elderly patients with dementia who benefit from an SGA.[142] Subsequent estimates of NNH for individual medications have been as low as 25 to 50,[150] such that it would not be unreasonable to suggest that the modest benefits of APD treatment might be easily outweighed by considerable mortality risk.

Second, the risk of SGA treatment must be balanced against other available pharmacologic options. With initial concerns about SGAs in the elderly demented, the question of whether FGAs might be safer soon arose. Although a recent meta-analysis of short-term RCTs involving FGAs in elderly patients with dementia and delirium concluded no increased risk of mortality compared with placebo,[151] Schneider and colleagues[142] reported a relative risk of 2.07 for HAL and evidence from numerous longer-term cohort studies likewise indicates that the mortality risk with FGAs in this population is on par with if not higher than SGAs.[152–158] In 2008, the FDA extended the black box warning about risk of death among the demented elderly to all APDs, both FGAs and SGAs.[159] APD-associated death in this population seems both multifactorial and difficult to predict. Some studies have suggested the possibility that any differences in mortality risk between FGAs and SGAs might be related more to cardiovascular disease[155] than stroke risk[160] and that baseline respiratory disease increases mortality during treatment with APDs.[147] Because respiratory infection is one leading cause of APD-associated death, sedation leading to aspiration pneumonia may be a plausible mechanism. Sedation is, however, not a side effect limited to APDs. Valproate seems to have a mortality risk comparable with SGAs among the elderly demented.[158] Even antidepressants, which seem to have a lower mortality risk in this population compared with APDs, are associated with a statistically significant increase in mortality.[150] Consequently, it may be that any psychotropic sedation – often a desired outcome when treating agitated patients – may come at the expense of mortality risk.

In the absence of FDA-approved medications for behavioral disturbances in dementia, FDA warnings about APDs for dementia seem to have had limited effect on prescribing patterns.[161] In the final analysis, clinicians must maximize the benefits of evidence-based nonpharmacologic intervention among the elderly demented,[162,163] weighing the potential benefits of APD pharmacotherapy with considerable caution. Clinicians should also consider the utility of APD withdrawal, following evidence from controlled discontinuation studies. Two meta-analyses of such studies agree that overall, discontinuation has few detrimental effects[164,165] and may be associated with a decreased risk of death.[165] Discontinuation seems, however, associated with symptomatic worsening in certain patients whose severe symptoms have previously benefitted from APD medication.[164]

For elderly patients with schizophrenia where APD therapy is more clearly indicated, benefits must still be weighed against the risk of mortality detected in dementia studies. Because those patients with schizophrenia who live into their geriatric years have defied the odds in terms of longevity, however, it is possible that they may be less susceptible to the risks of APD-associated death.

HYPERPROLACTINEMIA

Drug-induced hPRL is a side effect commonly associated with FGAs, occurring in up to 70% of patients receiving APDs overall.[166] Estrogen's effects on prolactin (PRL) gene expression regulate PRL synthesis. Elevated PRL levels associated with APDs are greater in women than in men. In 1 study, the prevalence of hPRL was more common in premenopausal women taking FGAs (48%–93%) compared with men (42%–47%).[167] Another study found a similar prevalence range of hPRL for women (42%–93%); however, the prevalence range was wider for men (18%–72%).[168]

Since the introduction of SGAs into the treatment landscape in the 1990s for schizophrenia and other psychiatric disorders, there has been a decrease in the reporting of hPRL-associated side effects. With the exception of RIS and PAL, other SGAs do not seem to significantly increase PRL levels or have variable effects on PRL release.[168] hPRL is dose related and can be asymptomatic in some individuals. When it occurs as a bothersome side effect, it manifests as acne, hirsutism, gynecomastia, galactorrhea, oligomenorrhea, amenorrhea, sexual dysfunction, and infertility. Chronic hPRL may lead to osteopenia and osteoporosis.[169,170]

Mechanisms

Dopamine inversely regulates PRL secretion in the pituitary gland. Mechanistically, prolonged potent dopamine receptor 2 (D2) blockade on lactotroph cell membranes by FGAs, RIS, and their active metabolites can increase PRL. APDs have different binding affinities for dopamine receptors on pituitary lactotrophs, which may explain the weaker influence of most SGAs on PRL release.[170] In addition, PRL secretion is also stimulated by serotonin release,[171] mediated through serotonin 1A and serotonin 2A receptor stimulation. Many APDs have serotonin 1A agonist activities that could increase PRL, whereas the potent serotonin 2A antagonism many SGAs may decrease PRL levels.[172] Antidepressants with serotonergic properties can also cause mild hPRL. The severity of hPRL-associated effects can be attributed to the APDs and its receptor affinity profile, dose, and treatment duration.

The variable relationship between SGAs and PRL level changes may also be explained by individual patient factors, including age, gender, and genetic factors. Polymorphisms in the D2 receptor (D2DR) genes may also affect PRL release. Studies suggest that individuals with the DRD2 Taq1A polymorphism may have twice the increase in PRL levels when taking CLZ, OLZ, and RIS.[173]

Prevalence

A meta-analysis studying the safety and tolerability of 15 APDs revealed that RIS and PAL were associated with significantly higher PRL levels compared with some FGAs, such as HAL. OLZ was associated with a transient increase in PRL levels, whereas CLZ and QTP rarely increased PRL levels. PRL changes with ILP and ASE were similar to placebo.[23] A comprehensive review yielded similar findings, with RIS and PAL associated with a significant increase in PRL levels, OLZ with a moderate increase, and other SGAs with insignificant change in PRL. The investigators cautioned, however, against use of the term, *PRL sparing*, to avoid conclusions that these medications are never associated with hPRL.[174]

Unlike other SGAs, RIS behaves like FGAs with respect to significantly increasing PRL levels, which may be attributed to prolonged D2 blockade by its active metabolite, 9-hydroxy-RIS (PAL). PAL increases PRL levels because of its similar receptor profile (D2 and serotonin 2A receptor antagonism), longer half-life, and hydrophilic chemical structure, which explains the higher dose needed to achieve central effects.[169] Increased peripheral D2 blockade on the pituitary gland, located outside of the blood-brain barrier, can lead to increased PRL.[175] The increase in blood PRL levels is produced after a few hours of initiating acute treatment with RIS and PAL. Berwaerts and colleagues[176] observed similar elevations in serum PRL levels when PAL extended-release (12 mg) and RIS immediate-release (4 mg) were administered over 6 days. The 80% to 90% rate of hPRL associated with RIS in female subjects was consistently greater than any of the other APDs, including the FGAs. As a reference, hPRL was found in 71% of patients treated with FGAs with a mean PRL level of 42.1 ng/mL.[177]

The extent of SGA effects on PRL release was demonstrated in the CATIE and CAFE studies. In both phases of the CATIE study, patients receiving RIS had higher increases in PRL levels compared with patients on CLZ, OLZ, QTP, and ZIP. Moreover, when patients were switched from RIS to CLZ, OLZ, or QTP, their PRL levels dropped significantly.[178,179] In phase I, between 2% to 4% of patients receiving RIS experienced gynecomastia or galactorrhea. Patients receiving RIS in phase II of the study also had higher rates of gynecomastia or galactorrhea (5%) compared with other treatment groups (<1%). Episodes of menstrual irregularities were observed in 6% to 18% of female patients (mean age 40 years) on RIS and were common among those on QTP.[179] The CAFE study followed patients (16–40 years old) with first-episode of psychosis treated with OLZ, RIS, or QTP. Patients who received RIS had significantly elevated PRL levels from baseline (mean of 32.7 ng/mL). PRL levels dropped from baseline when they received either OLZ (by 16 ng/mL) or QTP (by 18 ng/mL). Gynecomastia was more commonly reported in the RIS group (9.8%) than in the QTP group (2.2%). Menstrual irregularities were also more commonly observed in patients on RIS (47%) compared with those on QTP (24%).[180]

There is little evidence reporting clinically significant PRL-related adverse effects associated with these 3 newest SGAs, ASE, ILP, and LUR.[181] ASE seems to have the lowest propensity for increasing PRL levels, with modest PRL elevation with ILP and LUR. ASE has lesser affinity for D2, with fewer hPRL-related adverse effects than HAL.[182] In 1 short-term clinical study comparing ASE with HAL, both the placebo and ASE groups had reduced PRL levels compared with the HAL group. The percentages of patients with abnormal postbaseline PRL levels (greater than 4 times the upper limit of normal) were 4%, 5%, 2%, and 10% in the ASE (10 mg/d), ASE (20 mg/d), placebo, and HAL groups, respectively.[183] For patients in whom PRL-related side effects may be bothersome, ASE may be a good alternative. The adverse effect profile of ILP is similar to RIS with regard to metabolic side effects (eg, weight gain, lipid, and glycemic changes) but with less hPRL. Greater increases in PRL concentrations are observed in patients receiving RIS and HAL than ILP.[118] LUR has a propensity to increase PRL levels in a dose-dependent manner with a slightly greater effect in women than men. hPRL may occur during the early phase of LUR treatment (3.6%) compared with placebo (0.6%).[121] Nakamura and colleagues[184] demonstrated a statistically significant PRL increase compared with placebo (+2.4 ng/mL vs −0.3 ng/mL; $P<.05$). In spite of the PRL increase, study participants did not experience bothersome side effects associated with LUR.

In contrast to other APDs, ARI seems PRL sparing and has been used as an adjunctive agent to decrease PRL levels in patients with hPRL associated with other APDs. ARI's PRL lowering effect seems to derive from its partial agonism of D2 receptors.[185] ARI has been reported to decrease hPRL associated with RIS and relieve associated menstrual disorders.[186] It can also normalize hPRL caused by other APDs, even at a low dose of 5 mg/d.[187] Shim and colleagues[188] evaluated the effects of ARI as adjunctive therapy in an 8-week double-blind RCT involving 56 patients with schizophrenia (18–45 years old) who developed hPRL while receiving HAL (mean dose 23 mg/d). Female patients who experienced menstrual disturbances had higher PRL levels than those with normal menstruation (114 ng/mL and 58.6 ng/mL, respectively). Patients treated with adjunctive ARI had PRL levels reduced by 84.2% compared with baseline levels; 88.5% of patients had PRL levels return to normal by week 8 compared with

3.6% in the placebo group. In the ARI group, 7 of 11 women with oligomenorrhea or amenorrhea resumed menstruation compared with none in the placebo group. Mir and colleagues[189] performed an observational study with 27 patients who received ARI as a second APD or were switched to ARI. Within 12 weeks, patients experienced improvement in libido that correlated with significant reductions in PRL levels. Men experienced improvement with erectile and ejaculatory difficulties, whereas women experienced improvements with menstrual dysfunction. The utility of ARI in reducing PRL is also supported by a trial in which PRL levels were reduced in patients with symptomatic hPRL associated with oral PAL.[190]

Monitoring and Management

Patients may be hesitant to discuss concerns about sexual function; in particular, men may be embarrassed by symptoms, such as gynecomastia, galactorrhea, or impotence. Clinicians must, therefore, inquire about these signs of hPRL as part of routine clinical examinations. Normal plasma PRL levels are typically less than or equal to 20 ng/mL for women and less than or equal to 25 ng/mL for men. Although patients with elevated PRL levels are often asymptomatic, clinical symptoms may manifest in patients experiencing unusually elevated PRL levels. For premenopausal women, excessively high PRL levels (>100 ng/mL) are associated with amenorrhea, galactorrhea, and hypogonadism, whereas moderately high PRL levels (51–75 mg/mL) are associated with oligomenorrhea. Mildly elevated levels (31–50 ng/mL) are associated with decreased libido, short luteal phase, and infertility.[174] Similarly, chronic estrogen deficiency from hPRL in women may lead to osteopenia and osteoporosis. Clinical symptoms of hPRL in men include reduced libido, erectile dysfunction, gynecomastia, decreased sperm production, infertility, and galactorrhea.[170] With published evidence of APD-induced hPRL and related side effects, some investigators have recommended that patients have PRL checked on initiation of APD treatment and at 3 months,[191,192] although this is not a consensus guideline.[38]

In terms of intervention, dopamine agonists in the treatment of APD-induced hPRL are not well studied and could pose a risk of worsening psychosis. In patients with drug-induced hPRL, sex steroid replacement can be considered to treat hypogonadism, particularly if there is evidence of osteoporosis. ARI can be considered as a replacement for other APD agents, if the clinical situation allows, or as an adjunctive therapy in patients with psychotropic-induced hPRL.[193]

SEXUAL DYSFUNCTION
Mechanisms

APDs have been associated with all phases of sexual dysfunction, such as decreased sexual desire, sexual arousal, anorgasmia, and delayed or retrograde ejaculation.[194,195] Dopamine exerts a positive influence on libido, whereas serotonin has negative effects. PRL can decrease testosterone, which is an important hormone for healthy libido in both men and women. As D2 antagonists, APDs can, therefore, decrease libido. Norepinephrine, acetylcholine, and dopamine facilitate sexual arousal, whereas serotonin has a negative effect. APDs with strong anticholinergic effects can, therefore, cause sexual arousal issues (decreased vaginal lubrication and erectile dysfunction). Orgasm is facilitated by norepinephrine and inhibited by serotonin, whereas dopamine may have weak positive influences. Strong adrenergic antagonists can cause priapism.[196–198]

PRL can affect sexual function through its actions on the hypothalamus-pituitary-gonad axis and by altering sex hormone release. PRL levels exceeding twice the upper limit of normal may suppress the hypothalamus-pituitary-gonad axis, whereas less than 2-fold elevations may not cause any sexual side effects.[199] Elevated PRL levels directly inhibit the release of gonadotropin-releasing hormone from the hypothalamus, resulting in a decrease in secretion of follicle-stimulating hormone and luteinizing hormone from the anterior pituitary gland and reduced levels of gonadal hormones, such as estrogen and testosterone.

Effects on different phases of sexual arousal may be interdependent, with phase-specific side effects rarely observed in isolation. For example, many patients who report anorgasmia admit to having milder difficulties in arousal if asked. Furthermore, secondary side effects, such as decreased libido, may result from arousal dysfunction and/or anorgasmia.[196,200]

Prevalence

In the general population, 31% of men and 42% of women have reported sexual dysfunction.[201] Evidence suggests, however, that both psychotic illness and its treatment can contribute to sexual dysfunction. Both medication-free men with schizophrenia and men with schizophrenia on APD treatment have been found to have lower libido compared with normal controls.[166] In 1 study, men taking APDs complained of more erectile and orgasmic difficulties and lower levels of sexual satisfaction than those who were medication-free.[166]

Rates of APD-induced sexual dysfunction are high but variable. Studies showed that patients taking APDs experienced significant sexual dysfunction with rates of 30% to 52% in women and 50% to 68% in men.[202,203] Baggaley[194] reported a wide range of female (between 30% and 80%) and male (between 45% and 80%) patients with schizophrenia experienced impaired sexual functioning. The variation in prevalence rates may be due to different sexual questionnaires, interviews, and methodological approaches used in studies.[195]

The prevalence of sexual dysfunction in patients taking FGAs is approximately 60% and is often attributed to elevated PRL levels arising from dopamine blockade.[204] Among the FGAs, thioridazine had been frequently reported as causing the highest rate of sexual dysfunction, especially retrograde ejaculation.[200] A 2014 review concluded that FGAs and RIS had the most reports of sexual dysfunction in clinical studies but noted an inconsistent association between PRL and sexual side effects and the presence of many other confounding factors.[205] The investigators noted that APDs with minimal potential to increase PRL, like CLZ, are also associated with sexual side effects. Although CLZ may not increase PRL, sexual arousal issues could arise through anticholinergic mechanisms.

A meta-analysis concluded that ARI, QTP, perphenazine, and ZIP were associated with relatively low rates of sexual dysfunction, between 16% and 27%, compared with higher rates of sexual dysfunction associated with CLZ, HAL, OLZ, RIS, and thioridazine at 40% to 60%.[195] Other earlier reviews reported similar conclusions, with the highest rate of sexual side effects associated with RIS and the lowest with ARI.[194,204] As yet, few data are available regarding sexual dysfunction with the newer APDs ILP, ASE, and LUR. Additional well-designed studies that investigate the incidence of APD-induced sexual dysfunction and its management are needed.[198,206,207]

Priapism

Drug-induced priapism, or prolonged (4–6 hours) and painful penile erection, has occurred in patients treated with APDs. The proposed mechanism involves antagonist effects at the adrenergic α-receptor in the corpora cavernosa, causing arteriodilatation and inhibition of detumescence. Although priapism may be a rare occurrence, it can result in severe clinical consequences, such as permanent erectile dysfunction and penile damage through infarction. Most of the reported cases with APDs have been associated with strong adrenergic antagonists.[208] Among the SGAs, CLZ, OLZ, QTP, RIS, and ILP have been reported to cause priapism. ILP has the strongest adrenergic blockade among the APD agents, with common associated side effects, like orthostatic hypotension.[209,210] Medications with the greatest incidence of orthostasis may be more likely to have a higher risk of priapism.

Monitoring and Management

The impact of APD-induced sexual dysfunction can negatively affect a patient's quality of life as well as APD treatment adherence. Discussions about these risks prior to treatment and inquiries about symptoms of these adverse effects during treatment are advised. Recommended approaches to managing APD-induced sexual dysfunction include completing a thorough clinical evaluation to rule out other possible etiologies (eg, physical or psychiatric) or secondary factors (eg, alcohol, illicit drug use, or other medications) that may cause sexual dysfunction, modifying risk factors (eg, avoiding the use of medications with high sexual dysfunction potential or controlling hypertension and dyslipidemia), obtaining serum PRL levels in patients with symptoms suggestive of hPRL, and switching to another APDs with a more benign sexual side effect profile. Sildenafil may be a useful option for men with drug-induced erectile dysfunction.

OSTEOPOROSIS

Like many chronic diseases, osteoporosis is more prevalent among people with schizophrenia than the general population.[211] Stubbs and colleagues[212] performed a meta-analysis of 19 cross-sectional studies examining bone mineral density (BMD) in patients with schizophrenia and found that 51.7% of patients had low bone mass, 40.0% had osteopenia, and 13.2% had osteoporosis. The prevalence of low bone mass was twice that of age-matched and gender-matched controls (OR = 1.9), whereas osteoporosis was nearly 3 times more prevalent (OR = 2.86).

Mechanisms

The increased prevalence of osteoporosis in schizophrenia is thought to be due to genetic risk along with risks associated with other conditions potentially overrepresented in schizophrenia, such as lack of exercise, poor nutrition, diabetes, smoking, alcohol use, insufficient sun exposure, and vitamin D deficiency.[211,213] Although low BMI is a risk factor in the general population, such that being obese is thought to have a protective effect, with schizophrenia, low bone mass seems associated with elevated BMI.[212]

Based on the observation that chronic hPRL is associated with decreased BMD due to both estrogen deficiency and osteoclast-mediated bone resorption, APD therapy has been proposed as an important modifiable risk factor for osteoporosis.[211] Over the past decade, several small, cross-sectional studies have attempted to explore the role of APDs in low BMD and osteoporosis. These studies have varied considerably with respect to different sizes, genders, ethnicities, and postmenopausal status of their samples as well as the measurement technique of BMD, such that results have been inconsistent.[213,214] A review by Kishimoto and colleagues[213] noted that 8 of 13 studies have demonstrated a relationship between hPRL and low BMD. For example, low BMD has been correlated with hPRL in some studies involving young women, with medications, such as FGAs and RIS, associated with greater risk of bone mineral loss than PRL-sparing antipsychotics.[215–217] Studies including men have been more variable, with some demonstrating an association between APD-induced hPRL and low BMD,[218,219] but others showing no such correlation.[220,221] Additional studies comparing BMD among patients taking different APDs as well as those taking no APDs are needed to better understand the osteoporosis risk of individual APDs.

Because osteoporosis is a clinical concern due in large part to its association with fractures, several large, epidemiologic studies have examined the prevalence of this particular outcome in schizophrenia. A meta-analysis of 8 such studies involving approximately 50,000 individuals with schizophrenia found a significantly greater risk of fractures compared with controls (incident rate ratio = 1.72).[222] A Danish study found that APDs were a significant predictor of hip fracture among individuals with schizophrenia.[223] As with osteoporosis, however, there are numerous explanations of the increased prevalence of hip fractures in schizophrenia beyond the possible contribution of APDs, including inactivity and deconditioning, diabetes, and the use of other medications associated with sedation and orthostasis that might predispose to falls.[222] Antidepressants, anticholinergics, benzodiazepines, and corticosteroids have been found significant predictors of hip fractures in this population as well.[223] Among elderly patients not limited to those with schizophrenia, FGAs, SGAs, and antidepressants are all associated with an increased risk of hip fracture.[224] Such findings caution against the assumption that the elevated risk of fracture in schizophrenia is mediated solely by APD-induced hPRL and osteoporosis.

Monitoring and Management

In the absence of better evidence regarding a link between APD treatments, bone mineral loss, osteoporosis, and fractures, clear clinical guidelines remain elusive. Patients can be screened for symptoms of osteoporosis, such as a decrease in height or recent falls or visits to emergency rooms for broken bones. Although some investigators have advised routine monitoring of PRL levels during APD therapy independent of osteoporosis risk,[192] it is well recognized that PRL levels are not well correlated with clinical symptoms; this was not recommended in the authors' previous review.[1] Based on the current state of evidence, there remains limited utility to the routine monitoring of PRL levels during APD therapy.[214] The potential link between APD therapy, osteoporosis, and hip fractures does add, however, to the rationale of encouraging good dietary habits, smoking cessation, regular exercise, and sun exposure among patients with schizophrenia.[213,222] Likewise, the importance of preventative maintenance care in schizophrenia, including the age-appropriate assessment for osteoporosis along with testing and treatment of vitamin D deficiency, is underscored.[211] For patients with other risk factors for bone mineral loss, including low BMI, women with amenorrhea, patients taking corticosteroids, and those with a history of family history of fractures, clinicians should maintain a low threshold for BMD testing. In the presence of low BMD and hPRL, clinicians should consider switching patients who require APD therapy to a PRL-sparing SGA.

SUMMARY

This article provides an extensive review of many of the nonextrapyramidal side effects of APDs. Given a multitude of APD options, clinicians must weigh the relative risks and benefits of medications with collaborative decision making with patients to optimize recovery. Patients should be informed of potential adverse effects, with each visit representing an opportunity to review both positive and negative experiences associated with APD treatment. Optimal care requires that clinicians be adept at recognizing and monitoring APD side effects. Ideally, clinicians should be attuned to the whole patient, with patients and prescribers partnering to minimize risks and maximize benefits of APD therapy. It is hoped that this article provides clinicians with detailed information about APD side effects that will guide informed treatment decisions.

ACKNOWLEDGMENTS

The authors wish to thank Alissa Myer, Christine Canilao, Thien Nguyen, and Zachary Erickson for article preparation assistance.

REFERENCES

1. Wirshing DA, Pierre JM, Erhart S, et al. Understanding the new and evolving profile of adverse drug effects in schizophrenia. Psychiatr Clin North Am 2003;26:165–90.
2. De Hert M, Correll CU, Bobes J, et al. Physical illness in patients with severe mental disorders. I. Prevalence, impact of medications and disparities in health care. World Psychiatry 2011;1:52–77.
3. Maina G, Salvi V, Vitalucci A, et al. Prevalence and correlates of overweight in drug-naïve patients with bipolar disorder. J affective Disord 2008;1-2:149–55.
4. Colton CW, Manderscheid RW. Congruencies in increased mortality rates, years of potential life lost, and causes of death among public mental health clients in eight states. Preventing Chronic Dis 2006;2:A42.
5. Perez-Iglesias R, Vazquez-Barquero JL, Amado JA, et al. Effect of antipsychotics on peptides involved in energy balance in drug-naive psychotic patients after 1 year of treatment. J Clin Psychopharmacol 2008;3:289–95.
6. Wirshing DA, Wirshing WC, Kysar L, et al. Novel Antipsychotics: Comparison of Weight Gain Liabilities. J Clin Psychiatry 1999;60(6):358–63.
7. Stahl SM, Mignon L, Meyer JM. Which comes first: atypical antipsychotic treatment or cardiometabolic risk? Acta Psychiatr Scand 2009;3:171–9.
8. Deng C, Weston-Green K, Huang XF. The role of histaminergic H1 and H3 receptors in food intake: a mechanism for atypical antipsychotic-induced weight gain? Prog Neuropsychopharmacol Biol Psychiatry 2009;1:1–4.
9. Lett TA, Wallace TJ, Chowdhury NI, et al. Pharmacogenetics of antipsychotic-induced weight gain: review and clinical implications. Mol Psychiatry 2012; 17(3):242–66.
10. Correll CU. Antipsychotic use in children and adolescents: minimizing adverse effects to maximize outcomes. J Am Acad Child Adolesc Psychiatry 2008;1: 9–20.
11. Cuerda C, Velasco C, Merchan-Naranjo J, et al. The effects of second-generation antipsychotics on food intake, resting energy expenditure and physical activity. Eur J Clin Nutr 2013;2:146–52.
12. Blouin M, Tremblay A, Jalbert ME, et al. Adiposity and eating behaviors in patients under second generation antipsychotics. Obesity 2008;8:1780–7.
13. Kluge M, Schuld A, Himmerich H, et al. Clozapine and olanzapine are associated with food craving and binge eating: results from a randomized double-blind study. J Clin Psychopharmacol 2007;6:662–6.
14. De Hert M, Detraux J, Winkel RV, et al. Metabolic and cardiovascular adverse effects associated with antipsychotic drugs. Nat Rev Endocrinol 2011;8:114–26.

15. Kahn RS, Fleischhacker WW, Boter H, et al. Effectiveness of antipsychotic drugs in first-episode schizophrenia and schizophreniform disorder: an open randomised clinical trial. Lancet (London, England) 2008;9618:1085–97.

16. Lieberman JA, Stroup TS, McEvoy JP, et al. Effectiveness of antipsychotic drugs in patients with chronic schizophrenia. N Engl J Med 2005;12:1209–23.

17. Newcomer JW. Second-generation (atypical) antipsychotics and metabolic effects: a comprehensive literature review. CNS Drugs 2005;19(Suppl 1):1–93.

18. Patel JK, Buckley PF, Woolson S, et al. Metabolic profiles of second-generation antipsychotics in early psychosis: findings from the CAFE study. Schizophr Res 2009;1-3:9–16.

19. Deng C. Effects of antipsychotic medications on appetite, weight, and insulin resistance. Endocrinol Metab Clin North Am 2013;42(3):545–63.

20. Paliperidone [package insert]. In: Janssen Pharmaceuticals I, editor. Titusville, NJ: 2011.

21. Lurasidone [package insert]. In: Inc SP, editor. Marlborough, MA: 2013.

22. Asenapine [package insert]. In: Co M, editor. Whitehouse Station, NJ: 2013.

23. Leucht S, Cipriani A, Spineli L, et al. Comparative efficacy and tolerability of 15 antipsychotic drugs in schizophrenia: a multiple-treatments meta-analysis. Lancet 2013;382:951–62.

24. Pai N, Deng C, Vella SL, et al. Are there different neural mechanisms responsible for three stages of weight gain development in anti-psychotic therapy: temporally based hypothesis. Asian J Psychiatr 2012;4:315–8.

25. Zipursky RB, Gu H, Green AI, et al. Course and predictors of weight gain in people with first-episode psychosis treated with olanzapine or haloperidol. Br J Psychiatry 2005;187:537–43.

26. Henderson DC, Nguyen DD, Copeland PM, et al. Clozapine, diabetes mellitus, hperlipidemia, and cardiovascular risks and mortality: results of a 10-year naturalistic study. J Clin Psychiatry 2005;66(9):1116–21.

27. Bak M, Fransen A, Janssen J, et al. Almost All Antipsychotics Result in Weight Gain: A Meta-Analysis. PLoS One 2014;9(4):e94112.

28. Kinon BJ, Kaiser CJ, Ahmen S, et al. Association between early and rapid weight gain and change in weight over one year of olanzapine therapy in patients with schizophrenia and related disorders. J Clin Psychopharmacol 2005;3:255–8.

29. Simon V, van Winkel R, De Hert M. Are weight gain and metabolic side effects of atypical antipsychotics dose dependent? A literature review. J Clin Psychiatry 2009;7:1041–50.

30. Perry PJ, Argo TR, Carnahan RM, et al. The association of weight gain and olanzapine plasma concentrations. J Clin Psychopharmacol 2005;3:250–4.

31. Citrome L, Stauffer VL, Chen L, et al. Olanzapine plasma concentrations after treatment with 10, 20, and 40 mg/d in patients with schizophrenia: an analysis of correlations with efficacy, weight gain, and prolactin concentration. J Clin Psychopharmacol 2009;3:278–83.

32. Kane JM, Detke HC, Naber D, et al. Olanzapine long-acting injection: a 24-week, randomized, double-blind trial of maintenance treatment in patients with schizophrenia. Am J Psychiatry 2009;2:181–9.

33. Neovius M, Eberhard J, Lindstrom E, et al. Weight development in patients treated with risperidone: a 5-year naturalistic study. Acta Psychiatr Scand 2007;4:277–85.

34. Saddichha S, Manjunatha N, Ameen S, et al. Diabetes and schizophrenia - effect of disease or drug? Results from a randomized, double-blind, controlled

prospective study in first-episode schizophrenia. Acta Psychiatr Scand 2008;5: 342–7.

35. Kinon BJ, Basson BR, Gilmore JA, et al. Long-term olanzapine treatment: weight change and weight-related health factors in schizophrenia. J Clin Psychiatry 2001;2:92–9100.

36. Gebhardt S, Haberhausen M, Heinzel-Gutenbrunner M, et al. Antipsychotic-induced body weight gain: predictors and a systematic categorization of the long-term weight course. J Psychiatr Res 2008;6:620–6.

37. Perez-Iglesisas R, Martinez-Garcia O, Pardo-Garcia G, et al. Course of weight gain and metabolic abnormalities in first treated episode of psychosis: the first year is a critical period for development of cardiovascular risk factors. Int J Neuropsychopharmacol 2014;17(1):41–51.

38. American Diabetes Association, American Psychiatric Association, American Association of Clinical Endocrinologists, et al. Consensus development conference on antipsychotic drugs and obesity and diabetes. Diabetes Care 2004; 27(2):596–601.

39. Chen Y, Bobo WV, Watts K, et al. Comparative effectiveness of switching antipsychotic drug treatment to aripiprazole or ziprasidone for improving metabolic profile and atherogenic dyslipidemia: a 12-month, prospective, open-label study. J Psychopharmacol (Oxford, England) 2012;9:1201–10.

40. Rosen J, Wirshing D. Diabetes and the metabolic syndrome in mental health. Philadelphia: Lippincott; 2008.

41. Guzik L, Wirshing D. Behavioral weight loss classes for patients with severe mental illness. Psychiatr Serv 2007;58(11):1.

42. Wirshing D, Smith R, Erickson Z, et al. A wellness class for inpatients with psychotic disorders. J Psychiatr Pract 2006;12(1):5.

43. Kwan C, Gelberg H, Rosen J, et al. Nutritional counseling for adults with severe mental illness: key lessons learned. J Acad Nutr Diet 2014;114(3):5.

44. Das C, Mendez G, Jagasia S, et al. Second-generation antipsychotic use in schizophrenia and associated weight gain: a critical review and meta-analysis of behavioral and pharmacologic treatments. Ann Clin Psychiatry 2012;3: 225–39.

45. Baptista T, Rangel N, Fernandez V, et al. Metformin as an adjunctive treatment to control body weight and metabolic dysfunction during olanzapine administration: a multicentric, double-blind, placebo-controlled trial. Schizophr Res 2007; 93(1–3):99–108.

46. Wu RR, Zhao JP, Guo XF, et al. Metformin addition attenuates olazapine-induced weight gain in drug-naive first-episode schizophrenia patients: a double-blind, placebo-controlled study. Am J Psychiatry 2008;3:352–8.

47. Wu RR, Zhao JP, Jin H, et al. Lifestyle intervention and metformin for treatment of antipsychotic-induced weight gain: a randomized controlled trial. JAMA 2008;2: 185–93.

48. Jarskog LF, Hamer RM, Catellier DJ, et al. Metformin for weight loss and metabolic control in overweight outpatients with schizophrenia and schizoaffective disorder. AM J Psychiatry 2013;170(9):1032–40.

49. Ko YH, Joe SH, Jung IK, et al. Topiramate as an adjuvant treatment with atypical antipsychotics in schizophrenic patients experiencing weight gain. Clin neuropharmacology 2005;4:169–75.

50. Joffe G, Takala P, Tchoukhine E, et al. Orlistat in clozapine- or olanzapine-treated patients with overweight or obesity: a 16-week randomized, double-blind, placebo-controlled trial. J Clin Psychiatry 2008;69(5):706–11.

51. Baptista T, Uzcategui E, Rangel N, et al. Metformin plus sibutramine for olanzapine-associated weight gain and metabolic dysfunction in schizophrenia: a 12-week double-blind, placebo-controlled pilot study. Psychiatry Res 2008; 159(1–2):250–3.

52. Henderson DC, Copeland PM, Daley TB, et al. A double-blind, placebo-controlled trial of sibutramine for olanzapine-associated weight gain. Am J Psychiatry 2005;5:954–62.

53. Henderson DC, Fan X, Copeland PM, et al. A double-blind, placebo-controlled trial of sibutramine for clozapine-associated weight gain. Acta Psychiatr Scand 2007;2:101–5.

54. Holt RI, Bushe C, Citrome L. Diabetes and schizophrenia 2005: are we any closer to understanding the link? J Psychopharmacol 2005;6:56–65.

55. Holt RI, Mitchell AJ. Diabetes mellitus and severe mental illness: mechanisms and clinical implications. Nature reviews. Endocrinology 2014;2:79–89.

56. Annamalai A, Tek C. An overview of diabetes management in schizophrenia patients: office based strategies for primary care practitioners and endocrinologists. Int J Endocrinol 2015;2015:969182.

57. Spelman LM, Walsh PI, Sharifi N, et al. Impaired glucose tolerance in first-episode drug-naive patients with schizophrenia. Diabet Med 2007;5:481–5.

58. Lindenmayer JP, Czobor P, Volavka J, et al. Changes in glucose and cholesterol levels in patients with schizophrenia treated with typical or atypical antipsychotics. Am J Psychiatry 2003;2:290–6.

59. Citrome LL, Holt RI, Zachry WM, et al. Risk of treatment-emergent diabetes mellitus in patients receiving antipsychotics. Ann Pharmacother 2007;41(10): 1593–603.

60. Holt RI, Peveler RC. Association between antipsychotic drugs and diabetes. Diabetes Obes Metab 2006;2:125–35.

61. Wirshing DA, Spellberg BJ, Erhart SM, et al. Novel antipsychotics and new onset diabetes. Biol Psychiatry 1998;44:778–83.

62. Westphal SA. Obesity, abdominal obesity, and insulin resistance. Clin cornerstone 2008;1:23–9.

63. Allison DB, Mentore JL, Heo M, et al. Antipsychotic-induced weight gain: a comprehensive research synthesis. Am J Psychiatry 1999;11:1686–96.

64. Teff KL, Rickels MR, Grudziak J, et al. Antipsychotic-induced insulin resistance and postprandial hormonal dysregulation independent of weight gain or psychiatric disease. Diabetes 2013;9:3232–40.

65. Wu RR, Zhao JP, Zhai JG, et al. Sex difference in effects of typical and atypical antipsychotics on glucose-insulin homeostasis and lipid metabolism in first-episode schizophrenia. J Clin Psychopharmacol 2007;4:374–9.

66. Smith RC, Lindenmayer JP, Davis JM, et al. Effects of olanzapine and risperidone on glucose metabolism and insulin sensitivity in chronic schizophrenic patients with long-term antipsychotic treatment: a randomized 5-month study. J Clin Psychiatry 2009;11:1501–13.

67. Gautam D, Han SJ, Hamdan FF, et al. A critical role for beta cell M3 muscarinic acetylcholine receptors in regulating insulin release and blood glucose homeostasis in vivo. Cell Metab 2006;6:449–61.

68. Starrenburg FC, Bogers JP. How can antipsychotics cause Diabetes Mellitus? Insights based on receptor-binding profiles, humoral factors and transporter proteins. Eur Psychiatry 2009;24(3):164–70.

69. Correll CU. From receptor pharmacology to improved outcomes: individualising the selection, dosing, and switching of antipsychotics. Eur Psychiatry 2010;25: S12–21.

70. Wirshing DA, Boyd JA, Meng LR, et al. The effects of novel antipsychotics on glucose and lipid levels. J Clin Psychiatry 2002;10:856–65.

71. Wani RA, Dar MA, Margoob MA, et al. Diabetes mellitus and impaired glucose tolerance in patients with schizophrenia, before and after antipsychotic treatment. J neurosciences Rural Pract 2015;1:17–22.

72. Mitchell AJ, Malone D, Doebbeling CC. Quality of medical care for people with and without comorbid mental illness and substance misuse: systematic review of comparative studies. Br J Psychiatry 2009;6:491–9.

73. Standards of medical care in diabetes–2015: summary of revisions. Diabetes care 2015;38:S4.

74. Nasrallah HA, Meyer JM, Goff DC, et al. Low rates of treatment for hypertension, dyslipidemia and diabetes in schizophrenia: data from the CATIE schizophrenia trial sample at baseline. Schizophr Res 2006;86(1–3):15–22.

75. Skrede S, Steen VM, Ferno J. Antipsychotic-induced increase in lipid biosynthesis: activation through inhibition. J Lipid Res 2013;54:307–9.

76. Meyer JM, Koro CE. The effects of antipsychotic therapy on serum lipids: a comprehensive review. Schizophr Res 2004;70(1):1–17.

77. Saari K, Koponen H, Laitinen J. Hyperlipidemia in persons using antipsychotic medication: a general population-based birth cohort study. J Clin Psychiatry 2004;65(4):547–50.

78. Procyshyn R, Wasan K, Thorton A, et al. Changes in serum lipids, independent of weight, are associated with changes in symptoms during long-term clozapine treatment. J Psychiatry Neurosci 2007;32(5):331–8.

79. Spivak B, Lamschtein C, Talmon Y, et al. The impact of clozapine treatment on serum lipids in chronic schizophrenic patients. Clin Neuropharmacol 1999; 22(2):98–101.

80. Leitão-Azevedo CL, Guimarães LR, Abreu MGD. Increased dyslipidemia in schizophrenic outpatients using new generation antipsychotics. Rev Bras Psiquiatr 2006;28(4):301–4.

81. Sasaki J, Funakoshi M, Arakawa K. Lipids and apolipoproteins in patients treated with major tranquilizers. Clin Pharmacol Ther 1985;37:684.

82. de Leon JD, Susce MT, Johnson M, et al. A clinical study of the association of antipsychotics with hyperlipidemia. Schizophr Res 2007;92:95–102.

83. Olfson M, Marcus SC, Corey-Lisle P, et al. Hyperlipidemia following treatment with antipsychotic medications. Am J Psychiatry 2006;163:1821–5.

84. Meltzer HY, Bobo WV, Nuamah IF, et al. Efficacy and tolerability of oral paliperidone extended-release tablets in the treatment of acute schizophrenia: pooled data from three 6-week, placebo-controlled studies. J Clin Psychiatry 2008; 69(5):817–29.

85. Weiden PJ, Cutler AJ, Polymeropoulos MH, et al. Safety profile of iloperidone: a pooled analysis of 6-week acute-phase pivotal trials. J Clin Psychopharmacol 2008;28(2 Suppl 1):S12–9.

86. Kemp D, Zhao J, Cazorla P, et al. Weight Change and Metabolic Effects of Asenapine in Patients With Schizophrenia and Bipolar Disorder. J Clin Psychiatry 2014;75(3):238–45.

87. Potkin SG, Ogasa M, Cucchiaro J, et al. Double-blind comparison of the safety and efficacy of lurasidone and ziprasidone in clinically stable outpatients with schizophrenia or schizoaffective disorder. Schizophr Res 2011;132(2–3):101–7.

88. Samalin L, Garnier M, Llorca P. Clinical potential of lurasidone in the management of schizophrenia. Ther Clin Risk Manag 2011;7:239–50.

89. Garman P, Ried L, Bengtson M, et al. Effect on lipid profiles of switching from olanzapine to another second-generation antipsychotic agent in veterans with schizophrenia. J Am Pharm Assoc 2007;47:373–8.

90. Ray W, Meredith S, Thapa P, et al. Antipsychotics and the risk of sudden cardiac death. Arch Gen Psychiatry 2001;58:1161–7.

91. Vieweg W, Schneider R, Wood M. Torsade de pointes in a patient with complex medical and psychiatric conditions receiving low-dose quetiapine. Acta Psychiatr Scand 2005;112:318–22.

92. Tei Y, Morita T, Inoue S, et al. Torsades de pointes caused by a small dose of risperidone in a terminally ill cancer patient. Psychosomatics 2004;45:450–1.

93. Heinrich TW, Biblo LA, Schneider J. Torsades de pointes associated with ziprasidone. Psychosomatics 2006;47:264–8.

94. Ray W, Chung C, Murray K, et al. Atypical antipsychotic drugs and the risk of sudden cardiac death. N Engl J Med 2009;360:225–35.

95. Sager P, Seltzer J, Turner J, et al. Cardiovascular safety outcomes trials: a meeting report from the cardiac safety research consortium. Am Heart J 2015;169:486–95.

96. Beach S, Celano C, Noseworthy P, et al. QTc interval prolongation, torsades de pointes, and psychotropic medications. Psychosomatics 2013;54:1–13.

97. Titier K, Girodet P, Verdoux H, et al. Atypical antipsychotics from potassium channels to torsade de pointes and sudden death. Drug Saf 2005;28:35–51.

98. Haddad P, Anderson I. Antipsychotic-related QTc interval prolongation, torsade de points and sudden death. Drugs 2002;62:1649–71.

99. Isbister G, Page C. Drug induced QT prolongation: the measurement and assessment of the QT interval in practice. Br J Clin Pharmacol 2012;76:48–57.

100. Crouch M, Limon L, Cassano A. Clinical relevance and management of drug-related QT interval prolongation. Pharmacotherapy 2003;23:881–908.

101. Niemeijer M, van den Berg ME, Eijgelsheim M, et al. Short-term QT variability markers for the prediction of ventricular arrhythmias and sudden cardiac death: a systematic review. Heart 2014;100:1831–6.

102. Alvarez P, Pahissa J. QT alterations in psychopharmacology: proven candidates and suspects. Curr Drug Saf 2010;5:97–104.

103. Wu C, Tsai Y, Tsai H. Antipsychotic drugs and the risk of ventricular arrhythmia and/or sudden cardiac death: a nation-wide case-crossover study. J Am Heart Assoc 2015;4:e001568.

104. Murray-Thomas T, Jones M, Patel D, et al. Risk of mortality (including sudden cardiac death) and major cardiovascular events in atypical and typical antipsychotic users: a study with the general practice research database. Cardiovasc Psychiatry Neurol 2013;2013:247486.

105. Weeke P, Jensen A, Folke F, et al. Antipsychotics and associated risk of out-of-hospital cardiac arrest. Clin Pharmacol Ther 2014;96:490–7.

106. Trinkley K, Page R, Lien H, et al. QT interval prolongation and the risk of torsades de pointes: essentials for clinicians. Curr Med Res Opin 2013;29:1719–26.

107. Koponen H, Alaraisanen A, Saari K, et al. Schizophrenia and sudden cardiac death - a review. Nord J Psychiatry 2008;62:342–5.

108. Shah A, Aftab A, Coverdale J. QTc interval prolongation with antipsychotics: is routine ECG monitoring recommended? J Psychiatr Pract 2014;20:196–206.

109. Khasawneh F, Shankar G. Minimizing cardiovascular adverse effects of atypical antipsychotic drugs in patients with schizophrenia. Cardiol Res Pract 2014; 2014:8.
110. Kato M, Chang C. Augmentation treatments with second-generation antipsychotics to antidepressants in treatment-resistant depression. CNS Drugs 2013;27:S11–9.
111. Wright B, Eiland E, Lorenz R. Augmentation with atypical antipsychotics for depression: a review of evidence-based support from the medical literature. Pharmacotherapy 2013;33:344–59.
112. Spina E, Leon JD. Clinically relevant interactions between newer antidepressants and second-generation antipsychotics. Expert Opin Drug Metab Toxicol 2014;10:721–46.
113. Baller J, McGinty E, Azrin S, et al. Screening for cardiovascular risk factors in adults with serious mental illness: a review of the evidence. BMC Psychiatry 2015;15:55.
114. Jensen K, Juul K, Fink-Jensen A, et al. Corrected QT changes during antipsychotic treatment of children and adolescents: a systematic review and meta-analysis of clinical trials. J Am Acad Child Adolesc Psychiatry 2015;54:25–36.
115. Khanna P, Suo T, Komossa K, et al. Aripiprazole versus other atypical antipsychotics for schizophrenia. Cochrane Database Syst Rev 2014;1:CD006569.
116. Asmal L, Flegar SJ, Wang J, et al. Quetiapine versus other atypical antipsychotics for schizophrenia. Cochrane Database Syst Rev 2013;11:CD006625.
117. Komossa K, Rummel-Kluge C, Schwarz S, et al. Risperidone versus other atypical antipsychotics for schizophrenia. Cochrane Database Syst Rev 2011;1: CD006626.
118. Marino J, Caballero J. Iloperidone for the treatment of schizophrenia. Ann Pharmacother 2010;44:863–70.
119. Citrome L. Asenapine review, part II: clinical efficacy, safety and tolerability. Expert Opin Drug Saf 2014;13:803–30.
120. Sanford M. Lurasidone in the treatment of schizophrenia. CNS Drugs 2013;27: 67–80.
121. Citrome L. Lurasidone for schizophrenia: a review of the efficacy and safety profile for this newly approved second-generation antipsychotic. Int J Clin Pract 2011;65:189–210.
122. Rauch A, Fleischhacker W. Long-acting injectable formulations of new-generation antipsychotics: a review from a clinical perspective. CNS Drugs 2013;27:637–52.
123. Gentile S. Adverse effects associated with second-generation antipsychotic long-acting injection treatment: a comprehensive systematic review. Pharmacotherapy 2013;33:1087–106.
124. Fusar-Poli P, Kempton M, Rosenheck R. Efficacy and safety of second-generation long-acting injections in schizophrenia: a meta-analysis fo randomized-controlled trials. Int Clin Psychopharmacol 2013;28:57–66.
125. Brennan M. Pharmacogenetics of second-generation antipsychotics. Pharmacogenomics 2014;15:869–84.
126. January C, Wann S, Alpert J. AHA/ACC/HRS practice guideline: 2014 AHA/ACC/HRS guideline for the management of patients with atrial fibrillation: executive summary. Circulation 2014;130(23):2071–104.
127. Tisdale J, Jaynes H, Kingery J, et al. Development and validation of a risk score to predict QT interval prolongation in hospitalized patients. Circ Cardiovasc Qual Outcomes 2013;6:479–87.

128. Goff DC Jr, Lloyd-Jones D, Bennett G, et al. 2013 ACC/AHA guideline on the assessment of cardiovascular risk: a report of the American College of Cardiology/American Heart Association Task Force on Practice Guidelines. Circulation 2014;129(25 Suppl 2):S49–73.

129. Laursen TM, Nordentoft M, Mortensen PB. Excess early mortality in schizophrenia. Annu Rev Clin Psychol 2014;10:425–48.

130. Saha S, Chant D, McGrath J. A systematic review of mortality in schizophrenia: is the differential mortality gap worsening over time? Arch Gen Psychiatry 2007; 64:1123–31.

131. Mittal D, Corrigan P, Sherman MD, et al. Healthcare providers' attitudes towards persons with schizophrenia. Psychiatr Res J 2014;37:297–303.

132. Isaac M, Koch A. The risk of death among adult participants in trials of antipsychotic drugs in schizophrenia. Eur Neuropsychopharmacol 2010;20:139–45.

133. Weinmann S, Read J, Aderhold V. Influence of antipsychotics on mortality in schizophrenia: systematic review. Schizophr Res 2009;113:1–11.

134. Tiihonen J, Lonnqvist J, Whalbeck K, et al. 11-year follow-up of mortality in patients with schizophrenia: a population-based cohort study (FINA11 study). Lancet 2009;374:620–7.

135. De Hert M, Correll CU, Cohen D. Do antipsychotic medications reduce or increase mortality in schizophrenia? A critical appraisal of the FIN-11 study. Schizophr Res 2010;117:68–74.

136. Jones ME, Campbell G, Patel D, et al. Risk of mortality (including sudden cardiac death) and major cardiovascular events in users of olanzapine and other antipsychotics: a study with the General Practice Research Database. Cardiovasc Psychiatry Neurol 2013;2013:647476.

137. Khan A, Faucett J, Morrison S, et al. Comparative mortality risk in adult patients with schizophrenia, depression, bipolar disorder, anxiety disorders, and attention-deficit/hyperactivity disorder participating in psychopharmacology trials. JAMA Psychiatry 2013;70:1091–9.

138. Torniainen M, Mittendorfer-Rutz E, Tanskanen A, et al. Antipsychotic treatment and mortality in schizophrenia. Schizophr Bull 2015;41:656–63.

139. Tenback D, Pijl B, Smeets H, et al. All-cause mortality and medication risk factors in schizophrenia: A prospective cohort study. J Clin Psychopharmacol 2012;32:31–5.

140. Leonard CE, Freeman CP, Newcomb CW, et al. Antipsychotics and the risks of sudden cardiac death and all-cause death: cohort studies in medicaid and dually eligible medicaid-medicare beneficiaries of five states. J Clinic Exp Cardiol 2013;10(6):1–9.

141. Herrmann N, Lanctôt KL. Do atypical antipsychotics cause stroke? CNS Drugs 2005;19:91–103.

142. Schneider LS, Dagerman KS, Insel P. Risk of death with atypical antipsychotic drug treatment for dementia: meta-analysis of randomized placebo-controlled trials. JAMA 2005;294:1934–43.

143. FDA. Public health advisory: deaths with antipsychotics in elderly patients with behavioral disturbances. 2005. Available at: http://www.fda.gov/Drugs/DrugSafety/PostmarketDrugSafetyInformationforPatientsandProviders/ucm053171.htm. Accessed February 23, 2016.

144. Maher AR, Maglione M, Bagley S, et al. Efficacy and comparative effectiveness of atypical antipsychotic medications for off-label uses in adults: a systematic review and meta-analysis. JAMA 2011;306:1359–69.

145. Tan L, Tan L, Wang H, et al. Efficacy and safety of atypical antipsychotic drug treatment for dementia: a systematic review and meta-analysis. Alzheimers Res Ther 2015;7:20.
146. Gill SS, Bronskill SE, Normand ST, et al. Antipsychotic drug use and mortality in older adults with dementia. Ann Intern Med 2007;146:775–86.
147. Gisev N, Hartikainen S, Chen TF, et al. Effect of comorbidity on the risk of death associated with antipsychotic use among community-dwelling older adults. Int Psychogeriatr 2012;24:1058–64.
148. Pratt N, Roughead EE, Salter A, et al. Choice of observational study design impacts on measurement of antipsychotic risks in the elderly: a systematic review. BMC Med Res Methodol 2012;12:72.
149. Sultzer DL, Davis SM, Tariot PN, et al. Clinical symptom responses to atypical antipsychotic medications in Alzheimer's disease: phase 1 outcomes from the CATIE-AD effectiveness trial. Am J Psychiatry 2008;165:844–54.
150. Maust DT, Kim HM, Seyfried LS, et al. Antipsychotics, other psychotropics, and the risk of death in patients with dementia: number needed to harm. JAMA Psychiatry 2015;72:438–45.
151. Hulshof TA, Zuidema SU, Ostelo RW, et al. The mortality risk of conventional antipsychotics in elderly patients: a systematic review and meta-analysis of randomized placebo-controlled trials. J Am Med Dir Assoc 2015;16(10):817–24.
152. Wang PS, Schneeweiss S, Avorn J, et al. Risk of death is elderly users of conventional vs. atypical antipsychotic medications. N Engl J Med 2005;113:1–11.
153. Schneeweiss S, Setoguichi S, Brookhart A, et al. Risk of death associated with the use of conventional versus atypical antipsychotic drugs among elderly patients. CMAJ 2007;176:627–32.
154. Liperoti R, Onder G, Landi R, et al. All-cause mortality associated with atypical and conventional antipsychotic among nursing home residents with dementia: a retrospective cohort study. J Clin Psychiatry 2009;70:1340–7.
155. Setoguchi S, Wang PS, Brookhart MA, et al. Potential causes of higher mortality in elderly users of conventional and atypical antipsychotic medications. J Am Geriatr Soc 2008;56:1644–50.
156. Huybrechts KF, Gerhard T, Crystal S, et al. Differential risk of death in older residents in nursing homes prescribed specific antipsychotic drugs: population based cohort study. BMJ 2012;344:e977.
157. Aparasu RR, Chatterjee S, Mehta S, et al. Risk of death in dual-eligible nursing home residents using typical or atypical antipsychotic agents. Med Care 2012; 50:961–9.
158. Kales HC, Kim HM, Zivin K, et al. Risk of mortality among individual antipsychotics in patients with dementia. Am J Psychiatry 2012;169:71–9.
159. FDA. Information for healthcare professionals: conventional antipsychotics. 2008. Available at: http://www.fda.gov/Drugs/DrugSafety/PostmarketDrugSafetyInformationforPatientsandProviders/ucm124830.htm. Accessed February 23, 2016.
160. Jackson JW, VanderWee TJ, Viswanathan A, et al. The explanatory role of stroke as mediator of the mortality risk difference between older adults who initiate first-versus second-generation antipsychotic drugs. Am J Epidemiol 2014;180:847–52.
161. Desai VC, Heaton PC, Kelton CM. Impact of the Food and Drug Administration's antipsychotic black box warning on psychotropic drug prescribing in elderly patients with dementia in outpatient and office-based settings. Alzheimers Dement 2012;8:453–7.

162. Keenmon C, Sultzer D. The role of antipsychotic drugs in the treatment of neuro-psychiatric symptoms of dementia. Focus 2013;11:32–8.

163. Livingston G, Kelly L, Lewis-Holmes E, et al. Non-pharmacologic interventions for agitation in dementia: systematic review of randomized controlled trials. BR J Psychiatry 2015;205:436–42.

164. Declercq T, Petrovic M, Azermai M, et al. Withdrawal versus continuation of chronic antipsychotic drugs for behavioural and psychological symptoms in older people with dementia. Cochrane Database Syst Rev 2013;(3):CD007726.

165. Pan Y, Wu C, Gau SS, et al. Antipsychotic discontinuation in patients with dementia: a systematic review and meta-analysis of published randomized controlled studies. Dement Geriatr Cogn Disord 2014;37:125–40.

166. Inder WJ, Castle D. Antipsychotic-induced hyperprolactinemia. Aust N Z J Psychiatry 2011;68:361–7.

167. Kinon BJ, Gilmore JA, Liu H, et al. Prevalence of hyperprolactinemia in schizophrenic patients treated with conventional antipsychotic medications or risperidone. Psychoneuroendocrinology 2003;28:55–68.

168. Bushe C, Shaw M, Peveler RC. A review of the association between antipsychotic use and hyperporolactinaemia. J Psycholpharmacol 2008;22:46–55.

169. Alpak G, Unal A, Bulbul F, et al. Hyperprolactinemia due to paliperidone palmitate and treatment with aripiprazole. Bull Clin Psychopharmacol 2014;24(3): 253–6.

170. Cookson J, Hodgson R, Wildgust H. Prolactin, hyperprolactinema and antipsychotic treatment: a review and lessons for treatment of early psychosis. J Psychopharmacol 2012;26:42–51.

171. Haddad PM, Wieck A. Antipsychotic-induced hyperprolactinemia: mechanisms, clinical features and management. Drugs 2004;64:2291–314.

172. Madhusoodanan S, Parida S, Jimenez C. Hyperprolactinemia associated with psychotropics: a review. Hum Psychopharmacol 2010;25:281–97.

173. Lopez-Rodriguez R, Roman M, Novalbos J, et al. DRD2 Taq1A polymorphism modulates prolactin secretion induced by atypical antipsychotics in healthy volunteers. J Clin Psychopharmacol 2011;31:555–62.

174. Peuskens J, Pani L, Detraux J, et al. The effects of novel and newly approved antipsychotics on serum prolactin levels: a comprehensive review. CNS Drugs 2014;28:421–53.

175. Knegtering R, Baselmans P, Castelein S, et al. Predominant role of the 9-hydroxy metabolite of risperidone in elevating blood prolactin levels. Am J Psychiatry 2005;162:1010–2.

176. Berwaerts J, Cleton A, Rossenu S, et al. A comparison of serum prolactin concentrations after administration of paliperidone extended-release and risperidone tables in patients with schizophrenia. J Psychopharmacol 2010;24: 1011–8.

177. Montgomery J, Winterbottom E, Jessani M, et al. Prevalence of hyperprolactinemia in schizophrenia: association with typical and atypical antipsychotic treatment. J Clin Psychiatry 2004;65:1491–8.

178. McEvoy JP, Lieberman JA, Stroup TS, et al. Effectivness of clozapine versus olanzapine, quetiapine, and risperidone in patients with chronic schizophrenia who did not respond to prior atypical antipsychotic treatment. Am J Psychiatry 2006;163:600–10.

179. Stroup TS, Lieberman JA, McEvoy JP, et al. Effectiveness of olanzapine, quetiapine, and risperidone in patients with chronic schizophrenia after discontinuing perphenazine: A CATIE study. Am J Psychiatry 2007;164:415–27.

180. McEvoy JP, Lieberman JA, Perkins DO, et al. Efficacy and tolerability of olanzapine, quetiapine, and risperidone in the treatment of early psychosis: a randomized, double-blind 52-week comparison. Am J Psychiatry 2007;164:1050–60.

181. Bobo WV. Asenapine, iloperidone and lurasidone: critical appraisal of the most recently approved pharmacotherapies for schizophrenia in adults. Expert Rev Clin Pharmacol 2013;6:61–91.

182. Shahid M, Walker GB, Zorn SH, et al. Asenapine: a novel psychopharmacologic agent with a unique human receptor signature. J Psychopharmacol 2009;23: 65–73.

183. Citrome L. Role of sublingual asenapine in treatment of schizophrenia. Neuropsychiatr Dis Treat 2011;7:325–39.

184. Nakamura M, Ogasa M, Guarino J, et al. Lurasidone in the treatment of acute schizophrenia: a double-blind, placebo-controlled trial. J Clin Psychiatry 2009; 70:829–36.

185. Shapiro DA, Renock S, Arrington E, et al. Aripiprazole, a novel atypical antipsychotic drug with a unique and robust pharmacology. Neuropsychopharmacology 2003;28:1400–11.

186. Kooten MV, Arends J, Cohen D. Preliminary report: a naturalistic study of the effect of aripiprazole addition on risperidone-related hyperprolactinemia in patients treated with risperidone long-acting injection. J Clin Psychopharmacol 2011;31:126–8.

187. Basterreche N, Zumárraga M, Arrue A, et al. Aripiprazole reverses paliperidone-induced hyperprolactinemia. Actas Esp Psiquiatr 2012;40(5):90–2.

188. Shim JC, Shin JG, Kelly DL, et al. Adjunctive treatment with a dopamine partial agonist, aripiprazole, for antipsychotic-induced hyperprolactinemia: a placebo-controlled trial. Am J Psychiatry 2007;164:1404–10.

189. Mir A, Shivakumar K, Williamson RJ, et al. Change in sexual dysfunction with aripiprazole: a switching or add-on study. J Psychopharmacol 2008;22:244–53.

190. Rocha FL, Hara C, Ramos MG. Using aripiprazole to attenuate paliperidone-induced hyperprolactinemia. Prog Neuropsychopharmacol Biol Psychiatry 2010;34:1153–4.

191. Citrome L. Current guidelines and their recommendations for prolactin monitoring in psychosis. J Psychopharmacol 2008;22:90–7.

192. Peveler RC, Branford D, Citrome L, et al. Antipsychotics and hyperprolactinemia: clinical recommendations. J Psychopharmacol 2008;22(2 Suppl):98–103.

193. Ajmal A, Joffe H, Nachtigall LB. Psychotropic-Induced Hyperprolactinemia: a clinical review. Psychosomatics 2014;55(1):29–36.

194. Baggaley M. Sexual dysfunction in schizophrenia: focus on recent evidence. Hum Psychopharmacol 2008;23:201–9.

195. Serretti A, Chiesa A. A meta-analysis of sexual dysfunction in psychiatric patients taking antipsychotics. Int Clin Psychopharmacol 2011;26:130–40.

196. Gutierrez MA, Mushtaq R, Stimmel G. Sexual dysfunction in women with epilepsy: role of antiepileptic drugs and psychotropic medications. Int Rev Neurobiol 2008;83:157–67.

197. Stahl SM. Stahl's essential psychopharmacology: Neuroscientific basis and practical applications. 4th edition. New York: Cambridge University Press; 2013. p. 129–236.

198. Torre AL, Duffy ACD. Sexual dysfunction related to psychotropic drugs: a critical review part II: antipsychotics. Pharmacopsychiatry 2013;46:201–8.

199. Inder WJ, Castle D. Antipsychotic-induced hyperprolactinemia. Aust N Z J Psychiatry 2011;45(10):830–7.

200. Gitlin M. Sexual dysfunction with psychotropic drugs. Expert Opin Pharmacother 2003;4(12):2259–69.
201. Laumann EO, Paik A, Rosen RC. Sexual dysfunction in the United States. JAMA 1999;281:537–44.
202. Smith S, O'Keane V, Murray R. Sexual dysfunction in patients taking conventional antipsychotic medication. Br J Psychol 2002;181:49–55.
203. Howes OD, Wheeler MJ, Pilowsky LS, et al. Sexual function and gonadal hormones in patients taking antipsychotic treatment for schizophrenia or schizoaffective disorder. J Clin Psychiatry 2007;68:361–7.
204. Knegtering H, Bosch RVD, Castelein S, et al. Are sexual side effects of prolactin-raising antipsychotics reducible to serum prolactin? Psychoneuroendocrinology 2008;33:159–74.
205. De Hert M, Detraux J, Peuskens J. Second-generation and newly approved antipsychotics, serum prolactin levels and sexual dysfunctions: a critical literature review. Expert Opin Drug Saf 2014;13(5):605–24.
206. Nunes LV, Moreira HC, Razzouk D, et al. Strategies for the treatment of antipsychotic-induced sexual dysfunction and/or hyperprolactinemia among patients of the schizophrenia spectrum: a review. J Sex Marital Ther 2012; 38(2):281–301.
207. Schmidt HM, Hagen M, Kriston L, et al. Management of sexual dysfunction due to antipsychotic drug therapy. Cochrane Database Syst Rev 2012;(11): CD003546.
208. Andersohn F, Schmedt N, Weinmann S, et al. Priapism associated with antipsychotics: role of alpha1 adrenoreceptor affinity. J Clin Psychopharmacol 2010;30: 68–71.
209. Kirshner A, Davis RR. Priapism associated with the switch from oral to injectable risperidone. J Clin Psychopharmacol 2006;26:626–8.
210. Rodriguez-Cabezas L, Kong B, Agarwal G. Priapism associated with iloperidone: a case report. Gen Hosp Psychiatry 2014;36:451.
211. Wu H, Deng L, Zhao L, et al. Osteoporosis associated with antipsychotic treatment in schizophrenia. Int J Endocrinol 2013;2013:167138.
212. Stubbs B, De Hert M, Sepehry AA, et al. A meta-analysis of prevalence estimates and moderators of low bone mass in people with schizophrenia. Acta Psychiatr Scand 2014;130:470–86.
213. Kishimoto T, De Hert M, Carlson HE, et al. Osteoporosis and fracture risk in people with schizophrenia. Curr Opin Psychiatry 2012;25:415–29.
214. Crews MPK, Howes OD. Is antipsychotic treatment linked to bone mineral density and osteoporosis? A review of the evidence and the clinical implications. Hum Psychopharmacol 2012;27:15–23.
215. O'Keane V, Meaney A. Antipsychotic drugs: a new risk factor for osteoporosis in young women with schizophrenia? J Clin Psychopharmacol 2005;25:26–31.
216. Meaney AM, O'Keane V. Bone mineral density changes over a years in young females with schizophrenia: relationship to medication and endocrine variables. Schizophr Res 2007;93:136–43.
217. O'Keane V. Antipsychotic-induced hyperprolactinemia, hypogonadism and osteoporosis in the treatment of schizophrenia. J Psychopharmacol 2008; 22(2 suppl):70–5.
218. Abraham G, Halbreich U, Friedman RH, et al. Bone mineral desnity and prolactin assocations in patients with chronic schizophrenia. Schizophr Res 2003;59: 17–8.

219. Kishimoto T, Watanabe K, Shimada N, et al. Antipsychotic-induced hyperprolactinaemia inhibits the hypothalamo-pituitary-gonadal axis and reduces bone mineral desnity in male pateints with schizophrenia. J Clin Psychiatry 2008;69:382–91.
220. Howes OD, Wheeler MJ, Meaney AM, et al. Bone mineral density and its relationship to prolactin levels in patients taking antipsychotic treatment. J Clin Psychopharmacol 2005;25:259–61.
221. Lee TY, Chung MY, Chung HK, et al. Bone density in chronic schizophrenia with long-tern antipsychotic treatment: Preliminary study. Psychiatry Investig 2010;7:278–84.
222. Stubbs B, Gaughran F, Mitchell AJ, et al. Schizophrenia and the risk of fractures: a systematic review and comparative meta-analysis. Gen Hosp Psychiatry 2015;37:126–33.
223. Sorenson HJ, Jensen SOW, Nielson J. Schizophrenia, antipsychotics and risk of hip fracture: A population-based analysis. Eur Neuropsychopharmacol 2013;23:872–8.
224. Oderda LH, Young JR, Asche CV, et al. Psychotropic-related hip fractures: Meta-analysis of first-generation and second-generation antidepressant and antipsychotic drugs. Ann Pharmacother 2012;46:917–28.

Recovery in Schizophrenia

What Consumers Know and Do Not Know

Anthony O. Ahmed, PhD[a],*, Brielle A. Marino, MA[a], Elizabeth Rosenthal, MA[a], Alex Buckner, MS[a], Kristin M. Hunter, MS[b], Paul Alex Mabe, PhD[b], Peter F. Buckley, MD[b]

KEYWORDS

- Recovery model • Peer support • Illness self-management • Supported housing
- Supported employment • Strengths model • Shared decision making
- Advance directives

KEY POINTS

- The view that recovery is a personal, experiential process has permeated mental health systems in North America.
- There are areas of philosophic synergy between recovery and evidence-based practice that serve as impetus for practical convergence.
- The recovery model has led to innovative treatments and services for people with schizophrenia that support their pursuit of goals, aspirations, independence, and meaning.
- There is growing empirical support for the benefits and cost-effectiveness of recovery-oriented interventions for people with schizophrenia.
- Ongoing challenges include advancing recovery-oriented training to practitioners and combating negative provider attitudes about the prospects of care recipients and the recovery model.

INTRODUCTION

Recovery is "a deeply personal, unique process of changing one's attitudes, values, feelings, goals, skills, and/or roles. It is a way of living a satisfying, hopeful, and contributing life even with the limitations caused by illness".
—William Anthony[1(p527)]

For more than 3 decades, there has been an increased interest among mental health policy makers in North America, Europe, Australia, and New Zealand to adopt and promote the recovery model of mental health.[2–4] To foster the vision of recovery, mental

Disclosures: None.
[a] Department of Psychiatry, Weill Cornell Medical College, 21 Bloomingdale Road, White Plains, NY 10605, USA; [b] Department of Psychiatry and Health Behavior, Augusta University, 997 Saint Sebastian Way, Augusta, GA 30904, USA
* Corresponding author.
E-mail address: aoa9001@med.cornell.edu

health systems in several countries are putting in significant effort to transform their programs into care systems with recovery-oriented outcomes as their central aim.[5–7] Representing a deviation from the medical model that underscored the reduction or remission of psychiatric symptoms and disability, recovery-oriented systems promote a restoration to full citizenship.[1,8] That is, regardless of the status of psychiatric symptoms, people with mental illness pursue personal goals, engage in valued social roles, and live and remain in a community of their own choosing.[9,10] This newer view of recovery has recently been extended to incorporate elements of citizenship in which systems enable care recipients to be full participants in their community through active knowledge of, influence on, and involvement in their community.[11]

It is recognized that the recovery model does not espouse a treatment approach per se; rather, as a guiding philosophy or vision, recovery redefines the parameters of psychiatric care. The goal of treatment is centered not on a restoration of symptom-free state but on the promotion of the care recipient's wellness, independence, and the subjective experience of personalized experiential recovery.[9,12] Its status as a guiding philosophy situates recovery in such a way that it can be confluent and synergistic with traditional, clinic-based treatments for psychiatric illnesses.[10] On the one hand, consumers of mental health services and advocates have criticized the traditional medical model as impinging on the civil rights of care recipients while fostering disability and dependency.[13,14] Some advocates have gone as far as to call for a complete eradication of traditional care and a replacement with recovery-oriented services that they view as more inclusive and sensitive to choices and autonomy. Conversely, many practitioners and consumers who promote recovery while considering the benefits and empirical basis of psychiatric interventions advocate for a complementary relationship.[10,15]

Notwithstanding opposing views regarding the prospects of synergy between recovery and traditional practice, recovery has found its way into mainstream psychiatric practice. This review sets out to describe recovery-based advances in contemporary psychiatric services for people with schizophrenia. The review underscores system-wide measures, treatments, and services that promote recovery for people with schizophrenia. The current review also highlights ongoing challenges that have continued to plague the full adoption of the recovery model in the care of people with schizophrenia.

RECOVERY AND TRADITIONAL PRACTICES: FINDING PHILOSOPHIC SYNERGY

To establish the prospects of synergy between recovery and traditional psychiatric practice, some philosophic confluences are first considered. In particular, areas of philosophic convergence between recovery and evidence-based practice and areas where their goals are complementary are considered.

Intervention targets in schizophrenia care often extend beyond its well-recognized positive, negative, and affective symptoms. In many cases, people with schizophrenia also experience the challenge of limited social supports, unemployment, homelessness, societal stigma, and limited community resources. Traditional providers may depend on available evidence to inform many aspects of their psychiatric practice. This includes reviewing the empirical status of psychopharmacologic, somatic, psychosocial, and system-based interventions. Traditional care relies on the dissemination of knowledge accrued through clinical trials of interventions that have garnered empirical support. Practitioners, however, also consider person-level variables in clinical decision making, often drawing from their own clinical experience with the care recipient or others to whom they have provided services.[16,17] As illuminated by

Davidson and colleagues,[10] evidence-based medicine advocates a consideration of the care recipient's own cultural context, available supports, goals, and preferences in clinical decisions, particularly when there is equivocal evidence favoring alternatives.

Contemporary evidence-based medicine strongly advocates *personal medicine* — a personalized approach to treatment that goes beyond the empirical support for a particular intervention and, rather, considers the impact of variables unique to the individual in medical decision making.[18] The principles of knowledge dissemination, informed decision making, a consideration of an individual's own preferences, and a personalized approach to care are consistent with principles espoused by the recovery model. Practitioners, care recipients, and families are interested in and want access to the most efficacious treatments to address presenting problems. Consumer choice and the availability of options with demonstrable benefits through empirical support are consistent with recovery. It is often the case that parties differ with regard to their decisional criteria for an effective intervention. In a subsequent section, the process of shared decision making as an innovation that capitalizes on shared and disparate yet compatible guiding principles for optimal treatment decision making is described.

The shared philosophic underpinnings of recovery and evidence-based practices might suggest to some practitioners that evidence-based practice is equivalent to recovery-oriented care or that recovery-oriented care simply implies a directed implementation of evidence-based care. This supposition is in error, however, because recovery denotes specific outcome dimensions that have hardly been the targets of treatment in the traditional care of people with schizophrenia. Recovery-oriented care underscores outcomes that include hope and optimism, empowerment, meaning, connectedness, and citizenship.[19,20] The recovery movement has influenced the thinking of some traditional providers to reorient the goals of medication management and psychosocial interventions toward recovery. The greater impact of recovery, however, is on the development of new evidence-based interventions targeted toward fostering recovery-oriented outcomes as alternatives or adjuncts to the traditional care of people with schizophrenia.

THE ADVANCEMENT OF RECOVERY-ORIENTED PRACTICES

The recovery model has led to the development of several recovery-oriented interventions in the mental health system. In contrast to traditional clinical care, with a central focus on decreasing symptoms and disability, the recovery dimensions — hope, empowerment, meaning, identity, and connectedness/citizenship — represent the treatment target of recovery-oriented interventions for schizophrenia. Given their advent within the zeitgeist of evidence-based practice, there is growing effort to study the empirical support for these interventions.[21] Some of the recovery-oriented practices that have permeated traditional care systems are reviewed.

Peer-led Interventions

A more extensive discussion of peer-led interventions can be found elsewhere.[22,23] Peer-led interventions are a collection of mental health programs inspired by the consumer/survivor movement for recovery but have become recognized as an important complement to standard psychiatric care. In these interventions, people dealing with the challenge of psychiatric illnesses foster the experience of recovery for others dealing with similar challenges by providing support, encouragement, mentorship, and serving as coping models.[22] Peer-led interventions are classified into

3 forms—mutual support/self-help groups, consumer-operated services, and peer support services.[22–32] These programs differ in the degree to which they have been integrated into standard psychiatric care, with peer support provided within traditional clinics being the most integrated. All peer-led interventions are experiencing increased continuity with traditional care by

- Seeking referrals from traditional providers and mental health settings[24–26]
- Partnering with traditional providers to develop program curriculum[24]
- Offering adjunctive services to those provided in traditional clinics and decreasing the burden on traditional settings[27–29]
- Providing consultation to traditional providers about recovery-oriented practice[30–32]
- Partnering with traditional providers to conduct clinical trials of the benefits of peer-led interventions

There has been concerted effort since the 2000s to rigorously investigate the benefits of peer-led interventions using clinical trial designs.[30,33] Many of these studies have investigated the benefits of peer-led interventions clinical outcomes, such as psychiatric symptoms, functioning, and hospitalization.[34–40] Studies have also evaluated peer-led interventions in relation to recovery-oriented outcomes, such as hope, empowerment, recovery, and user satisfaction.[41,42] Several selective reviews of the empirical status of peer-led interventions have been favorable, with many suggesting that peer-led interventions contribute to improvements in clinical and recovery-oriented outcomes.[22,30] A recent meta-analysis, however, of 18 randomized control trials of such interventions targeted toward people with severe mental illnesses was less enthusiastic about the empirical support for peer-led interventions.[43] The review included 4 comparisons of mutual support, 11 of peer support, and 3 of consumer-operated programs to treatment as usual. Although peer-led interventions did not produce significant benefits on symptoms, hospitalization, and satisfaction over treatment as usual, peer-led services did seem to have significant small to medium effects on hope, empowerment, and recovery. Therefore, in this small-sampled meta-analysis, peer-led interventions contribute to the outcomes they are exactly targeted to address.[44] The meta-analysis makes a case for the complementary contribution of peer-led interventions to traditional care by contributing to outcomes unaddressed by the latter. In particular, studies show that peer-led self-management interventions demonstrate benefits for people with severe mental illnesses by contributing to decreased symptoms, improved quality of life, and greater endorsement of recovery attitudes.[45,46] In addition, a systematic review of 11 several randomized clinical trials demonstrated that peer providers are able to provide certain services, such as case management, with efficacy that was comparable to those of traditional providers.[47] One consideration of the benefits of peer-led interventions that has received little attention in research studies is the impact of serving in a provider role on peer specialists themselves. In a sample of peer specialists, a recent study demonstrated that hiring people with schizophrenia and other severe mental illness in peer specialist roles seemed to contribute to feelings of hope and empowerment and to greater social engagement and psychosocial competence.[31,48] The degree to which peer specialists embraced the recovery philosophy also predicted the degree to which life stressors contributed to psychiatric symptoms.

Peer-led interventions have seen significant growth and integration within the US and Canadian mental health systems. Policy advancements within both countries have fostered increased feasibility of implementation. Peer-led interventions in the United States are Medicare/Medicaid reimbursable in most states, and guidelines for certification and standard practice have been developed in both countries.

There are currently no recent (past 5 years) estimates of the number of peer-led services/providers in the country. The last estimate, published in 2002, however, suggested that there were close to 7500 self-help or consumer-operated services in the United States, an estimate that did not include traditional care settings that provided peer support services.[49,50] It is reasonable to expect that policy allowances and increased popularity of peer-led interventions in the past 13 years have allowed even greater growth of these interventions.

Self-management Interventions

The recovery model has led to the advancement of the principle of self-management in contemporary psychiatric care. One of the guiding principles of recovery is that it involves care recipients in collaboration with family members and the community, increasing their level of engagement treatment. This principle underscores the existing strengths and resources that care recipients have that can be recruited as they contribute to their own wellness. The recovery focus on strengths intersects with the principles of self-determination and personal responsibility as individuals with schizophrenia and other severe mental illnesses collaborate with others in their own self-care. Self-management interventions have a long-standing legacy in chronic medical illnesses where they have been found to contribute to improved medical outcomes, function, and quality of life.[51,52] In psychiatric care, self-management programs have been developed to

1. Improve coping skills and decrease risk for relapse
2. Enhance subjective well-being
3. Foster greater autonomy of self-care
4. Increase psychosocial and role functioning
5. Increase self-direction, self-efficacy, and overall experiential recovery.

Two of the most recognized self-management interventions for people with schizophrenia are the Illness Management and Recovery (IMR) program and the Wellness Recovery Action Plan (WRAP).

The IMR program was developed and is usually delivered by traditional providers (case managers, social workers, nurses, and so forth) in individual or group psychotherapy formats.[53] The goals of the intervention include helping people with schizophrenia develop problem-solving skills, improve their understanding of symptoms and treatment, improve medication adherence, develop social support, and set personal goals. Participants are exposed to the recovery philosophy early in the intervention and skills acquired during the treatment are justified in the context of personal recovery goals established early in the IMR program. IMR practitioners use several evidence-based strategies that include psychoeducation and cognitive behavioral, motivational, and social skills training to accomplish IMR goals. IMR underscores the setting and accomplishment of recovery goals. IMR's emphasis on psychiatric diagnosis and medication adherence in its modules as well as its use of several traditional interventions may promote confluence with traditional interventions. To some practitioners in the recovery movement, however, IMR may overly emphasize symptom severity and medication adherence. The rejoinder is that taking medications is not inconsistent with recovery as long as these are considered tools that may support recovery rather than primary steps to recovery.[54,55] Moreover, IMR practitioners work collaboratively with care recipients to identify targets for treatment and preferred coping strategies and to develop recovery goals, all of which are consistent with recovery.

The WRAP is a self-management tool that originated within the recovery movement and currently represents the most widely used self-management intervention among care recipients. The WRAP is usually taught by peer specialists in workshops using materials authored by Mary Ellen Copeland.[56,57] Using the WRAP, people with schizophrenia and other severe mental illnesses develop a personal wellness plan that comprises

1. The creation of a daily maintenance strategy
2. The identification of triggers and early warning signs of crises
3. Development of a crises action plan
4. Establishment of a healthy/nurturing lifestyle
5. Social support and self-advocacy planning
6. Fostering and building self-esteem
7. Managing tension and stress

Care recipients draw on coping skills included in a "wellness toolbox" that is informed by examples from peer facilitators, other peers, and their own personal experiences of successful coping. Unlike IMR, the WRAP de-emphasizes psychiatric diagnosis and medication management at a primary coping strategy, although it may be discussed as one of many tools in the wellness toolbox. Given that the WRAP groups are facilitated by peer specialists, care recipients benefit from active peer modeling, mentoring, and support.

There have been several studies of the benefits of IMR that suggest that it contributes to improvements in psychiatric symptoms, functional status, and knowledge of and engagement with recovery goals in people with severe mental illnesses.[58–60] Fewer studies have evaluated the WRAP.[61,62] A recent multisite clinical trial of 519 people with severe mental illnesses, including 105 with schizophrenia, however, found that peer-led training and use of the WRAP contributed to significant improvements in psychiatric symptoms, hopefulness, and quality of life.[61] The WRAP has been widely incorporated into mental health programs in the United States, Canada, New Zealand, Australia, Japan, and the United Kingdom.[63] In the United States, a February 2011 estimate suggested that more than 2000 people had been trained as WRAP peer facilitators and more than 10,000 copies of the WRAP had been distributed by the Copeland Center for Wellness and Recovery and Wellness. Moreover, WRAP programs have been initiated and funded in most US states.[61,63]

Strength-based Case Management

The recovery model purports that care recipients, their families, and the immediate environment possess strengths and resources that can be channeled to overall well-being and recovery. A similar perspective evolved and gained traction in the traditional care of people with severe mental illnesses. This strength-based perspective has become important particularly in the provision of case management services.[64] Strength-based case management focuses on helping people with schizophrenia and other severe mental illnesses reclaim their lives and achieve personally established goals. Goals are attained through the securing of personal and environmental resources that are necessary for optimal interdependent community living. The resources in view include a care recipient's own external resources (competencies, aspirations, and sense of efficacy) and internal resources (social relationships and community resources). Unlike traditional case management, which focuses on the brokering of services (benefits assistance, treatment coordination, referrals, and so forth), the strength-based approach focuses on enhancing and bridging between both external and internal resources.

The strength-based model originated in the 1980s independent of the recovery perspective but seems based on similar philosophic assumptions. For example, both advocate for niches that support an individual's aspirations and competencies. The goal of strength-based case management has come to be viewed as promoting recovery by supporting achievement and improved quality of life. Much like the recovery model, strength-based case management underscores the importance of supporting community integration—such that care recipients have housing, satisfactory employment and income, social support, and advocacy. Rapp and Goscha[65] highlight 6 principles of strength-based case management:

1. Recovery is possible; the goal of case management is to create conditions that support recovery.
2. An emphasis is on strengths and resources rather than psychiatric symptoms or deficits.
3. The community can be channeled to support the individual as a source of well-being.
4. The care recipient is involved in case management decisions and exercises full self-determination.
5. Case management is community oriented in that it occurs within the care recipient's environment.
6. A strong and trusting relationship between the case manager and the care recipient is necessary to mobilize resources for personalized recovery.

There have been 4 randomized studies of the benefits of strengths-based case management.[66–69] Examined outcomes include symptoms, well-being, psychosocial functioning variables, and consumer satisfaction. The studies overall demonstrated that the case management approach was associated with reductions in psychiatric symptoms, improvements in psychosocial functioning, and greater consumer satisfaction. Moreover, in a large multicenter study, Fukui and colleagues[70] demonstrated that high case manager fidelity to the strength-based model predicted decreased risk of hospitalization and greater employment and vocational attainment on the part of care recipients. Strength-based case management has permeated mental health services in the United States; however, estimates are currently unavailable.

Supported Housing

Recovery principles advocate for the full support and integration of people with psychiatric illnesses in communities of their choice. Housing is considered a prerequisite for full social integration. Epidemiologic studies have shown that people with schizophrenia and other severe mental illnesses are at high risk for homelessness, and, consequently, they represent a substantial proportion (20%–40%) of homeless individuals.[71,72] Several systems-level factors have contributed to the high rate of homelessness, including a legacy of poor social planning, limited availability of community resources to aid the transition from hospital to the community, rising cost, and discrimination. Coupled with the possible disruptions caused by acute psychotic episodes, substance use, psychosocial stressors, and cognitive impairments, people with schizophrenia are at particularly high risk of homelessness.[72]

Supported housing is an approach to addressing housing needs in people with schizophrenia and other severe mental illnesses.[73,74] Supported housing approaches work with care recipients to find safe and permanent placements that support their recovery. These placements become the platform for the integration of supportive services and psychiatric care. The supported housing model is at its heart a recovery-oriented model and subscribes to assumptions that echo principles espoused by recovery advocates[74]:

- Housing is a basic right: care recipients have a right to safe and affordable housing.
- Choices and options: housing choices and options, including location and whom to live with, should be provided.
- Individualized flexible support: all care recipients regardless of the status of illness can live successfully in flexible supported housing. The level of support provided should be malleable to the amount needed.
- Citizenship: care recipients should be provided with placements that are fully integrated rather than segregated from the community.
- Social activities, roles, and lifestyle: care recipients should be supported as they embark on activities and roles of their own choosing. Care recipients have a right to determine the level of support they need.
- Autonomy: housing should be provided for as long as it is desired. Community supports provided in the context of the program should be provided as long as they are needed. Supports should not be a prerequisite for housing.

The mental health systems in the United States and Canada have witnessed a proliferation of supported housing programs, such as Housing First, Tenancy Support, At Home, Projects for Assistance in Transition from Homelessness. Many programs integrate support services drawn from traditional psychiatric interventions, such as case management, psychotherapy services, and psychopharmacologic treatment, and from other recovery-oriented services, such as peer-led interventions and leisure activities. In this way, the housing program serves to integrate traditional and recovery-oriented services in the advancement of a care recipient's experiential recovery. Studies have examined the benefits of the supported housing model by comparing it to a prior housing situation or homelessness.[75–80] These studies have found that supported housing programs contribute to greater reductions in homelessness, hospitalization, jail confinement, and psychiatric symptoms. Moreover, supported housing programs also contributed to improved psychosocial outcomes, life satisfaction, and quality of life.

Supported Employment

People with schizophrenia and other severe mental illnesses experience a high rate of unemployment.[81,82] The experience of psychotic symptoms and schizophrenia-related functional impairments might have initially contributed to vocational impairments. Systemic factors, however, such as employment discrimination and prejudice against people with severe mental illnesses, have contributed to high rates of unemployment.[83] In addition, traditional providers often assumed that employment would be overly stressful for people with schizophrenia and contribute to decompensation.[84] Consequently, many who might have otherwise enjoyed the benefits of employment—financial independence, recreation, and community life—are discouraged from seeking gainful employment.

Supported employment programs, such as individual placement and support, encourage and assist care recipients seeking competitive employment—that is, part-time or full-time jobs that are open to anyone regardless of their psychiatric status.[85] Care recipients receive wages and employment benefits comparable to those of employees without a psychiatric diagnosis. Care recipients are provided with an employment specialist who provides support with job search and the management of work demands. The employment specialist and the care recipient work collaboratively with traditional providers to coordinate the provision of psychiatric care around work schedule. Supported employment programs echo recovery principles in their assumptions and practice.[86] These include

- Care recipient's self-determination and preferences: unlike traditional vocational rehabilitation programs that screen care recipients to determine their employment readiness, supported employment programs do not exclude any prospective participants. Rather, care recipients who express interest in employment are eligible to participate. Care recipients are also encouraged to express preferences about type of work, schedule, and the level of supports that they would receive.
- Individualized: the supports provided along with employment include benefits counseling and continuous follow-along supports. Benefits counseling is tailored to individual care recipients to help them understand social security benefits, Medicaid health insurance, and other sources of income that may be impacted by employment income. Follow-along supports needed are individualized to the care recipient and are determined by the care recipient in collaboration with the employment specialist and traditional care providers.
- Inclusion: traditional vocational rehabilitation programs usually provide employment to people with schizophrenia in segregated settings—jobs specifically created and for people with psychiatric illnesses. In contrast, supported employment seeks competitive employment in settings that foster the care recipient's community integration.

A recent systematic review of 18 randomized clinical trials of supported employment was favorable regarding its benefits at improving vocational outcomes in people with schizophrenia and other severe mental illnesses.[87] Care recipients who participated in supported employment were often approximately 3 times more likely to be employed at 12-month, 18-month, and 24-month follow-up intervals than those who participated in other forms of vocational rehabilitation. Employment rates for supported employment, however, were on average only approximately 34% at follow-up intervals. Moreover, studies suggest that people with schizophrenia may gain less from supported employment than people with other severe mental illnesses.[88–90] They do, however, demonstrate better vocational outcomes in supported employment than other vocational programs.[90] It seems that the degree of cognitive impairment experienced by the care recipient may be a critical moderating variable, with people who experience more severe impairments likely to have poorer work outcomes.[91] Recent studies have shown that cognitive remediation therapy, a behavioral intervention that seeks to reduce cognitive impairments through repeated training, may enhance outcomes from supported employment for people with schizophrenia.

Recovery Meets Psychopharmacology

Even as antipsychotic management represents the primary intervention for symptoms of schizophrenia, the recovery model has implications for aspects of standard medication practice. Recovery-oriented psychopharmacology is a recently proposed model of medication management that places recovery as the central focus of medication management.[92–94] Recovery informs the process of treatment decision making in a way that aligns the objectives and process of medication management to the life goals, aspirations, growth, and overall well-being of the care recipient. Recovery-oriented medication management involves

- Recovery goals: the goal of antipsychotic medication management is reframed from the reduction of psychiatric symptoms to promoting experiential recovery and the pursuit of meaningful goals. Medication evaluation includes a discussion of progress around accomplishing social, vocational, educational, and other plans. Medication adjustments are informed by a collaborative discussion of the extent to which they support or detract from a care recipient's own goals and wishes.

- Compliance versus engagement: traditional medication management emphasizes treatment compliance and adherence to accomplish the goal of symptom reduction. In contrast, a recovery-oriented approach underscores the engagement of the care recipient in defining treatment goals, deciding on treatment course, and taking medications. Although the focus on engagement, which seeks an increased involvement of care recipients and their family members, may have an impact on how readily care decisions are made, this has been argued as an ethical imperative.[95] Moreover, the autonomy of the care recipient and the principles of empowerment and self-direction should be weighed heavily when care decisions involve alternatives that are equivocal or situations that are controversial.[96]
- Shared decision making: shared decision making is an innovation in medicine that has recently seen discussion and application in medication management decision making. Shared decision making engages the care recipient in every aspect of the treatment decision making in a way that significantly influences the final medication decision.[97] The care recipient is provided with information about options and alternatives and both parties weigh options in terms of their decisional criteria. The essential features of shared decision making include
  ○ Shared expertise and information exchange: an acknowledgment of the shared expertise of the practitioner and the care recipient contributes to bidirectional information exchange.[98,99] With expertise in medicine, the practitioner is situated to educate the care recipient about treatment options. Care recipients' expertise lies with knowledge of their own goals, preferences, values, and life circumstances that may be impacted by or consequential to treatment decisions.[100] This process may be enhanced through the involvement of family members and other caretakers.
  ○ Shared deliberation: the practitioner and the care recipient discuss treatment options in terms of their preferences while weighing their decisional criteria. Criteria important to both practitioner and patient are weighed equally and actively for each available option.[99] For practitioners, the amount of evidence may weigh heavily in their decision and they may be interested in sharing this information with the care recipient.[101,102] The selection of the final option, however, is negotiated between practitioner and patient, with a goal of identifying an option consistent with the patient's values and preferences.
  ○ Shared acceptance: the treatment course is mutually negotiated and accepted by both parties and may not necessarily conform to either's idea of the best choice.[98] What is, therefore, crucial in shared decision making is not whether a practitioner acquiesces or persuades the patient but that the practitioner ensures that there is agreement on the final decision.

The need for shared decision making is apparent when considering the high rates of nonadherence to traditional antipsychotic care.[103–105] High rates of dissatisfaction with treatment, skepticism about the benefits of treatment, and a wish to maintain independence have been cited as common reasons for nonadherence.[106–108] Recent studies have demonstrated that more than 70% people with schizophrenia demonstrate a preference of for shared decision making.[97,109] Studies found that most care recipients with schizophrenia who experienced decisional impairments benefited from interventions aimed at supporting their decisional capacity (ie, decisional aids).[110] In all, shared decision making contributed to greater adherence, knowledge, treatment satisfaction, and quality of decisions made, as rated by practitioners.[111–113] In addition, shared decision making contributed to decreased hospitalization in a sample of people with schizophrenia.[113]

Advance Directives

Advance directives have seen recent application in psychiatric settings where they allow people with severe mental illnesses to anticipate and control the care they receive during periods of decisional impairment.[114] Advance directives are particularly useful for people with schizophrenia who are susceptible to emotional crises. With this tool, care recipients can specify actions that are acceptable during episodes or who could serve as a proxy decision maker. Advance directives can be developed in collaboration with the traditional providers in the form of joint crises plans.[115] Studies have shown that advance directives contribute to a sense of control and a decreased need for forced treatment.[116–118]

FUTURE CHALLENGES

Although recovery has permeated mainstream psychiatric practice, challenges abound for the sustained advancement of the recovery model. Ensuring that providers in traditional psychiatric settings are educated and influenced by the recovery model is critical. Recovery has been mostly an endeavor within mental health settings but has yet to permeate the training of mental health practitioners, in particular the training of psychiatrists and psychologists. Training programs maintain a medical conception of schizophrenia and residents, trainees, and attending physicians are often reluctant to adopt a recovery-based perspective. In a survey of trainees, Buckley and colleagues[119] found that psychiatry and psychology residents often held assumptions that were consistent with the medical model and also expressed skepticism about the recovery model in their practice. The Georgia Recovery-Based Educational Approach to Treatment (Project GREAT) is an example of an initiative to provide recovery-based education to traditional providers.[119,120] The Project GREAT team includes peer specialists and doctoral-level providers. Project GREAT helps trainees and practitioners transform their practices into recovery-oriented ones by

1. Developing curriculums geared toward increasing provider knowledge about recovery
2. Developing and disseminating recovery practice tools
3. Providing consultation services to programs seeking to transform their services
4. Conducting outreach visits

Advancing recovery education requires that many more training programs develop and adopt recovery-based curricula in their training of future practitioners.

Many mental health providers continue to harbor attitudes that detract from the experiential recovery-of-care recipients. These include skepticism about their expressed preferences, goals, and perspectives about care, which are more often dismissed or discounted as indicative of poor reality testing, noncompliance, and limited insight. Many traditional providers who continue to view the goal of psychiatric treatment as primarily the reduction of symptoms and disability may be more apt to discount the relevance of recovery principles to care recipients whom they view as very symptomatic.[19] Skepticism about the salience of recovery for people with schizophrenia continues to contribute to the use of seclusion, restraint, and forced psychiatric treatment. The continued use of these interventions remains a significant challenge for the advancement of recovery in inpatient settings.[121,122] Several successful hospital-based initiatives suggest that inpatient programs can realistically eliminate the use of seclusion and restraints and all forms of mandatory interventions.[123–125]

SUMMARY

The recovery model is wielding a welcome influence on the care of people with schizophrenia and other severe mental illnesses. The philosophic underpinnings of recovery are evident in several next-generation psychiatric interventions, many of which have been shown to contribute to positive clinical and recovery-oriented outcomes. New ideas that reframe the focus of traditional psychiatric practices, such as medication treatment and case management, as more recovery oriented are also permeating psychiatric clinics. Challenges remain, particularly around advancing recovery-based training and combating the skepticism many traditional providers may harbor about recovery. Greater awareness and dissemination of recovery-oriented curricula are warranted to further advance the knowledge of recovery.

REFERENCES

1. Anthony WA. Recovery from mental illness: the guiding vision of the mental health service system in the 1990s. Psychosoc Rehabil J 1993;16(4):11–23.
2. Jacobson N, Curtis L. Recovery as policy in mental health services: Strategies emerging from the states. Psychiatr Rehabil J 2000;23(4):333.
3. Slade M, Amering M, Oades L. Recovery: an international perspective. Epidemiol Psichiatr Soc 2008;17(2):128–37.
4. Ahmed AO, Buckley PF, Mabe PA. International efforts at implementing and advancing the recovery model. Int Psychiatry 2012;9(1):4–6.
5. Bradstreet S, Mcbrierty R. Recovery in Scotland: beyond service development. Int Rev Psychiatry 2012;24(1):64–9.
6. Peebles SA, Mabe PA, Davidson L, et al. Recovery and systems transformation for schizophrenia. Psychiatr Clin North Am 2007;30(3):567–83.
7. Ahmed AO, Serdarevic M, Mabe PA, et al. Triumphs and challenges of transforming a state psychiatric hospital in Georgia. Int J Ment Health Promot 2013;15(2):68–75.
8. Farkas M. The vision of recovery today: what it is and what it means for services. World Psychiatry 2007;6(2):68.
9. Davidson L, Roe D. Recovery from versus recovery in serious mental illness: one strategy for lessening confusion plaguing recovery. J Ment Health 2007;16(4):459–70.
10. Davidson L, Drake RE, Schmutte T, et al. Oil and water or oil and vinegar? Evidence-based medicine meets recovery. Community Ment Health J 2009;45(5):323–32.
11. Ware NC, Hopper K, Tugenberg T, et al. Connectedness and citizenship: redefining social integration. Psychiatr Serv 2007;58(4):469–74.
12. Bellack AS. Scientific and consumer models of recovery in schizophrenia: concordance, contrasts, and implications. Schizophr Bull 2006;32(3):432–42.
13. Haan M. The evolution of the consumer movement. Psychiatr Serv 2006;57(8):1215 [author reply: 1216].
14. Sowers W. The evolution of the consumer movement. Psychiatr Serv 2006;57(8):1215 [author reply: 1216].
15. Frese FJ, Stanley J, Kress K, et al. Integrating evidence-based practices and the recovery model. Psychiatr Serv 2001;52(11):1462–8.
16. Whitley R. Cultural competence, evidence-based medicine, and evidence-based practices. Psychiatr Serv 2007;58(12):1588–90.
17. Cox JL. Towards an evidence-based "medicine of the person": the contribution of psychiatry to health care provision. J Eval Clin Pract 2008;14(5):694–8.

18. Ozomaro U, Wahlestedt C, Nemeroff CB. Personalized medicine in psychiatry: problems and promises. BMC Med 2013;11(1):132.
19. Slade M, Amering M, Farkas M, et al. Uses and abuses of recovery: implementing recovery-oriented practices in mental health systems. World Psychiatry 2014;13(1):12–20.
20. Bird V, Leamy M, Tew J, et al. Fit for purpose? Validation of a conceptual framework for personal recovery with current mental health consumers. Aust N Z J Psychiatry 2014;48(7):644–53.
21. Silverstein SM, Bellack AS. A scientific agenda for the concept of recovery as it applies to schizophrenia. Clin Psychol Rev 2008;28(7):1108–24.
22. Ahmed AO, Doane NJ, Mabe PA, et al. Peers and peer-led interventions for people with schizophrenia. Psychiatr Clin North Am 2012;35(3):699–715.
23. Duckworth K, Halpern L. Peer support and peer-led family support for persons living with schizophrenia. Curr Opin Psychiatry 2014;27(3):216–21.
24. What is schizophrenics anonymous? [Internet]. Available at: http://www.sardaa.org/schizophrenics-anonymous/what-is-sa/. Accessed September 25, 2015.
25. Dixon L, Lucksted A, Stewart B, et al. Outcomes of the peer-taught 12-week family-to-family education program for severe mental illness. Acta Psychiatr Scand 2004;109(3):207–15.
26. Dixon LB, Lucksted A, Medoff DR, et al. Outcomes of a randomized study of a peer-taught Family-to-Family Education Program for mental illness. Psychiatr Serv 2011;62(6):591–7.
27. Hardiman ER. Networks of caring A qualitative study of social support in consumer-run mental health agencies. Qual Soc Work 2004;3(4):431–48.
28. Segal SP, Hardiman ER, Hodges JQ. Characteristics of new clients at self-help and community mental health agencies in geographic proximity. Psychiatr Serv 2002;53(9):1145–52.
29. Solomon P. Peer support/peer provided services underlying processes, benefits, and critical ingredients. Psychiatr Rehabil J 2004;27(4):392–401.
30. Davidson L, Chinman M, Sells D, et al. Peer support among adults with serious mental illness: a report from the field. Schizophr Bull 2006;32(3):443–50.
31. Ahmed AO, Hunter KM, Mabe AP, et al. The professional experiences of peer specialists in the Georgia Mental Health Consumer Network. Community Ment Health J 2015;51(4):424–36.
32. Cook JA, Steigman P, Pickett S, et al. Randomized controlled trial of peer-led recovery education using Building Recovery of Individual Dreams and Goals through Education and Support (BRIDGES). Schizophr Res 2012;136(1–3): 36–42.
33. Ahmed AO, Mabe PA, Buckley PF. Peer specialists as educators for recovery-based systems transformation. Psychiatr Times 2012;29(2):1–7.
34. Repper J, Carter T. A review of the literature on peer support in mental health services. J Ment Health 2011;20(4):392–411.
35. Posner CM, Wilson KG, Kral MJ, et al. Family psychoeducational support groups in schizophrenia. Am J Orthopsychiatry 1992;62(2):206–18.
36. Castelein S, Bruggeman R, van Busschbach JT, et al. The effectiveness of peer support groups in psychosis: a randomized controlled trial. Acta Psychiatr Scand 2008;118(1):64–72.
37. Ochocka J, Nelson G, Janzen R, et al. A longitudinal study of mental health consumer/survivor initiatives: part 3—A qualitative study of impacts of participation on new members. J Community Psychol 2006;34(3):273–83.

38. Rogers ES, Teague GB, Lichenstein C, et al. Effects of participation in consumer-operated service programs on both personal and organizationally mediated empowerment: results of multisite study. J Rehabil Res Dev 2007; 44(6):785–99.

39. Barber JA, Rosenheck RA, Armstrong M, et al. Monitoring the dissemination of peer support in the VA Healthcare System. Community Ment Health J 2008; 44(6):433–41.

40. Resnick SG, Rosenheck RA. Integrating peer-provided services: a quasi-experimental study of recovery orientation, confidence, and empowerment. Psychiatr Serv 2008;59(11):1307–14.

41. Corrigan PW, Sokol KA, Rüsch N. The impact of self-stigma and mutual help programs on the quality of life of people with serious mental illnesses. Community Ment Health J 2013;49(1):1–6.

42. van Gestel-Timmermans H, Brouwers EPM, van Assen MALM, et al. Effects of a peer-run course on recovery from serious mental illness: a randomized controlled trial. Psychiatr Serv 2012;63(1):54–60.

43. Lloyd-Evans B, Mayo-Wilson E, Harrison B, et al. A systematic review and meta-analysis of randomised controlled trials of peer support for people with severe mental illness. BMC Psychiatry 2014;14:39.

44. Ahmed AO, Buckley PF. Review tempers expectations for peer-led services but further studies are required. Evid Based Ment Health 2014;17(4):123.

45. van Gestel-Timmermans JA, Brouwers EPM, van Nieuwenhuizen C. Recovery is up to you, a peer-run course. Psychiatr Serv 2010;61(9):944–5.

46. Fukui S, Davidson LJ, Rapp CA. Pathways to recovery, a peer-led group intervention. Psychiatr Serv 2010;61(9):944.

47. Pitt V, Lowe D, Hill S, et al. Consumer-providers of care for adult clients of statutory mental health services. Cochrane Database Syst Rev 2013;(3):CD004807.

48. Ahmed AO, Birgenheir D, Buckley PF, et al. A psychometric study of recovery among Certified Peer Specialists. Psychiatry Res 2013;209(3):721–31.

49. Goldstrom ID, Campbell J, Rogers JA, et al. National estimates for mental health mutual support groups, self-help organizations, and consumer-operated services. Adm Policy Ment Health 2006;33(1):92–103.

50. Ahmed AO, Mabe PA, Buckley PF. Recovery in schizophrenia: perspectives, evidence, and implications. In: Ritsner MS, editor. Handbook of schizophrenia spectrum disorders, volume III. Dordrecht, Netherlands: Springer; 2011. p. 1–22.

51. Bodenheimer T, Lorig K, Holman H, et al. Patient self-management of chronic disease in primary care. JAMA 2002;288(19):2469–75.

52. Coleman MT, Newton KS. Supporting self-management in patients with chronic illness. Am Fam Physician 2005;72(8):1503–10.

53. Mueser KT, Corrigan PW, Hilton DW, et al. Illness management and recovery: a review of the research. Psychiatr Serv 2002;53(10):1272–84.

54. Deegan P. Recovery as a journey of the heart. Psychiatr Rehabil J 1996; 19(3):91–7.

55. Frese FJ, Knight EL, Saks E. Recovery from schizophrenia: with views of psychiatrists, psychologists, and others diagnosed with this disorder. Schizophr Bull 2009;35(2):370–80.

56. Copeland ME. Wellness recovery action plan. Occup Ther Ment Health 2002; 17(3–4):127–50.

57. Copeland ME. Wellness recovery action plan: a system for monitoring, reducing and eliminating uncomfortable or dangerous physical symptoms and emotional feelings. Rev edition. West Dummerston, VT: Peach Press; 2000.

58. Färdig R, Lewander T, Melin L, et al. A randomized controlled trial of the illness management and recovery program for persons with schizophrenia. Psychiatr Serv 2011;62(6):606–12.
59. Lin EC-L, Chan CH, Shao W-C, et al. A randomized controlled trial of an adapted Illness Management and Recovery program for people with schizophrenia awaiting discharge from a psychiatric hospital. Psychiatr Rehabil J 2013; 36(4):243–9.
60. Lin EC-L, Shao W-C, Chan CH, et al. A pilot study of an illness management and recovery program in discharged patients with schizophrenia. J Nurs Res 2013; 21(4):270–7.
61. Cook JA, Copeland ME, Jonikas JA, et al. Results of a randomized controlled trial of mental illness self-management using Wellness Recovery Action Planning. Schizophr Bull 2012;38(4):881–91.
62. Cook JA, Jonikas JA, Hamilton MM, et al. Impact of Wellness Recovery Action Planning on service utilization and need in a randomized controlled trial. Psychiatr Rehabil J 2013;36(4):250–7.
63. Roberts G, Wolfson P. The rediscovery of recovery: open to all. Adv Psychiatr Treat 2004;10(1):37–48.
64. Rapp CA. The strengths model: case management with people suffering from severe and persistent mental illness. New York: Oxford University Press; 1998.
65. Rapp CA, Goscha RJ. The strengths model: case management with people with psychiatric disabilities. New York: Oxford University Press; 2006.
66. Modrcin M, Rapp CA, Poertner J. The evaluation of case management services with the chronically mentally ill. Eval Program Plann 1988;11(4):307–14.
67. Macias C, Kinney R, Farley OW, et al. The role of case management within a community support system: partnership with psychosocial rehabilitation. Community Ment Health J 1994;30(4):323–39.
68. Macias C, Farley OW, Jackson R, et al. Case management in the context of capitation financing: an evaluation of the strengths model. Adm Policy Ment Health 1997;24(6):535–43.
69. Stanard RP. The effect of training in a strengths model of case management on client outcomes in a community mental health center. Community Ment Health J 1999;35(2):169–79.
70. Fukui S, Goscha R, Rapp CA, et al. Strengths model case management fidelity scores and client outcomes. Psychiatr Serv 2012;63(7):708–10.
71. Hopper K, Jost J, Hay T, et al. Homelessness, severe mental illness, and the institutional circuit. Psychiatr Serv 1997;48(5):659–65.
72. Foster A, Gable J, Buckley J. Homelessness in Schizophrenia. Psychiatr Clin 2012;35(3):717–34.
73. Rog DJ. The Evidence on Supported Housing. Psychiatr Rehabil J 2004;27(4): 334–44.
74. Ridgway P, Zipple AM. The paradigm shift in residential services: from the linear continuum to supported housing approaches. Psychosoc Rehabil J 1990;13(4): 11–31.
75. Montgomery P, Forchuk C, Duncan C, et al. Supported housing programs for persons with serious mental illness in rural northern communities: a mixed method evaluation. BMC Health Serv Res 2008;8:156.
76. Gilmer TP, Stefancic A, Ettner SL, et al. Effect of full-service partnerships on homelessness, use and costs of mental health services, and quality of life among adults with serious mental illness. Arch Gen Psychiatry 2010;67(6): 645–52.

77. Stergiopoulos V, Gozdzik A, Misir V, et al. Effectiveness of housing first with intensive case management in an ethnically diverse sample of homeless adults with mental illness: a randomized controlled trial. PLoS One 2015;10(7): e0130281.

78. Henwood BF, Matejkowski J, Stefancic A, et al. Quality of life after housing first for adults with serious mental illness who have experienced chronic homelessness. Psychiatry Res 2014;220(1–2):549–55.

79. Wolf J, Burnam A, Koegel P, et al. Changes in subjective quality of life among homeless adults who obtain housing: a prospective examination. Soc Psychiatry Psychiatr Epidemiol 2001;36(8):391–8.

80. Evensen S, Wisløff T, Lystad JU, et al. Prevalence, employment rate, and cost of schizophrenia in a high-income welfare society: a population-based study using comprehensive health and welfare registers. Schizophr Bull 2015. [Epub ahead of print].

81. Ramsay CE, Stewart T, Compton MT. Unemployment among patients with newly diagnosed first-episode psychosis: prevalence and clinical correlates in a U.S. sample. Soc Psychiatry Psychiatr Epidemiol 2012;47(5):797–803.

82. Marwaha S, Johnson S, Bebbington P, et al. Rates and correlates of employment in people with schizophrenia in the UK, France and Germany. Br J Psychiatry 2007;191:30–7.

83. Grove B, Secker J, Seebohm P. New thinking about mental health and employment. Radcliffe Publishing; 2005.

84. Bailey J. I'm just an ordinary person. Psychiatr Rehabil J 1998;22(1):8–10.

85. Bond GR, Drake RE, Becker DR. Generalizability of the Individual Placement and Support (IPS) model of supported employment outside the US. World Psychiatry 2012;11(1):32–9.

86. Marshall T, Rapp CA, Becker DR, et al. Key factors for implementing supported employment. Psychiatr Serv 2008;59(8):886–92.

87. Crowther R, Marshall M, Bond G, et al. Vocational rehabilitation for people with severe mental illness. Cochrane Database Syst Rev 2001;(2):CD003080.

88. Wewiorski NJ, Fabian ES. Association between demographic and diagnostic factors and employment outcomes for people with psychiatric disabilities: a synthesis of recent research. Ment Health Serv Res 2004;6(1):9–21.

89. Fabian ES. Longitudinal outcomes in supported employment: a survival analysis. Rehabil Psychol 1992;37(1):23.

90. Cook JA, Leff H, Blyler CR, et al. Results of a multisite randomized trial of supported employment interventions for individuals with severe mental illness. Arch Gen Psychiatry 2005;62(5):505–12.

91. McGurk SR, Mueser KT, Harvey PD, et al. Cognitive and symptom predictors of work outcomes for clients with schizophrenia in supported employment. Psychiatr Serv 2003;54(8):1129–35.

92. McGurk SR, Mueser KT, Pascaris A. Cognitive training and supported employment for persons with severe mental illness: one-year results from a randomized controlled trial. Schizophr Bull 2005;31(4):898–909.

93. Noordsy DL, Torrey WC, Mead S, et al. Recovery-oriented psychopharmacology: redefining the goals of antipsychotic treatment. J Clin Psychiatry 2000; 61(Suppl 3):22–9.

94. Jakovljević M. Creativity, mental disorders and their treatment: recovery-oriented psychopharmacotherapy. Psychiatr Danub 2013;25(3):311–5.

95. Buckley PF, Ahmed AO. Principles and practices of medication management for people with schizophrenia: evolution within a recovery-based framework of

care. In: Yeager K, Cutler D, Svendsen D, et al, editors. Modern community mental health: an interdisciplinary approach. New York: Oxford University Press; 2013. p. 337–57.

96. Drake RE, Deegan PE. Shared decision making is an ethical imperative. Psychiatr Serv 2009;60(8):1007.
97. Mistler LA, Drake RE. Shared decision making in antipsychotic management. J Psychiatr Pract 2008;14(6):333–44.
98. Adams JR, Drake RE, Wolford GL. Shared decision-making preferences of people with severe mental illness. Psychiatr Serv 2007;58(9):1219–21.
99. Charles C, Gafni A, Whelan T. Shared decision-making in the medical encounter: what does it mean? (or it takes at least two to tango). Soc Sci Med 1997;44(5):681–92.
100. Kriston L, Scholl I, Hölzel L, et al. The 9-item Shared Decision Making Questionnaire (SDM-Q-9). Development and psychometric properties in a primary care sample. Patient Educ Couns 2010;80(1):94–9.
101. Godolphin W. Shared decision-making. Healthc Q 2009;12 Spec No Patient: e186–90.
102. Adams JR, Drake RE. Shared decision-making and evidence-based practice. Community Ment Health J 2006;42(1):87–105.
103. Barratt A. Evidence based medicine and shared decision making: the challenge of getting both evidence and preferences into health care. Patient Educ Couns 2008;73(3):407–12.
104. Kreyenbuhl J, Nossel IR, Dixon LB. Disengagement from mental health treatment among individuals with schizophrenia and strategies for facilitating connections to care: a review of the literature. Schizophr Bull 2009;35(4):696–703.
105. Stowkowy J, Addington D, Liu L, et al. Predictors of disengagement from treatment in an early psychosis program. Schizophr Res 2012;136(1–3):7–12.
106. Doyle R, Turner N, Fanning F, et al. First-episode psychosis and disengagement from treatment: a systematic review. Psychiatr Serv 2014;65(5):603–11.
107. O'Brien A, Fahmy R, Singh SP. Disengagement from mental health services. A literature review. Soc Psychiatry Psychiatr Epidemiol 2009;44(7):558–68.
108. Priebe S, Watts J, Chase M, et al. Processes of disengagement and engagement in assertive outreach patients: qualitative study. Br J Psychiatry 2005; 187:438–43.
109. Rossi A, Amaddeo F, Sandri M, et al. What happens to patients seen only once by psychiatric services? Findings from a follow-up study. Psychiatry Res 2008; 157(1–3):53–65.
110. Hamann J, Kruse J, Schmitz FS, et al. Patient participation in antipsychotic drug choice decisions. Psychiatry Res 2010;178(1):63–7.
111. Carpenter WT, Gold JM, Lahti AC, et al. Decisional capacity for informed consent in schizophrenia research. Arch Gen Psychiatry 2000;57(6):533–8.
112. Hamann J, Langer B, Winkler V, et al. Shared decision making for in-patients with schizophrenia. Acta Psychiatr Scand 2006;114(4):265–73.
113. Loh A, Simon D, Wills CE, et al. The effects of a shared decision-making intervention in primary care of depression: a cluster-randomized controlled trial. Patient Educ Couns 2007;67(3):324–32.
114. Hamann J, Cohen R, Leucht S, et al. Shared decision making and long-term outcome in schizophrenia treatment. J Clin Psychiatry 2007;68(7):992–7.
115. Srebnik DS, La Fond JQ. Advance directives for mental health treatment. Psychiatr Serv 1999;50(7):919–25.

116. Campbell LA, Kisely SR. Advance treatment directives for people with severe mental illness. Cochrane Database Syst Rev 2009;(1):CD005963.
117. Farrelly S, Lester H, Rose D, et al. Barriers to shared decision making in mental health care: qualitative study of the Joint Crisis Plan for psychosis. Health Expect 2015. [Epub ahead of print].
118. Thornicroft G, Farrelly S, Szmukler G, et al. Clinical outcomes of Joint Crisis Plans to reduce compulsory treatment for people with psychosis: a randomised controlled trial. Lancet 2013;381(9878):1634–41.
119. Buckley P, Bahmiller D, Kenna CA, et al. Resident education and perceptions of recovery in serious mental illness: observations and commentary. Acad Psychiatry 2007;31(6):435–8.
120. Mabe PA, Ahmed AO, Duncan GN, et al. Project GREAT: immersing physicians and doctorally-trained psychologists in recovery-oriented care. Prof Psychol Res Pract 2014;45(5):347.
121. Peebles SA, Mabe PA, Fenley G, et al. Immersing practitioners in the recovery model: an educational program evaluation. Community Ment Health J 2009; 45(4):239–45.
122. Ashcraft L, Anthony W. Eliminating seclusion and restraint in recovery-oriented crisis services. Psychiatr Serv 2008;59(10):1198–202.
123. Ashcraft L, Anthony WA, Jaccard S. Rein in seclusion and restraints. They are not compatible with recovery-oriented services. Behav Healthc 2008; 28(12):6–7.
124. Smith GM, Davis RH, Bixler EO, et al. Pennsylvania State Hospital system's seclusion and restraint reduction program. Psychiatr Serv 2005;56(9):1115–22.
125. Madan A, Borckardt JJ, Grubaugh AL, et al. Efforts to reduce seclusion and restraint use in a state psychiatric hospital: a ten-year perspective. Psychiatr Serv 2014;65(10):1273–6.

What Does Mental Health Parity Really Mean for the Care of People with Serious Mental Illness?

John Bartlett, MD, MPH[a],*, Ron Manderscheid, PhD[b]

KEYWORDS

- Parity • Affordable Care Act • MHPAEA Act • SMI population
- Mental health and substance abuse benefits • Essential health benefits
- Medicaid expansion • Non-quantitative treatment limitations

KEY POINTS

- Achievement of parity, equality for both what is covered and also how and when it is covered, for mental health and substance abuse benefits is a major step forward in providing more comprehensive care for individuals living with SMI and psychosis.
- However, parity is a *relative* concept and does not necessarily provide access to the full set of recovery-oriented benefits, such as supported housing and employment, required by many of the SMI population for their full recovery.
- The path to parity for mental health/substance use disorder (MH/SUD) benefits has been marked by many often seemingly minor, incremental changes, which over the past 50 years have resulted in positive quantitative and qualitative changes to the reach and scope of parity.
- The combined requirements of the 2008 Mental Health Parity and Addiction Equity Act and the 2010 Patient Protection and Affordable Care Act have greatly expanded access to parity MH/SUD benefits, but major gaps in parity coverage and major challenges to its expansion still exist.
- The path to parity in many respects parallels the civil rights movement, in that full integration of benefits, rather than separate but equal ones, should be the ultimate goal.

INTRODUCTION

Over the past six decades, one, if not the most important, policy issue in behavioral health has been the establishment of benefit and coverage parity for the prevention and treatment of mental illness and addiction. Beginning with the directives of

[a] The Carter Center Mental Health Program, One Coppenhill, 453 Freedom Parkway, Atlanta, GA 30307, USA; [b] 25 Massachusetts Avenue Northwest, Suite 500, Washington, DC 2001, USA
* Corresponding author.
E-mail address: John.bartlett@cartercenter.org

Psychiatr Clin N Am 39 (2016) 331–342
http://dx.doi.org/10.1016/j.psc.2016.01.010
0193-953X/16/$ – see front matter © 2016 Elsevier Inc. All rights reserved.

psych.theclinics.com

President John F. Kennedy to the Civil Service Commission in the early 1960s to provide parity coverage within the Federal Employees Health Benefit Program and continuing on over the next 50 years to the recent passage of the Patient Protection and Affordable Care Act (ACA), this movement toward parity has been perhaps the most important strategic guide for policy within our field. However, as has been pointed out by Grob and Goldman in their 2006 book "*The Dilemma of Federal Mental Health Policy: Radical Reform or Incremental Change?*" the path to parity has been neither quick nor direct.[1] Instead, it has been a guiding principle for a set of many incremental, sequential improvements over a long period.

With the passage of the ACA in 2010, many in the behavioral health care field saw its commitment to behavioral health prevention and treatment as the final step to parity. However, as so often proves true, the passage of legislation is not the same as its successful implementation. The thesis of this paper is that effective implementation of parity as originally envisioned by Senator Ted Kennedy of Massachusetts and Representative Patrick Kennedy of Rhode Island would be a major step forward for improving the care and outcomes for persons with serious mental illness (SMI), especially those persons living with schizophrenia. In fact, a number of roadblocks to the full achievement of that vision have occurred during the implementation process. In this article, we describe the original vision, review the obstacles and challenges to its successful implementation to date, and finally, indicate additional steps that will be necessary to implement fully the potential of parity for the SMI population.

One needs only to look back less than a decade to view a less than optimal situation for people living with SMIs and addictions. For these adults, only 50% to 60% actually received any care at that time.[2] The remainder were either part of the homeless population, in and out of local and county jails, or were being cared for by family members.[2] At the same time, state mental health agency budgets were being cut by about $4.5 billion after 2008 as a result of the Great Recession, which made the community care situation for persons with SMI even more precarious.[3] The community mental health system was very poorly funded, offered inadequate services in many places, and simply did not extend into many rural areas. Little or nothing was done to address initial psychosis at that time, and many persons with SMI were not enrolled in Medicaid.

But how, one might ask, could such a situation exist, especially after the passage of the Mental Health Parity and Addiction Equity Act (MHPAEA) in 2008. This legislation sped through the Congress and the White House, because it was the legislative vehicle used to pass the Emergency Economic Stabilization Act of 2008 in response to the Great Recession. Moreover, the MHPAEA was landmark behavioral health legislation because it required parity with medical benefits for both mental health and substance use disorder (MH/SUD) care in all private health insurance plans that offered coverage for behavioral health conditions and insured 50 or more persons. The legislation also required parity in the management of benefits, so that behavioral health care benefits could not be managed more stringently than medical benefits.[4] However, while requiring parity for insurance plans that offered mental health and substance abuse benefits, it in no way required a plan to offer them. The reach of parity under the MHPAEA was still a limited one (**Box 1**).

However, many have seen MHPAEA as the vehicle that leveled the playing field for behavioral health care so that it could participate fully in the development and implementation of the ACA.[5] The ACA extended parity's reach by requiring that MH/SUD benefits be offered in all insurance plans offered through the state health insurance marketplaces, to all insurance plans offered through the individual and small group markets, and to all new coverage offered through the state Medicaid Expansions.

Box 1
Overview of parity protections

Mental Health Parity and Addiction Equity Act of 2008

Applied to large (>50 enrollees) private plans that offered behavioral health services

Applied to both mental health and substance use benefits

Applied to management of benefits

Patient Protection and Affordable Care Act of 2010

Required that mental health and substance use benefits be offered as part of new insurance plans as Essential Health Benefits

Extended parity to all insurance plans offered through the state health insurance marketplaces, to insurance offered through the individual and small group markets, and to new coverage offered through the state Medicaid Expansions

---

The US Department of Health and Human Services (HHS) has estimated that approximately 84 million persons now have parity protections as a result of these changes,[6] including, in theory at least, a large proportion of those living with SMI largely through the extension of Medicaid.

In the following pages, we examine how all of these legislative changes are, in fact, being implemented, and what impact they are having for adults with SMI. This examination includes consideration of issues that have been encountered along the way, as well as new opportunities that remain to be explored.

THE PATH TO PARITY

As described previously, parity applies to health insurance benefits as well as to the management of health insurance benefits, namely, to both *what* is covered as well as to *when and if* it is covered. Taking a step back from this fundamental notion, it also is very important to say that parity is a *relative* standard. In other words, if a health insurance plan has weak medical benefits, then parity requires only that the MH/SUD benefits be no less than the weak medical benefits. The clear implication is that we need to advocate for both good medical *and* behavioral health benefits.

After the passage of MHPAEA in 2008, it took almost 2 years for HHS to develop and finalize implementing regulations for private sector health insurance plans.[7] Subsequently, it took almost 5 additional years for the department to finalize implementing regulations in 2015 for state Medicaid plans operated by private sector managed care entities, which also were covered by the 2008 legislation (**Fig. 1**).[8]

Thus far, although an 800 number is available to report parity violations to the federal government, little direct action has been taken by HHS or the US Department of Labor, the actual enforcement entity, to make it easy to report parity violations or to actually engage in field enforcement when violations do occur. Further, the consensus would be that parity has been difficult to enforce for several key reasons:

- Health insurance purchasers have not been educated regarding what to look for when they purchase health insurance.
- Many health insurance plans do not provide sufficient information in advertising materials so that consumers actually can understand the specifics of behavioral health and medical benefits in their plans.[9]

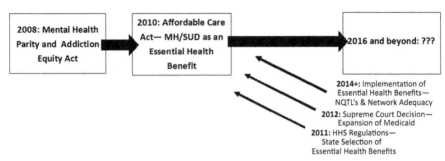

Fig. 1. Policy path to parity.

- Many state health insurance commissioners and their staffs lack the detailed knowledge needed to assess parity in a plan submitted for state approval.
- Similarly, many private plan developers and administrators lack this knowledge as well.

For almost 2 years, the Coalition for Whole Health, which represents 165 national and state MH/SUD advocacy organizations, has been seeking better federal enforcement of the 2008 MHPAEA. More recently, the Coalition also has been supporting the efforts of the Kennedy Forum, organized by former representative Patrick Kennedy, to track parity developments in the states. In June 2015, the Kennedy Forum introduced www.ParityTrack.org. Through a review of legislation, regulation, and litigation, the Forum already has completed parity analyses for 13 states: California, Connecticut, Florida, Idaho, New York, Maryland, Kansas, Illinois, Massachusetts, Pennsylvania, Texas, Tennessee, and Minnesota. These analyses are available at the Forum Web site, www.thekennedyforum.org.

An assessment of how the MHPAEA of 2008 has had an impact on insurance coverage and care for persons with SMI shows that, considered alone, we believe that the effect of MHPAEA has been relatively minor. Most adults with SMI do not have private insurance. Those who were covered through state Medicaid programs operated by private managed care entities likely experienced some improvement in the management of their Medicaid benefits as a result of the legislation. However, Medicaid benefits in these programs already were reasonably good before the passage of MHPAEA.

As noted previously in a passing reference, the MHPAEA set the stage for behavioral health care to be included in the 2010 ACA. And, unlike the MHPAEA, the ACA as passed in 2010 required *both* mental health and substance use insurance coverage *and* parity between medical and behavioral health benefits. Hence, the effect of the ACA as originally envisioned is potentially much more dramatic vis-à-vis parity.

PARITY UNDER THE AFFORDABLE CARE ACT: THE VISION

The ACA requires that all Americans have health insurance, and it provides 2 mechanisms through which this goal can be achieved:

- Private insurance offered through state health insurance marketplaces (whether operated by the state directly or by HHS in lieu of a state) for persons at or above 138% of the Federal Poverty Level (FPL). Tax subsidies are offered for all persons up to 400% FPL purchasing private insurance, and those up to 250% FPL also receive cost-sharing for their care.
- State Medicaid Expansions for those with incomes less than 138% FPL. For the state Medicaid Expansions, the federal government will pay 100% of the cost for

FY2014 to FY2016, and a decreasing amount thereafter, with a floor of 90% in FY2020 and beyond.

All private insurance offered through the ACA is guided by an Essential Health Benefit (EHB) requirement, which mandates that any benefit package covered under the ACA must encompass 10 areas, including MH/SUD, pharmacy, and prevention and promotion. In addition, EHB mental health and substance use benefits must be at parity with medical benefits. Similarly, the state Medicaid Expansions are guided by an Alternative Medicaid Benefit that encompasses the same 10 areas, with the same requirement for parity.

The original vision for mental health and addiction coverage under the ACA, as defined by the Substance Abuse and Mental Health Services Administration of the US Department of Health Human Services, was that the benefits should correspond to a "good and modern system."[10] This type of coverage would include the full range of services beginning with primary prevention and moving through screening and early intervention onward to acute care and ultimately to chronic care management, including such interventions as digitally based care by telephone, e-mail, or even text messaging. Such a "good and modern" system for the SMI population also would include coverage for "a continuum of effective treatment and support services that span health care, employment, housing and educational sectors."

Although it is still early, as of the writing of this article (August to September 2015), we can begin to get some indication of what is happening for adults with SMI as a result of these insurance transformations. To date, approximately 11.4 million persons have enrolled in health insurance through the state health insurance marketplaces.[11] If we assume conservatively that the rate of SMI is the same in this population as in the US population as a whole, approximately 5.8%, then approximately 660,000 adults with SMI have enrolled in health insurance through this mechanism. If we assume that the new Medicaid enrollees are similar to current Medicaid enrollees who enrolled previously via disability qualification for Supplemental Security Income (a good proxy for SMI), then approximately 2.5% of new enrollees (1.5 million/60 million × 100) are adults with SMI. Because approximately 6.4 million persons have enrolled in the state Medicaid Expansions, we would estimate that approximately 160,000 are adults with SMI. Thus, to date, we would estimate that approximately 820,000 adults with SMI have enrolled in one of these insurance programs. In addition, because access to benefits under any Medicaid expansion or exchange product does not require a prior determination of disability, for the first time access to coverage for early and first-break psychoses is available to many.

PARITY UNDER THE AFFORDABLE CARE ACT: THE REALITY

It is clear that the vision for parity under the ACA was one that was intended, if not to actually achieve, then certainly to move well down the path to full equality of health benefits and coverage. This achievement of full parity for most Americans, including those living with SMI and substance abuse, was based on the following assumptions:

- The ACA, including its provision for the conversion of Medicaid from a targeted program for defined subpopulations of the poor (such as single mothers with young children) to full coverage for all people whose income fell below 138% FPL, would be implemented in all 54 states and other jurisdictions (eg, Puerto Rico). Based on income levels alone, the ACA would provide access to new coverage for a significant number of persons with SMI, such as young single men, without their having to suffer multiple psychotic episodes and develop severe disabilities.

- The mental health and substance abuse benefit provided under the ACA to the Medicaid expansion population, to all insured through so-called "qualified" health plans (meaning those not grandfathered, not large group, and not self-insured plans), and those insured through all individual and small employer plans, would be a full set of benefits for a "good and modern" behavioral health system covering the full range of treatment and preventive services, including services such as housing, which had not traditionally been covered under health insurance in the past.
- Access to primary care services for those living with SMI and addictions would be enhanced through both targeted increased reimbursement to primary care providers, as well as through the funding of demonstration projects to increase accessibility to evidence-based integrated care, such as patient-centered medical homes and health homes for the chronically mentally ill under Section 2703 of the ACA.

However, the reality of the implementation of parity that has transpired over the 5 years since the ACA was passed differs in many respects from the vision described earlier. In some cases, these differences are due to political and even philosophic opposition to the ACA; in others, they are due to missteps and failed opportunities on the part of the Obama Administration, including HHS.

CHALLENGE NUMBER 1: THE ESSENTIAL HEALTH BENEFIT

Such was the case with the first major deviation from the vision described previously during the implementation of the ACA. In the spring of 2011, HHS released a set of interim regulations on the implementation of the essential benefits requirement of the ACA. Although this interim regulation continued the mandate that all 10 of the essential areas as defined in the ACA must be covered, it left the definition of the actual benefits to the individual states. Rather than go through another prolonged and perhaps even destructive fight with Congress over a so-called "national benefit plan," the department and the Obama Administration trusted, whether intentionally or not, the "new Federalism" to continue the implementation of the original vision for parity on a state-by-state basis. In so doing, they also followed the traditional approach of allowing individual states to regulate insurance activities.

This decision resulted in 2 major issues for parity implementation. The first was that this delegation of the decision to the individual states over the definition of the essential benefit package for mental health and substance abuse has led to significant variation in the benefits from state to state.[12] In turn, this has resulted in significant variation in the current benefits provided to persons with SMI and severe addictions from those originally envisioned under the "full and modern system" envisioned by the Substance Abuse and Mental Health Services Administration (SAMHSA) and HHS. Second, this decision has made the very assessment of whether or not parity is, in fact, being implemented nationally a tremendous challenge, as the process of doing so has now been "balkanized" and made even more complex by requiring a state-by-state evaluation and advocacy process.

In an attempt to bring some degree of standardization to the state-by-state definition process, in 2012 HHS released proposed regulations requiring states to choose a "benchmark" plan for the definition of its actual EHB from 1 of 10 potential existing private health plans within that state. These 10 included the following:

- One of the 3 largest Federal Employees Health Benefit plans
- One of the 3 largest state employee health benefit plans

- One of the 3 largest small group plans in the state
- The largest non-Medicaid health maintenance plan in the state

By October 2014, the vast majority of states had either chosen or defaulted to their largest small group plan as their benchmark for the determination of covered services.[13] This development is, of course, troubling, because traditionally small group plans have provided little to no coverage for mental health and substance abuse services. In fact, the reality of the few services they may have covered is far indeed from that "good and modern" system described by SAMHSA in 2009. Judging to what extent such a benchmark benefit may adhere to or deviate from the parity requirements outlined in the MHPAEA and the ACA is complicated because most evidence of coverage documents provided on the state and federal exchanges have only the most general categories listed, such as "outpatient mental health services." Two useful tools to track parity implementation on a state-by-state basis include the following:

- A recent online publication from HHS's Center for Consumer Information and Insurance Oversight (CCIIO), which includes the 2017 EHB plans for all 50 states and Washington, DC https://www.cms.gov/CCIIO/Resources/Data-Resources/ehb.html
- The Kennedy Forum's online blog on parity implementation https://www.thekennedyforum.org/blog/paritytrack-is-accountability-in-action

CHALLENGE NUMBER 2: THE INDIVIDUAL MANDATE AND THE SUPREME COURT

Central to the vision of greatly expanded health insurance coverage under the ACA, especially for those individuals and families at the lower end of the income scale, such as the SMI population, was the expansion of Medicaid to those with incomes less than 138% FPL. This expansion involved the transitioning of the Medicaid program from one targeted at very specific categories of beneficiaries, such as pregnant woman and children younger than 6 with incomes at or below 133% FPL, to one more widely available based solely on income levels below 138% FPL for all individuals younger than 65. Because Medicaid is a voluntary joint federal-state program, with cost-sharing between the 2 parties, the ACA offered an incentive to states for expansion by defining a transitional period, in which the federal government would cover 100% of the costs associated with these expanded Medicaid programs for several years, gradually decreasing to a still very generous 90% cost-sharing in 2020 and thereafter.

In addition, the ACA contained a minimum essential coverage provision, known as the individual mandate. This mandate requires all individuals to maintain a certain level of health insurance coverage for themselves and their family members beginning in January 2014 or, alternatively, to pay a tax penalty. This individual mandate was intended to address the possibility that healthy individuals would, without such a penalty in place, choose not to secure health insurance until they became ill (so-called adverse selection, in which the insured risk pool does not accurately reflect the overall health of the population, including the healthy).

In a suit accepted for review by the Supreme Court in 2011, *National Federation of Business v. Sebelius*, two related issues were raised. The first was the constitutionality of the individual mandate; the second was the constitutionality of the proposed Medicaid expansion as one of the remedies to increase access to health insurance coverage. In its ruling released in the spring of 2012, the individual mandate was upheld, but the proposed approach to Medicaid expansion was not. Therefore, the decision as to whether or not to expand Medicaid became a state-by-state decision.[14]

As of September 1, 2015, 20 states have not yet chosen to expand Medicaid, which leaves a significant coverage gap in those states for those whose income is less than 138% of the FPL, including potentially many persons in the SMI population.[15]

CHALLENGE NUMBER 3: THE DETERMINATION OF MEDICAL NECESSITY (AND OTHER NONQUANTITATIVE TREATMENT LIMITS)

It is extremely important to recognize that every study supporting the establishment of parity for mental health and substance abuse benefits since the days of the Clinton health care reform efforts has relied on a managed set of benefits so as to project costs associated with parity. Yet, even within the debates in the Congress over the ACA, this reliance on a "managed" benefit was seen as a double-edged sword. On the one hand, only a managed benefit would support the affordability of a parity MH/SUD benefit package; on the other hand, overly restrictive determinations of medical necessity could easily make the reality of parity disappear for the individual.

Before the release of the Final Rule for Parity implementation in November 2013 at the Carter Center in Atlanta, HHS conducted a study of parity implementation under a so-called Interim Final Rule. This study, overseen by the Office of the Assistant Secretary for Planning and Evaluation, found that the use of quantitative limitations (eg, limits on inpatient days, outpatient visits) and nonparity financial requirements (eg, separate deductibles, different coinsurance, co-pay levels) on mental health and substance abuse benefit levels in a representative national sample of employer plans, had largely been abandoned. However, the nonquantitative treatment limits (NQTLs), for mental health and substance abuse coverage, such as overly restrictive definitions of medically necessary treatment and harsh utilization review requirements, were generally stricter that the NQTLs used for medical/surgical care.[16]

The very determination of the definitions themselves of what is covered under a parity mental health and substance abuse benefit is problematic. First, it is important to recognize that parity is just that: equality. As was pointed out earlier, a poor or inadequate set of medical surgical benefits can lead to an equally poor set of mental health and substance abuse benefits that are, in fact, at parity. Even more problematic, especially for the SMI population, is the difficulty in determining the equivalency of clinically important services, such as Assertive Community Treatment, supported housing, and supported employment to possibly comparable medical/surgical benefits covered under a range of rehabilitative services.

Of equal concern to the proper care and support of the SMI population is the question of overly narrow provider networks. With all the concern about the individual states' decisions whether to expand Medicaid after the US Supreme Court decision cited previously, not enough attention has been given to the question of whether or not adequate numbers and representation by discipline for the providers exists in various networks and plans, including for Medicaid. For example, in many jurisdictions around the country (eg, Washington state), because of the extremely low rates paid by Medicaid, many psychiatrists have chosen not to accept Medicaid patients; in some cases, they are now refusing to see any insured patients and moving to "all cash" practices."[17] This issue of availability of the full range of appropriate and necessary providers is even worse in rural areas or other areas with large health disparities.

THE INDIVIDUAL'S PATH TO PARITY

Thus far, we have considered the impact of parity on policy and delivery system operations. Although by themselves these issues are exceptionally important, they clearly are not the complete picture vis-à-vis parity. The ultimate consideration is how both policy and system operations impact on the individual person's journey toward parity throughout his or her course of care. In this section, we explore this issue further through the use of a metaphor. As individuals living with SMI seek to achieve personal recovery and reconnection with their community, they must pass through a series of "gates" along the path to parity.

In all, there are 4 gates:

Gate 1: Capacity to pay for care
Gate 2: The ability to access care
Gate 3: The quality of the care they receive
Gate 4: The outcomes of care

Obviously, the inability of an individual to pass through any particular gate will interfere and even terminate his or her personal journey toward parity.

Gate 1: Capacity to Pay for Care

Once a need for behavioral health care has been identified by one's self, a peer, or a family member, an immediate consideration is whether the person has any insurance, and, if so, whether the insurance provides coverage for the condition. The person also needs to consider whether the insurance has affordable deductibles, co-pays, coinsurance, and so forth.

Parity can help with this gate. It requires that any MH/SUD benefits and their management be no different than for medical care. It also requires that there be only 1 deductible, a single co-pay, and 1 coinsurance for all benefits covered under any policy. For those with insurance provided under the ACA, federal law and policy also require that both MH/SUD care benefits actually be included as part of the EHB. Thus, parity and the ACA definitely can help a person negotiate gate 1. However, for many individuals living with SMI, the actual enrollment process in either Medicaid or an exchange product can be difficult at best. Some attention, but not enough in many jurisdictions, has been given to the role of trained "navigators" to assist with this process, but more evaluation of this approach's effectiveness needs to be conducted to ensure adequate enrollment from the SMI population.

Gate 2: Access to Care

A second major hurdle is access to care even when one actually has insurance coverage. Two major limitations may exist. First, local behavioral health care providers may refuse to accept insurance payments for care. Many providers in more affluent areas will not accept Medicaid or Medicare or even payment through private insurance.[17] In the former case, payment rates simply are too low; in the latter, benefit management and onerous payment practices are off-putting to many providers. Second, the local area may not have any behavioral health care providers to access. It is astonishing to note that fully 85% of the counties in the United States have either inadequate or no behavioral health care services.[18] In both of these cases, having access to insurance coverage does not equate to having access to actual care, never mind to parity care.

Gate 3: Quality of Care

A third gate is the nature of the care that a person actually receives. Again, 2 factors seem most relevant. The first is whether the care received actually addresses the condition for which care was sought. The second is whether the care delivered is an evidence-based or best field practice. Field reports suggest that one or the other of these 2 conditions is not met in many care episodes.[19] When this happens, the quality of the care is less than adequate.

Gate 4: Outcomes of Care

Even if the first 3 gates are negotiated successfully, no guarantee exists that a person will achieve the outcomes or effects of care that were sought in the first place. Because the person receiving care is focused on recovery and return to community life, whereas the provider is focused on symptom reduction, frequently a disconnect exists between the two.

From this brief analysis, it should be clear that parity can play a very important, yet often only a small role as the person negotiates gate 1 to gate 4 (**Fig. 2**). In a logical sense, good insurance coverage is a necessary, but not sufficient condition for achieving a good outcome from behavioral health care. Thus, we must put parity into a proper perspective as we consider the entire process of care-seeking by an individual person and clearly recognize that insurance reform is part of, but not the same as, health care delivery reform.

A FEW CONCLUDING REMARKS

As we were preparing this article, we came to recognize that a strong analogy exists between the phases of the civil rights movement and the phases of parity in health care.

Over time, the civil rights movement in the United States has evolved from "separate but equal" to "fully integrated." This transition has already taken more than half a century to achieve, and many areas of conflict still exist. In health care, our current parity efforts are directed at achieving "separate but equal" status in insurance benefits and benefit management. Yet, the ACA already is moving us toward "fully integrated care," as well as care that is paid for through "fully integrated financing."[20] Thus, at some future point, we may rejoice in being able to move beyond parity.

From all of this, we reach a number of conclusions. First, parity is a very important milepost on the way to another destination, which is the achievement of recovery and a meaningful life in the community for all individuals living with behavioral issues, including the SMI population. Second, we must view the current progress under the ACA, imperfect as it may be, in implementing parity for all as yet another step forward, with perhaps many more to come. Third, perhaps "separate but equal" for behavioral health benefits is not the final goal for which we should be striving, but rather the achievement of full integration, both financial and clinical. In the end, it is only when behavioral health is recognized fully as part of overall health and wellness, not as a "separate but equal" entity, that true equality will be reached and optimal health and wellness for all members of our national community will be achieved.

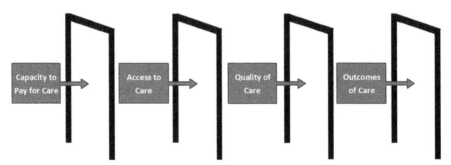

Fig. 2. The individual's path to parity.

REFERENCES

1. Grob GN, Goldman HH. The dilemma of federal mental health policy: radical reform or incremental change? New Brunswick (NJ): Rutgers University Press; 2006.
2. Duckworth K. Mental illness facts and numbers [Internet]. Arlington (VA): National Alliance on Mental Illness Website; 2013. Available at: http://www2.nami.org/factsheets/mentalillness_factsheet.pdf. Accessed September 20, 2015.
3. Glover RW, Miller JE, Sadowski SR. Proceedings on the state budget crisis and the behavioral health treatment gap: the impact on public substance abuse and mental health treatment systems. [Internet]. Washington, DC: 2012. Available at: http://www.nasmhpd.org/sites/default/files/Summary-Congressional%20Briefing_March%2022_Website%282%29.pdf.
4. US Department of Labor. Fact sheet. The mental health parity and addiction equity act of 2008 (MHPAEA). [Internet]. Employee Benefits Security Administration Newsroom. 2010. Available at: http://www.dol.gov/ebsa/newsroom/fsmhpaea.html. Accessed September 20, 2015.
5. Frank RG, Beronio K, Glied SA. Behavioral health parity and the Affordable Care Act [Internet]. J Soc Work Disabil Rehabil 2014;13(0):31–43. Available at: http://www.ncbi.nlm.nih.gov/pmc/articles/PMC4334111/pdf/nihms566563.pdf.
6. Beronio K, Po R, Skopec L, Glied S. Affordable Care Act will expand mental health and substance use disorder benefits and parity protections for 62 million Americans. ASPE Res Br [Internet]. Department of Health and Human Services, Office of the Assistant Secretary for Planning and Evaluation; 2013; p. 1–4. Available at: http://aspe.hhs.gov/report/affordable-care-act-expands-mental-health-and-substance-use-disorder-benefits-and-federal-parity-protections-62-million-americans. Accessed September 18, 2015.
7. The Center for Consumer Information & Insurance Oversight. The mental health parity and addiction equity act [Internet]. CCIIO Website. Available at: https://www.cms.gov/CCIIO/Programs-and-Initiatives/Other-Insurance-Protections/mhpaea_factsheet.html. Accessed September 20, 2015.
8. Centers for Medicare & Medicaid Services. Medicaid Fact Sheet: Mental Health Parity Proposed Rule for Medicaid and CHIP. [Internet]. Baltimore (MD): 2015. Available at: http://www.medicaid.gov/medicaid-chip-program-information/by-topics/benefits/downloads/medicaid-fact-sheet-parity.pdf. Accessed September 18, 2015.
9. Johns Hopkins Bloomberg School of Public Health. Despite federal law, some insurance exchange plans offer unequal coverage for mental health [Internet]. Baltimore (MD): Johns Hopkins News Releases; 2015. Available at: http://www.jhsph.edu/news/news-releases/2015/despite-federal-law-some-insurance-exchange-plans-offer-unequal-coverage-for-mental-health.html. Accessed September 20, 2015.
10. Colker A. The Affordable Care Act: how it expands coverage for those with behavioral health conditions. [Internet]. Available at: http://www.hhs.gov/partnerships/aca_act_and_community/aca_behavioral_health.pdf. Accessed September 15, 2015.
11. Young J. Obamacare signups top 11 million in second year, White House says. Huffington Post Online [Internet]. 2015 Feb 17; Available at: http://www.huffingtonpost.com/2015/02/17/obamacare-enrollment-2015_n_6701956.html. Accessed September 20, 2015.
12. Levitt L. Health reform and the art of federalism [Internet]. Menlo Park (CA): The Henry J. Kaiser Family Foundation Website; 2011. Available at: http://kff.org/health-reform/perspective/health-reform-and-the-art-of-federalism/. Accessed September 21, 2015.

13. Giovannelli J, Lucia KW, Corlette S. Realizing health reform's potential. Implementing the Affordable Care Act: revisiting the ACA's essential health benefits requirements [Internet]. Issue Brief (Commonw Fund) 2014;28:1–10. Available at: http://www.commonwealthfund.org/~/media/files/publications/issue-brief/2014/oct/1783_giovannelli_implementing_aca_essential_hlt_benefits_rb.pdf.

14. Musumeci M, Sobel L. The federal courts' role in implementing the Affordable Care Act [Internet]. Menlo Park (CA): The Henry J. Kaiser Family Foundation Website; 2014. Available at: http://kff.org/report-section/the-federal-courts-role-in-implementing-the-affordable-care-act-issue-brief/. Accessed September 12, 2015.

15. The Henry J. Kaiser Family Foundation. Status of state action on the Medicaid expansion decision [Internet]. Menlo Park (CA): The Henry J. Kaiser Family Foundation Website; 2015. Available at: http://kff.org/health-reform/state-indicator/state-activity-around-expanding-medicaid-under-the-affordable-care-act/. Accessed September 1, 2015.

16. Goplerud E. Consistency of large employer and group health plan benefits with requirements of the Paul Wellstone and Pete Domenici Mental Health Parity and Addiction Equity Act of 2008. [Internet]. 2013. Available at: http://www.dol.gov/ebsa/pdf/hhswellstonedomenicimhpaealargeemployerandghpbconsistency.pdf. Accessed September 18, 2015.

17. Galewitz P. Study: nearly a third of doctors won't see new Medicaid patients [Internet]. Washington DC: Kaiser Health News Online; 2012. Available at: http://khn.org/news/third-of-medicaid-doctors-say-no-new-patients/.

18. National Alliance on Mental Illness. President's New Freedom Commission on Mental Health. Achieving the promise: transforming mental health care in America [Internet]. National Alliance on Mental Illness Website. Available at: http://www2.nami.org/Template.cfm?Section=New_Freedom_Commission&Template=/ContentManagement/ContentDisplay.cfm&ContentID=28338. Accessed September 20, 2015.

19. Lehman AF, Goldman HH, Dixon LB, et al. Evidence-based mental health treatments and services: examples to inform public policy. [Internet]. New York: 2004. Available at: http://www.milbank.org/uploads/documents/2004lehman/2004lehman.html. Accessed September 18, 2015.

20. Manderscheid R, Kathol R. Fostering sustainable, integrated medical and behavioral health services in medical settings [Internet]. Ann Intern Med 2014;160(1):61–5. Available at: http://annals.org/article.aspx?articleid=1811029.

What's Hot in Schizophrenia Research?

Cynthia Shannon Weickert, PhD[a,b,c],*, Thomas W. Weickert, PhD[a,b,c],*

KEYWORDS

- Schizophrenia • Psychosis • Inflammation • Biomarkers • Cytokines
- Ultra-high risk • Microglia

KEY POINTS

- Evidence and interest are increasing for the role of inflammation in at least some people with schizophrenia.
- Inflammatory markers can be found in the peripheral blood of people at risk to develop psychosis and at the first episode of psychosis.
- Increased cytokines and microglia have been reliably reported in the brains of people with schizophrenia.
- Evidence from ultra-high-risk, brain imaging, post-mortem, animal models and genetic studies (genome-wide association studies) have converged to implicate neuroinflammation in the pathogenesis of at least some form of schizophrenia.

As schizophrenia research emerges halfway through the second decade of the twenty-first century, there have been some exciting findings that have confirmed and united 2 major lines of evidence regarding the cause of schizophrenia that were reported in the twentieth century. One line of evidence was that drugs that blocked the N-methyl D-aspartate receptor (NMDAR) could trigger a temporary delusional and/or hallucinatory state in otherwise healthy people.[1] The other line of evidence was that maternal infection during gestation or infection during postnatal life increased the risk of developing schizophrenia or psychosis by 2- to 3-fold in offspring.[2,3] The most recent lead into the mysteries of what causes schizophrenia could be viewed

Disclosures: The authors report no financial interests relevant to the content.
Funding sources: This work was supported by the University of New South Wales School of Psychiatry, Neuroscience Research Australia, the Schizophrenia Research Institute utilizing infrastructure funding from NSW Ministry of Health and the Macquarie Group Foundation. An Australian NHMRC Senior Research Fellowship (1021970) supported C.S. Weickert.
[a] Schizophrenia Research Institute, Barker Street, Randwick, New South Wales 2031, Australia; [b] School of Psychiatry, University of New South Wales, Hospital Road, Randwick, New South Wales 2031, Australia; [c] Neuroscience Research Australia, Barker Street, Randwick, New South Wales 2031, Australia
* Corresponding authors. Neuroscience Research Australia, Barker Street, Randwick, New South Wales 2031, Australia
E-mail addresses: cyndi@neura.edu.au; t.weickert@unsw.edu.au

as a fusion of the 2 lines of evidence referred to above. Indeed, an aberrant immune system response can cause NMDAR downregulation in the brain, which can lead to psychosis (hallucinations and delusions). Thus, what is considered to be really "hot" is the new awareness that anti-NMDAR encephalitis can result in a clinical manifestation that presents with psychosis[4] and can mimic schizophrenia. Furthermore, anti-NMDAR encephalitis can be "cured" by plasma immunotherapy, which can essentially eliminate psychotic symptoms. Observations like these are critical to the field because they demonstrate that schizophrenia symptoms or psychosis has a neurobiological basis and provides proof of principle that the psychotic symptoms can be abolished when treatment is aimed more directly at the underlying cause. Although some may argue that anti-NMDAR encephalitis is not "true" schizophrenia and that many of those cases can progress to paralysis and possibly death, milder or alternate forms of anti-NMDAR encephalitis may exist in a more chronic or relapsing and remitting fashion in some people with schizophrenia.

WHAT'S "HOT" IN BLOOD BIOMARKER STUDIES

Blood biomarker studies in general are a "hot" research area for schizophrenia. Blood is relatively easy to collect, and assays of thousands of different quantifiable factors can be performed fairly quickly and easily. Although some studies have focused on attempting to find blood biomarkers to distinguish Diagnostic and Statistical Manual of Mental Disorders (DSM)- or International Classification of Diseases (ICD)-defined schizophrenia compared with controls, or compared with bipolar illness or depression,[5] determining probability-based diagnostic categories is only one use of biomarkers.[6] Biomarkers can also be used to predict change over time, that is, prognosis (prognostic biomarkers). An important use of a prognostic biomarker is to predict who is more likely to transition to psychosis before they reach clear diagnostic criteria. Currently, the estimates of conversion to DSM-V/ICD-10 schizophrenia or psychotic bipolar illness from a prodormal state are around 22%.[7] In a recent paper from the North American Prodromal Longitudinal Study (NAPLS) group, increases in blood levels of several interleukins (IL), IL-1, IL-7, and IL-8, and molecules capable of modulating the blood-brain barrier (BBB) function could be used as part of a panel to predict conversion to psychotic illness, with blood levels of cytokines correlating with positive symptom severity (eg, delusional ideas), attentional dysfunction, and dysphoric moods.[8] Although an increase in inflammatory markers was also found concurrently with changes in markers of the hypothalamic-pituitary-adrenal axis dysregulation, these findings suggest that peripheral factors typically monitored by endocrinologists and immunologists may be useful for psychiatrists in monitoring risk for developing a psychotic mental illness.

Although predicting who will develop psychotic symptoms before manifestation of the illness is critical if the onset of major mental illness is to be prevented, many of the blood biomarker studies have been conducted in those that have already reached diagnostic criteria. One of the most highly cited meta-analyses on this topic is from Miller and colleagues,[9] which analyzes data combined from 40 studies and demonstrates clear increases in at least 9 proinflammatory cytokines (IL-1 beta, IL-6, IL-8, IL-12, IL-1RA [receptor antagonist], and tumor necrosis factor-α, transforming growth factor-β, interferon-γ, soluble IL-2 receptor) and decreases in an anti-inflammatory cytokine (IL-10) in chronically ill people with schizophrenia or people during a first psychotic episode relative to controls. Although this important analysis also suggests that antipsychotics can significantly decrease blood cytokine levels,[9] it is important to consider that although these peripheral cytokine levels may be reduced to some degree by antipsychotics, the peripheral cytokine levels can still be elevated in schizophrenia relative to healthy control levels.

Nonetheless, neuroinflammation could simply be a byproduct of chronic illness and poor lifestyles (ie, drug abuse and poor nutritional choices) rather than a causative factor in mental illness. However, as mentioned above, inflammation markers have been reported in people who are at high risk to develop psychosis, before reaching diagnostic criteria for mental illness. Thus, inflammation may be a primary cause of illness in some people, whereas it may be a byproduct of chronic illness in other people. In either case, chronic neuroinflammation would be detrimental to healthy neural and cognitive processes. Therefore, treatments aimed at reducing inflammation in general and neuroinflammation in particular in individuals within the mentally ill population who display signs of chronic inflammation would potentially be beneficial in reducing symptoms and improving cognitive processes.

In general, the validity of peripheral immune markers to reflect brain abnormalities has been questioned. Recent analysis of blood measures demonstrates that measures of chronic, low-grade, inflammation (ie, elevated C-reactive protein [CRP], IL6, and lymphocyte counts) are also predictive of metabolic syndrome or cardiovascular risk, which occur frequently in people with schizophrenia.[10] Thus, based on these examples, it seems that blood biomarkers may also be useful in predicting risk of developing other serious physical and metabolic problems in people with schizophrenia, that is, for prognosis of comorbid physical abnormalities/conditions.

One of the challenges in the field is to relate the more easily accessible peripheral measures of inflammation in the blood to other more difficult-to-assess brain abnormality measures in people with schizophrenia. In the authors' recent study, using recursive clustering methods from a panel of cytokines, it was found that approximately 40% of people with schizophrenia from their sample who had increased peripheral levels of proinflammatory cytokine messenger RNAs (mRNAs) derived from white blood cells, also had an 18% reduction in cortical (Broca's area) gray matter volume and significantly more impairment in verbal fluency.[11] Although elevated cytokines were found in a proportion of both people with schizophrenia (about 40%) and the healthy control group (about 20%), inflammation-associated decrease in brain (Broca's area) volume or cognitive (verbal fluency) impairment was not shown in the healthy controls. Thus, this differential finding between high "inflammatory" healthy and patient groups suggests that in the "healthy" control group with elevated peripheral cytokine levels the inflammatory target tissue may be outside the brain. In fact, it is estimated that around 30% of controls will have some level of increased inflammation because of a variety of nasal, lung, heart, gut, joint, or other ailments.[12] Thus, it is the combination of some overt brain dysfunction (psychiatric symptoms, cognitive impairment, and brain volumetric loss) and peripheral inflammation markers that may identify a subtype of neuroinflammatory schizophrenia. These same markers of peripheral inflammation would not be informative when they are used in isolation from clinical interview, patient history, cognitive assessment, and other biological measures.

WHAT'S "HOT" IN BLOOD BIOMARKER STUDIES CONTINUED: THERANOSTICS

Although using blood biological markers to subtype people with schizophrenia is considered a hot area of research and one that has great potential, clearly there is still much work to be done. One important area in blood biomarker development is to define blood biomarkers predictive of therapeutic response (theranostics) to both existing and novel drug therapies. One research area that is quite hot is "psychopharmacogenomics," in which an individual's genotype is used to predict response to common psychiatric drugs.[13] Indeed, a panel of biomarkers predicting metabolizer status is in current use by many psychiatrists to aid in choice of the optimal antipsychotic medication to prescribe to a given individual.[14] The authors suggest that mRNA and protein measures can complement DNA measures with regard to theranostics. For example, a subset of depressed people who responded best to an anti-inflammatory treatment expressed transcriptional changes in metabolism and the innate immune system in mRNA extracted from peripheral blood mononuclear cells.[15] The utility of a stratifying approach in which people with increased inflammation are defined with biomarkers has recently been demonstrated in major depression such that a significant improvement in depression was demonstrated with the anti-inflammatory infliximab only in those patients who displayed elevated CRP levels.[16] Further work showed that this therapy improved quality of sleep in depressed individuals who had elevated blood CRP levels.[17] Although only a few examples have been provided that were not from schizophrenia research, these examples provide a framework of how to conceptualize blood biomarker development for clinical benefit in psychiatry.

Although identification of a "high" inflammatory biotype may provide clues as to neuropathological changes or help to identify novel treatment options, it is not known if these biomarkers are directly related to the cause or causes of schizophrenia. There is some evidence that inflammation can be considered part of the primary cause of schizophrenia based on at least 2 lines of evidence: (1) autoimmunity against vascular or brain proteins results in psychosis, for example, anti-NMDAR encephalitis[4] or breakdown of the BBB is consistent with psychosis,[18] and (2) infections of the brain, for example, human immunodeficiency virus or *Toxoplasma gondi*, can trigger psychosis.[19] A "leaky" BBB may allow peripheral cytokines into the brain, or reactive microglia changes, already present in the brain, may produce cytokines and induce neural damage in response to excitatory glutamatergic neurotransmission. However, the cause of schizophrenia is unknown and most likely varied with many genes and environmental factors contributing to risk. That being said, the large-scale genetic genome-wide association studies have also provided evidence for neuroinflammation being a major factor in schizophrenia by consistently demonstrating the human leukocyte antigen locus, which contains multiple genes involved in immune function as being the top genetic region.[20,21] Thus, inflammation may be one point of potential convergence in at least a subset of people with the illness, which may provide more traction in terms of treatment than any single genetic or environmentally based intervention.

WHAT'S "HOT" IN BRAIN IMAGING STUDIES

Although human brain imaging can encompass structural MRI, functional MRI, magnetic resonance spectroscopy, and diffusion tensor imaging approaches, one of the "hottest" human brain imaging areas in schizophrenia research is currently brain imaging via PET studies. Several recent PET studies have identified an increase in the translocator protein (TSPO) binding (which is related to cytokine secretion and the inflammatory response) in the brains of people with schizophrenia compared with healthy controls.[22] This increase in binding has been interpreted to represent an increase in activated microglia. Although another recent study using a different TSPO ligand has challenged whether this finding applies to all patients with schizophrenia,[23] and others suggest that PK11195 is not specific for microglia, the original reports do appear to correspond to the increase in microglia density found by direct immunohistochemical measures in postmortem brains reported by the authors' group[24] and others.[25] However, any increase in microglia may be transient and more prominent early on in the course of schizophrenia, which may explain some of the inconsistencies reported when attempting to image microglia in the brains of chronically ill people with schizophrenia.[22,23] A very recent PET study[26] used the PBR28 ligand to monitor microglia activity in individuals from 2 cohorts: (1) an antipsychotic-naive, ultrahigh risk of developing schizophrenia group (mean age = 24, SD = 5.4) and (2) a chronically ill group of people with schizophrenia. Importantly, they found increased binding in both cohorts with large effects sizes, suggesting that these changes may be found throughout the course of schizophrenia. Furthermore, increases in actual microglial binding in the brains of those at high risk of developing psychosis were highly correlated with positive symptoms,[26] which was similar to the findings from the NAPLS high-risk study using peripheral blood biomarkers of inflammation and symptom assays.[8] Thus, these findings from the ultra-high-risk samples show that increases in brain microglia or immune activation are most likely not secondary to antipsychotic treatment. The inflammation relationship is further supported by preclinical and clinical work showing that antipsychotics decrease cytokine expression.[27,28] The exciting work performed to date suggests that neuroinflammation

1. is a part of the pathophysiology of some forms of schizophrenia,
2. may be directly related to the experience of psychosis, and
3. appears to be a factor that can be targeted with anti-inflammatory treatments before the first episode of psychosis.

WHAT'S "HOT" IN POSTMORTEM STUDIES

Early postmortem examinations of brains of people with schizophrenia were largely devoid of clear and consistent hallmarks of neuropathology, that is, neuronal loss or gliosis. These studies were limited by lack of brains (often <10/group), lack of sensitive measures, and lack of comprehensive screening tools. Presently, there is a dramatic change in the strategy of using postmortem brains in schizophrenia research, such that most current studies use relatively large samples sizes (>30, with some cohorts nearing 100 per group), and application of high-throughput technology to measure thousands of molecules at once, and use of more sensitive and specific molecular tools to track abnormality within cells of the brain. Using these more modern approaches, the field has identified that there is neuropathology in the brains of people with schizophrenia, including activation of neuroinflammatory pathways and gliosis.

High-throughput technology has been used effectively to identify molecular changes consistent with neuroinflammation. In early microarray studies, an upregulation of an inflammatory acute phase response molecule, SERPINA3 mRNA, and of other interferon-γ-induced transcripts, was reported in the brains of people with schizophrenia irrespective of antipsychotic treatment relative to controls.[29,30] In the authors' more recent study using RNA sequencing, they identified increases in proinflammatory molecules, including the prototypical IL mediators, IL-6 and IL-1 mRNAs, in the frontal cortex of people with schizophrenia,[24] which has recently been independently replicated.[31] Importantly, this increase in molecules consistent with neuroinflammation does not appear to be secondary to antipsychotic exposure, can be identified in individuals within a wide age range of 30 to 68 years, is found in a substantial subset ($\sim$40%) of people with schizophrenia, and appears to also be detectable in some people with bipolar illness.[32] Indeed, when people with schizophrenia are classified according to their neuroinflammatory status, an increase in glial fibrillary acidic protein and a hypertrophy of astrocytes can be detected, which are consistent with gliosis.[33] Because antipsychotics can suppress immune activation and reduce glia number in the cortex,[34,35] it is possible that attenuation of this astrocyte/inflammatory response may underlie some of the therapeutic action of antipsychotics. However, antipsychotics may not completely suppress neuroinflammation and neuroinflammation may be cyclic in nature in response to different environmental stressors. Microglial cells are also another possible source of proinflammatory cytokines, and some postmortem studies have found increased density of microglial cells in some people with psychosis.[24,25,36–38] However, the authors did not find that mRNA levels of proinflammatory cytokines correlated with their microglial markers in the same brains. At least some of the changes related to inflammation have been mapped to brain endothelial cells,[39] but further work to determine the cellular source of the increased SERPINA3 and the IL mRNAs is needed.

SUMMARY

Although there are many questions raised by all these findings described throughout this article, some of the most critical ones for the field are as follows:

1. Is the brain, the periphery or both the source of the neuroinflammatory profile found in schizophrenia?
2. If the brain is the source, then what is the neural damage that may precede the inflammatory response?
3. What is the cellular source of proinflammatory response mRNAs, and which brain cells are they impacting most?
4. What is the consequence to neurons when inflammatory changes are occurring in the brains of people with schizophrenia?
5. What is the timing of such inflammatory events, and how do they change over the course of the illness?

Although this last question is very difficult to answer with postmortem approaches and will require the use of blood biomarkers and neuroimaging in living people, some clues into timing can be provided by studying animal models in which type, duration, and timing of immune activation can be controlled. In this regard, Volk and colleagues[31] provided evidence that a peripheral immune challenge in adult animals (but not prenatal animals) could trigger a molecular immune signature in the brain of animals that recapitulated that found in adults with schizophrenia. How an adult inflammatory signal may interact with an earlier immune priming event to bring about a more exaggerated response would be an interesting question for future research given that the evidence for brain changes with maternal immune activation is arguably one of the "hottest" current animal models of schizophrenia used in research.[40,41]

REFERENCES

1. Krystal JH, Karper LP, Seibyl JP, et al. Subanesthetic effects of the noncompetitive NMDA antagonist, ketamine, in humans. Psychotomimetic, perceptual, cognitive, and neuroendocrine responses. Arch Gen Psychiatry 1994;51(3): 199–214.
2. Buka SL, Cannon TD, Torrey EF, et al, Collaborative Study Group on the Perinatal Origins of Severe Psychiatric Disorders. Maternal exposure to herpes simplex virus and risk of psychosis among adult offspring. Biol Psychiatry 2008;63(8): 809–15.
3. Brown AS. The environment and susceptibility to schizophrenia. Prog Neurobiol 2011;93(1):23–58.

4. Kayser MS, Dalmau J. Anti-NMDA receptor encephalitis, autoimmunity, and psychosis. Schizophr Res 2014. http://dx.doi.org/10.1016/j.schres.2014.10.007.
5. Schwarz E, Guest PC, Rahmoune H, et al. Identification of a biological signature for schizophrenia in serum. Mol Psychiatry 2012;17(5):494–502.
6. Weickert CS, Weickert TW, Pillai A, et al. Biomarkers in schizophrenia: a brief conceptual consideration. Dis Markers 2013;35(1):3–9.
7. Bechdolf A, Thompson A, Nelson B, et al. Experience of trauma and conversion to psychosis in an ultra-high-risk (prodromal) group. Acta Psychiatr Scand 2010; 121(5):377–84.
8. Perkins DO, Jeffries CD, Addington J, et al. Towards a psychosis risk blood diagnostic for persons experiencing high-risk symptoms: preliminary results from the NAPLS project. Schizophr Bull 2015;41(2):419–28.
9. Miller BJ, Buckley P, Seabolt W, et al. Meta-analysis of cytokine alterations in schizophrenia: clinical status and antipsychotic effects. Biol Psychiatry 2011; 70(7):663–71.
10. Miller BJ, Kandhal P, Rapaport MH, et al. Total and differential white blood cell counts, high-sensitivity C-reactive protein, and cardiovascular risk in nonaffective psychoses. Brain Behav Immun 2015;45:28–35.
11. Fillman SG, Weickert TW, Lenroot RK, et al. Elevated peripheral cytokines characterize a subgroup of people with schizophrenia displaying poor verbal fluency and reduced Broca's area volume. Mol Psychiatry 2015. http://dx.doi.org/10.1038/mp.2015.90.
12. Dakin SG, Martinez FO, Yapp C, et al. Inflammation activation and resolution in human tendon disease. Sci Transl Med 2015;7(311):311ra173.
13. Volpi S, Potkin SG, Malhotra AK, et al. Applicability of a genetic signature for enhanced iloperidone efficacy in the treatment of schizophrenia. J Clin Psychiatry 2009;70(6):801–9.
14. Hettige NC, Zai C, Hazra M, et al. Use of candidate gene markers to guide antipsychotic dosage adjustment. Prog Neuropsychopharmacol Biol Psychiatry 2014;54:315–20.
15. Mehta D, Raison CL, Woolwine BJ, et al. Transcriptional signatures related to glucose and lipid metabolism predict treatment response to the tumor necrosis factor antagonist infliximab in patients with treatment-resistant depression. Brain Behav Immun 2013;31:205–15.
16. Raison CL, Rutherford RE, Woolwine BJ, et al. A randomized controlled trial of the tumor necrosis factor antagonist infliximab for treatment-resistant depression: the role of baseline inflammatory biomarkers. JAMA Psychiatry 2013;70(1):31–41.
17. Weinberger JF, Raison CL, Rye DB, et al. Inhibition of tumor necrosis factor improves sleep continuity in patients with treatment resistant depression and high inflammation. Brain Behav Immun 2015;47:193–200.
18. Khandaker GM, Cousins L, Deakin J, et al. Inflammation and immunity in schizophrenia: implications for pathophysiology and treatment. Lancet Psychiatry 2015; 2(3):258–70.
19. Bergink V, Gibney SM, Drexhage HA. Autoimmunity, inflammation, and psychosis: a search for peripheral markers. Biol Psychiatry 2014;75(4):324–31.
20. Schizophrenia Working Group of the Psychiatric Genomics Consortium. Biological insights from 108 schizophrenia-associated genetic loci. Nature 2014; 511(7510):421–7.
21. Sekar A, Bialas AR, de Rivera H, et al. Schizophrenia risk from complex variation of complement component 4. Nature 2016;530(7589):177–83.

22. Kreisl WC, Jenko KJ, Hines CS, et al, Biomarkers Consortium PET Radioligand Project Team. A genetic polymorphism for translocator protein 18 kDa affects both in vitro and in vivo radioligand binding in human brain to this putative biomarker of neuroinflammation. J Cereb Blood Flow Metab 2013;33(1):53–8.

23. Kenk M, Selvanathan T, Rao N, et al. Imaging neuroinflammation in gray and white matter in schizophrenia: an in-vivo PET study with [18F]-FEPPA. Schizophr Bull 2015;41(1):85–93.

24. Fillman SG, Cloonan N, Catts VS, et al. Increased inflammatory markers identified in the dorsolateral prefrontal cortex of individuals with schizophrenia. Mol Psychiatry 2013;18(2):206–14.

25. Busse S, Busse M, Schiltz K, et al. Different distribution patterns of lymphocytes and microglia in the hippocampus of patients with residual versus paranoid schizophrenia: further evidence for disease course-related immune alterations? Brain Behav Immun 2012;26(8):1273–9.

26. Bloomfield PS, Selvaraj S, Veronese M, et al. Microglial activity in people at ultra high risk of psychosis and in schizophrenia: an [11C]PBR28 PET brain imaging study. Am J Psychiatry 2015;173(1):44–52.

27. Matsumoto A, Ohta N, Goto Y, et al. Haloperidol suppresses murine dendritic cell maturation and priming of the T helper 1-type immune response. Anesth Analg 2015;120(4):895–902.

28. Sobiś J, Rykaczewska-Czerwińska M, Świętochowska E, et al. Therapeutic effect of aripiprazole in chronic schizophrenia is accompanied by anti-inflammatory activity. Pharmacol Rep 2015;67(2):353–9.

29. Arion D, Unger T, Lewis DA, et al. Molecular evidence for increased expression of genes related to immune and chaperone function in the prefrontal cortex in schizophrenia. Biol Psychiatry 2007;62(7):711–21.

30. Saetre P, Emilsson L, Axelsson E, et al. Inflammation-related genes up-regulated in schizophrenia brains. BMC Psychiatry 2007;7:46.

31. Volk DW, Chitrapu A, Edelson JR, et al. Molecular mechanisms and timing of cortical immune activation in schizophrenia. Am J Psychiatry 2015;172(11): 1112–21.

32. Fillman SG, Sinclair D, Fung SJ, et al. Markers of inflammation and stress distinguish subsets of individuals with schizophrenia and bipolar disorder. Translational Psychiatry 2014;4:e365.

33. Catts VS, Wong J, Fillman SG, et al. Increased expression of astrocyte markers in schizophrenia: association with neuroinflammation. Aust N Z J Psychiatry 2014; 48(8):722–34.

34. Konopaske GT, Dorph-Petersen KA, Pierri JN, et al. Effect of chronic exposure to antipsychotic medication on cell numbers in the parietal cortex of macaque monkeys. Neuropsychopharmacology 2007;32(6):1216–23.

35. Konopaske GT, Dorph-Petersen KA, Sweet RA, et al. Effect of chronic antipsychotic exposure on astrocyte and oligodendrocyte numbers in macaque monkeys. Biol Psychiatry 2008;63(8):759–65.

36. Radewicz K, Garey LJ, Gentleman SM, et al. Increase in HLA-DR immunoreactive microglia in frontal and temporal cortex of chronic schizophrenics. J Neuropathol Exp Neurol 2000;59(2):137–50.

37. Steiner J, Bernstein HG, Bielau H, et al. S100B-immunopositive glia is elevated in paranoid as compared to residual schizophrenia: a morphometric study. J Psychiatr Res 2008;42(10):868–76.

38. Wierzba-Bobrowicz T, Lewandowska E, Lechowicz W, et al. Quantitative analysis of activated microglia, ramified and damage of processes in the frontal and temporal lobes of chronic schizophrenics. Folia Neuropathol 2005;43(2):81–9.
39. Siegel BI, Sengupta EJ, Edelson JR, et al. Elevated viral restriction factor levels in cortical blood vessels in schizophrenia. Biol Psychiatry 2014;76(2):160–7.
40. Vuillermot S, Weber L, Feldon J, et al. A longitudinal examination of the neurodevelopmental impact of prenatal immune activation in mice reveals primary defects in dopaminergic development relevant to schizophrenia. J Neurosci 2010; 30(4):1270–87.
41. Zuckerman L, Rehavi M, Nachman R, et al. Immune activation during pregnancy in rats leads to a postpubertal emergence of disrupted latent inhibition, dopaminergic hyperfunction, and altered limbic morphology in the offspring: a novel neurodevelopmental model of schizophrenia. Neuropsychopharmacology 2003; 28(10):1778–89.

Index

Note: Page numbers of article titles are in **boldface** type.

A

Psychiatr Clin N Am 39 (2016) 353–359
http://dx.doi.org/10.1016/S0193-953X(16)30009-0
0193-953X/16/$ – see front matter

psych.theclinics.com

Moving?

Make sure your subscription moves with you!

To notify us of your new address, find your **Clinics Account Number** (located on your mailing label above your name), and contact customer service at:

Email: **journalscustomerservice-usa@elsevier.com**

800-654-2452 (subscribers in the U.S. & Canada)
314-447-8871 (subscribers outside of the U.S. & Canada)

Fax number: **314-447-8029**

Elsevier Health Sciences Division
Subscription Customer Service
3251 Riverport Lane
Maryland Heights, MO 63043

Printed and bound by CPI Group (UK) Ltd, Croydon, CR0 4YY

03/10/2024

01040393-0020